NEUROLOGICAL EMERGENCIES
Effective Nursing Care

Jeanne Raimond, RN, BSN, CCRN
Grossmont District Hospital
La Mesa, California

Joyce Waterman Taylor, RN, MSN, FAAN
San Francisco General Hospital

AN ASPEN PUBLICATION®
Aspen Systems Corporation

1986

Rockville, Maryland
Royal Tunbridge Wells

Library of Congress Cataloging in Publication Data

Raimond, Jeanne.
Neurological emergencies.

"An Aspen publication."
Includes bibliographies and index.
1. Neurological nursing — Handbooks, manuals, etc. 2. Emergency nursing — Handbooks, manuals, etc. I. Taylor, Joyce Waterman. II. Title. [DNLM: 1. Critical Care — nurses' instruction. 2. Emergencies — nursing. 3. Nervous System Diseases — nursing. WY 160 R153n]
RC350.5.R35   1986   610.73'68   85-23027
ISBN: 0-87189-252-9

Editorial Services: Martha Sasser

Library of Congress Catalog Card Number: 85-23027
ISBN: 0-87189-252-9

Printed in the United States of America

1 2 3 4 5

Table of Contents

Preface

Nursing care can have a critical impact on the outcome of a patient's neurological illness. Proper nursing management begins with a basic understanding of the anatomy, physiology, and pathology involved in common neurological emergencies.

We have selected material that provides the nurse with a sound basis of knowledge for providing nursing care during the emergency phase of common neurological illnesses. Since our intent is to present the most common neurological emergencies, noticeably more space is devoted to intracranial disorders than to spinal cord disorders. We feel that nurses in emergency departments and critical care units encounter more patients with emergencies related to brain pathology than spinal cord disorders. Nevertheless, considerable space is devoted to the pathophysiology, clinical manifestations, and emergency nursing management of spinal cord injury in Chapter 8. Precautions in handling the spinal cord injury patient are discussed in Chapter 1.

The book is organized into three major parts. Part I, ''Introduction and Overview,'' centers on the most common neurological emergencies, with emphasis on the nurse's role. Neurological anatomy, physiology, and pathophysiology and nursing assessment are also included. These provide nurses a framework for making meaningful observations of their patients. Part II, ''Special Problems Related to Neurological Disease,'' addresses the dynamics of pathophysiology, and nursing management of patients with various neurological emergencies. Chapter 4, ''Intracranial Hypertension,'' stresses intensive nursing care of brain injured patients. These nursing principles are applicable to many chapters of this text, and frequent reference is made to Chapter 4. Part III, ''Quick Guide to Immediate Care of Patients with Neurological Emergencies,'' is based on the nursing process. As a quick reference guide, it will have practical on-the-job clinical application.

Although this book is intended primarily for emergency department nurses, it should also be of practical value to nurses in critical care units and to other paramedical personnel who encounter patients with neurological emergencies.

The practice of nursing as well as medicine is dynamic and ever-changing. The authors have made every effort to provide current information on medical and nursing therapies, drug dosages, etc., that are in keeping with standards accepted at the time of publication. Research and clinical experience will continually lead to changes in the understanding of neurological diseases and treatment regimens.

Part I

Introduction and Overview

Chapter 1

The Role of the Emergency Department Nurse in Neurological Emergencies

K. Sue Hoyt

Patients with neurological emergencies are among the most challenging encountered by the emergency department nurse. The cost for care of victims of neurological trauma and other neurological disorders runs into millions of dollars annually in the United States. Much worse than this is the cost in human suffering that accompanies those patients left with severe neurological deficits. Informed, intelligent, dedicated nursing can make a difference.

PRIORITY SETTING

Accurate triage and patient assessment, timely intervention, and reevaluation can greatly influence patient outcome. Prompt and appropriate interventions are essential to preventing transient neurological deficits from becoming permanent disabilities.

Nursing priorities consist of triage, performing primary and secondary surveys, obtaining brief histories, planning and implementing nursing interventions, assisting with therapeutic and diagnostic procedures, reevaluating, and documenting.

Triage

The role of the emergency department nurse begins with accurate triage of the neurological emergency patient. Triage facilitates rapid and efficient medical management. Triage is based on recognition of those patients most in need of urgent medical intervention, such as a patient with a rapidly evolving epidural hematoma, or the patient with an unstable cervical spine injury. Patients with the following problems need immediate attention:

- loss of airway
- severe blood loss
- unstable vital signs
- decreasing level of consciousness
- loss of motor/sensory function
- focal lesion as evidenced by a unilaterally dilated or oval pupil, etc.

The combative patient also requires a rapid work-up because the nature of the patient's disorder may not be known. Accurate triage often depends on the findings of the primary survey.

The Primary Survey

The primary survey is the most important component in the initial phase of emergency care because it determines subsequent methods of treatment. This initial examination must be brief but thorough, and should take no more than 60 seconds. The primary survey is performed on all emergency patients and can be summarized by the mnemonic device A through E (see Table 1–1).

A—Airway

Assessment for airway patency is the first consideration. Although this factor seems obvious, many clinicians have been seen starting intravenous lines without first assuring that the patient's airway is patent.

Effective airway management of the neurological patient begins with opening the airway if it is not patent while simultaneously maintaining the alignment of the cervical spine. The technique of using the jaw thrust to open the airway with little

---

Table 1–1 The Primary Survey[1]

Mnemonic	Assessment
A = Airway	Airway maintenance with C-spine precautions
B = Breathing	Ventilatory status
C = Circulation	Perfusion status with hemorrhage control
D = Disability	Neurological status
E = Expose	Complete examination of the undressed patient

or no movement of the cervical spine is depicted in Figure 1–1. In-line traction to the head and neck with minimal extension of the neck is acceptable if the neurological emergency does not involve the cervical spine.

Common causes of airway obstruction include foreign body, usually the tongue, improper head or jaw position, and secretions such as mucus or vomitus.

If the airway cannot be maintained with the methods described, including the use of an oropharyngeal or nasopharyngeal airway and proper positioning, and suctioning of secretions, then intubation or the surgical opening of the airway (tracheostomy or cricothyrotomy) is indicated.

The esophageal obturator airway (EOA) is still being used in some regions of the country as an alternative approach to prehospital airway maintenance. Because vomiting and aspiration can occur with EOA removal, its use is discouraged by many practitioners. With the advent of intubation in the prehospital setting, use of the EOA has diminished considerably.

Physician preference often dictates whether intubation or surgical intervention is the method of airway maintenance. Some physicians feel more skilled at nasotracheal intubation for patients with suspected cervical spine injury. Other physicians prefer to endotracheally intubate while maintaining the patient's head in a neutral or ''sniffing'' position using in-line traction to the head. Use of a fiberoptic bronchoscope facilitates placement of the endotracheal tube. Currently, Advanced Trauma Life Support (ATLS) guidelines recommend nasotracheal intubation for patients with suspected neck injuries and endotracheal intubation for patients with possible maxillofacial injuries.[1]

Those patients who cannot undergo intubation by either method should receive an immediate surgical opening for airway maintenance. A surgical cricothyrotomy is the recommended method of airway management; however, a skilled surgeon may be able to perform a tracheostomy just as quickly. Patients with severe neck swelling in whom the other approaches of needle or tracheostomy tube

---

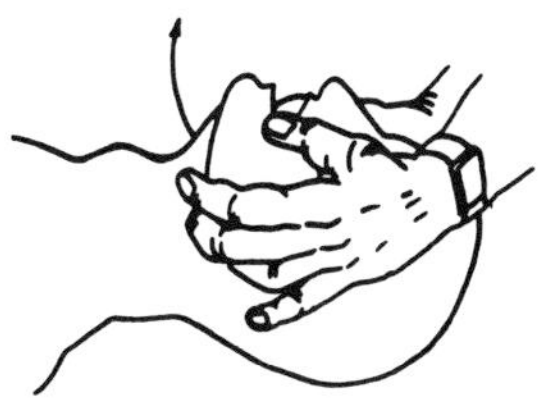

Fig. 1–1—Jaw thrust maneuver for opening an obstructed airway. The angle of the mandible is grasped with one hand on each side and pulled forward to open the airway.
Source: Adapted from Cardiac Arrest & CPR, ed 2 (p. 11) by PS Auerbach and SA Budassi (eds), Aspen Systems Corporation, © 1983.

placement have failed may need an opening made in the trachea through which an endotracheal tube can be placed.

Laryngospasm or combativeness in the neurologically injured patient may necessitate the administration of a barbiturate or a neuromuscular blocking agent, such as pancuronium or succinylcholine, prior to intubation. Intubation is best performed under controlled conditions (lidocaine, barbiturate, pancuronium) since harried and inexpert intubation will provoke coughing, increased intrathoracic pressure, and a subsequent rise in intracranial pressure (ICP). Ventilation will have to be controlled until the effects of the medication have worn off.

Some physicians follow the protocol that a patient with a Glasgow Coma Scale score (see Table 1–4) of 7 or less should be intubated and hyperventilated to a PaO_2 of 100 mm Hg and a $PaCO_2$ of 25–35 mm Hg.[2] Mild hypocarbia induces cerebral vasoconstriction and leads to a reduction in ICP.

Paramedics in the Seattle area are intubating patients that meet specific criteria. They also administer succinylcholine 0.5 mg/kg prior to intubation if necessary as part of their prehospital criteria.[3] This must be used with caution, however, as the paramedic may be unable to intubate even after the medication is given.

Airway management includes oxygen administration. The brain is very metabolically active and cannot store oxygen. In a recent national survey, 65 percent of all severe head injury patients were found to be hypoxemic upon arrival in the emergency department. These were patients who were assessed as having normal ventilatory patterns and no respiratory distress. This demonstrates the fact that one cannot assess the adequacy of respiratory function solely on the basis of physical observation.[2]

Neurological patients may require high-flow oxygen at 8–10 L/min by nonrebreather mask. Facial trauma or severe hypoventilation may necessitate intubation and ventilation to assure adequate airway and oxygenation. At no time should the patient be allowed to retain carbon dioxide which could occur in a hypoventilating patient receiving oxygen by mask. Carbon dioxide retention causes cerebral vasodilation and increases ICP.

Oxygen by mask at 10 L/min will deliver an FiO_2 of approximately .50–.60 (50–60 percent) to a patient with a normal respiratory pattern. FiO_2s of up to .90 (90 percent) can be obtained with the use of high-flow oxygen via a nonrebreather mask.[4]

The primary cause of death in trauma patients is inadequate airway,[2] and national data indicate that 70 percent of trauma patients have head injuries. Therefore, trauma patients must receive proper airway management from the moment of their injury if emergency nursing care is to make a difference in their morbidity and mortality.[2]

Regardless of whether the patient comes into the emergency department with an oxygen mask in place or intubated, the assessment of breathing is the next step in the primary survey.

B—Breathing

Methods of evaluation include assessment for:

- adequate rise and fall of the chest (to effectively move air)
- use of accessory muscles to breathe (claviculars and sternocleidomastoids)
- presence of nasal flaring or stridor (crowing sound indicative of obstructed airway)
- obvious deformity of the chest (flail chest or emphysema)
- tracheal deviation
- retraction (suprasternal, intercostal)

All of these assessments are made by visual observation. It may be necessary for the examiner to look at the patient's chest at eye level and stand at the side or the foot of the bed to assess shallow respirations or asymmetrical chest expansion.

The patient with a spinal cord injury above the C-4 level will have severely impaired respirations because of the loss of phrenic nerve innervation to the diaphragm. Shoulder girdle muscles may be all that the patient can move to effect minimal ventilation. Patients with lower C-spine injuries may have paralysis of all intercostal muscles and exhibit pure diaphragmatic breathing. No chest wall movement is seen. Only abdominal wall movement is observed with respirations.

Palpation is also important in the primary exam. By placing one's hands on the patient's chest, uneven chest expansion, asymmetry of the chest, crepitus, and deformity can be felt.

The quality of respirations is further assessed by auscultation of breath sounds. Diminished or absent breath sounds give important clues to the possibility of pneumothorax or profound hypoventilation. Respirations should be assessed for:

- rate (12–20 breaths per minute is normal)
- depth (full and effective, shallow, or deep)
- pattern (see Chapter 3, Figure 3–8)

If physical assessment or arterial blood gas (ABG) analysis reveals inadequate ventilation, then ventilatory assistance is required. Various ways to assist breathing include:

- mouth-to-mouth/mouth-to-nose ventilation
- positive pressure demand valve ventilation (watch for gastric distention)
- bag-valve resuscitation device (use with oral or nasopharyngeal airway in place)
- bag-valve device via endotracheal/tracheostomy tube

The methods of oxygen delivery and artificial ventilation should be guided by ABG analysis. Hypoxemia and hypercarbia must be prevented. Following the assurance of an adequate airway and effective breathing, the primary survey moves to the next step.

C—Circulation

Circulation or hemorrhage control refers to the assessment for and assurance of an adequate level of perfusion. A multiple trauma patient with a head injury is at increased risk for experiencing inadequate cerebral perfusion if associated injuries contribute to hypovolemic shock. Circulation involves more than the assessment of blood pressure (BP) and pulse. Perfusion is further assessed by evaluating:

- mental status (level of consciousness, LOC)
- skin vitals (color, temperature, moisture)
- capillary refill rate (normally two seconds or less)
- pulses (radial, femoral, carotid)
- urinary output (not performed on the primary survey)

When a blood pressure is inaudible, it can be estimated quickly using the following ATLS guidelines[1]:

- If the radial pulse is present, the blood pressure is at least 80 mm Hg.
- If the femoral pulse is present, the blood pressure is at least 70 mm Hg.
- If the carotid pulse is present, the blood pressure is at least 60 mm Hg.

The neurologically impaired or injured patient requires a more detailed but rapid assessment which probably takes an additional 30 seconds and includes disability.

D—Disability

Disability refers to the neurological component of the physical exam. Some of the parameters for the neurological component have already been assessed in the preceding ABCs of care. Assessment D of the primary survey focuses on the following:

- level of consciousness
- pupillary equality and reaction
- motor and sensory function

A frequently used mnemonic for assessing which stimuli the patient will respond to includes the following[1]:

- A = alert (and oriented to person, place, time)
- V = verbal (responds to verbal stimuli)
- P = painful (responds only to painful stimuli)
- U = unresponsive (flaccid, no response)

This is discussed in more detail in the mini-neurological examination presented later in this chapter. One must remember that this is a 30-second assessment. This information must be gathered prior to the administration of sedatives, analgesics, or neuromuscular blocking agents because future data gathered will not be reliable if a baseline is not first established. The D in disability also refers to cervical spine stabilization (Figure 1–2).

In A, the airway phase of the primary survey, the nurse assisted in the control of the C-spine. But now, cervical stabilization takes place if it has not already been done. This means full C-spine precautions that include:

- a stiff neck collar/hard collar (replace soft collar if present)
- long backboard placement (patient may be placed on board upon arrival if this procedure was not performed in the field)
- sandbags (to both sides of the head placed up against the shoulders and the sides of each ear)
- taping (wide adhesive tape across the forehead and down to both sides of the backboard to prevent rotation of the head or neck)

These four procedures will ensure total spinal immobilization. In case of vomiting, the patient and the backboard, as a unit, can be turned to the side to clear the airway. The final part of the primary survey involves the E of assessment.

E—Expose the Patient

The patient must be fully undressed to complete a head-to-toe examination.

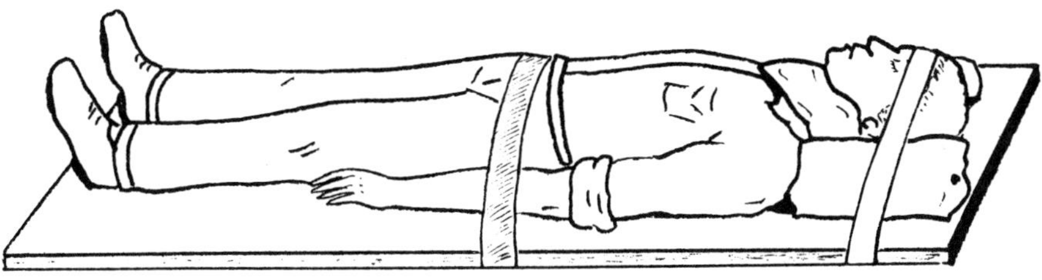

Fig. 1–2—Full cervical spine (C-spine) immobilization. This includes a stiff collar (if there is no neck swelling), a long backboard, sandbags to both sides of the head, and wide tape across the forehead and secured to each side of the backboard.

Secondary Survey

The secondary survey consists of a thorough head-to-toe examination. It does not matter whether one uses the head-to-toe approach or the systems approach. What does matter is that one is complete, systematic, thorough, and consistent and that a reevaluation is performed periodically. Most clinicians refer to this phase of assessment as the history and physical.

History

Obtaining a brief, pertinent history may aid in establishing a differential diagnosis. Use of the mnemonic A-M-P-L-E (see Table 1–2) helps prevent errors of omission in obtaining relevant historical data.[1] An attempt should be made to determine the mechanism of injury from information supplied by prehospital medical personnel.

An additional mnemonic that is helpful is establishing a differential diagnosis in the unconscious patient is A-E-I-O-U-T-I-P-S[5] (see Table 1–3). The secondary survey consists of an examination of the head, face, eyes, ears, nose, mouth, throat, neck, chest, abdomen, pelvis, back, and extremities.

Head and Neck

The head, face, and neck should be observed for symmetry and palpated for contusions, hematomas, lacerations, or fractures. One must also look for penetrating injuries, wounds, ecchymotic areas, or other occult injuries. One may feel a step-off fracture (fracture of the spinous process) in the cervical, thoracic, or lumbar spine prior to x-ray examination. Spinal palpation is done without disturbing the patient's spinal alignment. The neck should also be observed for flat or distended neck veins. One can also palpate for tracheal deviation if it is not readily observed.

Table 1–2 History Taking Guide[1]

Mnemonic	Questions to Ask
A = Allergies	Is the patient allergic to any medications?
M = Medications	Is the patient on any medications?
P = Past medical history	Is there any past serious illness or previous injury?
L = Last meal	When was the last meal?
E = Events	What were the events or occurrences surrounding the incident?

Table 1–3 Differential Diagnosis of Unconsciousness[5]

Mnemonic	*Questions to Ask*
A = Alcohol	Alcoholic odor to breath? History of alcoholic consumption? Blood alcohol level?
E = Epilepsy	History of seizures? Witnessed seizuring? Incontinent of urine? Medications found?
I = Insulin	Is patient a known diabetic? Response to intravenous dextrose? Dip stick urine result? Kussmaul's respirations? Skin vitals?
O = Overdose	Evidence of ingestion around mouth? Is patient breathing shallowly? Evidence of track marks? Difficulty starting intravenous fluids? Pupillary reaction? Response to intravenous Naloxone? Empty pill bottles?
U = Uremia (and other metabolic causes)	Endocrine disorder? Renal failure? Dialysis patient? Liver problems? Other metabolic causes?
T = Trauma	Evidence of trauma to head, chest, etc.? Results of C-spine x-ray? Clues at the scene? Mechanism of injury, if known? Hypotension? Capillary refill? Rapid pulse?
I = Infection	Recent infection? Signs of sepsis? Temperature? Oliguric? Blood pressure? Skin vitals?
P = Psychiatric	Verbal response? Painful response?

Table 1–3 continued

Mnemonic	Questions to Ask
	Eye opening?
	Motor response?
	Previous psychiatric history?
S = Stroke	Age of patient?
(and other cardiovascular causes)	Past cardiac/neurological history?
	Hemaparesis or paralysis?
	Hand grips?
	Vital signs?

Eyes. The eyes should be inspected externally for penetrating injuries, foreign bodies, swelling, contusions, orbital ecchymosis (raccoon eyes), or orbital fractures. The pupils are examined for size and equality, shape, and reaction to light and accommodation (pupillary constriction and convergence of the optical axes on focusing from a far to a near object). Opthalmoscopic examination may reveal retinal hemorrhages. One should always check for contact lenses and remove them if present.

Ears. The ears are inspected for clear or bloody drainage (otorrhea). Watery clear or blood stained otorrhea or hemotympanum (blood behind the ear drum) may indicate basal skull fracture with leakage of cerebrospinal fluid (CSF). The mastoid area should be inspected for ecchymosis (Battle's sign), which is also a sign of basal skull fracture.[5]

Nose. The external nares are also inspected for evidence of CSF or bloody drainage (rhinorrhea), which may indicate an anterior basal skull fracture. If a CSF leak is suspected, the halo test should be performed to confirm suspicions (see Chapter 8).

Mouth and Throat. The mucous membranes of the mouth and throat and the teeth are inspected. The larynx should be assessed for trauma or the presence of voice hoarseness, which could indicate blunt neck trauma or the presence of an aneurysm partially compressing the larynx.

Tongue. If the patient can say ''ah'' and stick out the tongue, any deviation to one side should be noted. With a neurological deficit, the tongue deviates toward the affected (paralyzed) side while the uvula deviates in the opposite direction.

Chest

More thorough assessment of the chest includes auscultation of the lungs and heart. Abnormalities should be noted and any electrocardiographic changes should be documented. Ischemic electrocardiographic changes and dysrhythmias may be seen in patients with intracranial disorders (see Chapter 11). Blunt chest trauma involving the heart can also cause T wave changes and dysrhythmias.

One should inspect and palpate the neck region of trauma patients for the appearance of subcutaneous emphysema. The chest should be inspected for wounds, hematomas, etc. The examiner should palpate and stress the rib cage for areas of deformity, pain, or tenderness.

Abdomen

The abdomen is checked for lesions, scars, abrasions, wounds, seat-belt marks (if automobile accident was involved), and distention. One should auscultate for bowel sounds, palpate for masses, tenderness, guarding, rigidity, or pain, and percuss the abdomen if distended.

Pelvis

The pelvis is examined for tenderness by performing the "shake" test after lumbosacral spinal injury has been ruled out. This is done by placing the examiner's hands on both sides of the patient's iliac crests and shaking or moving the pelvis firmly side to side. Assessment also includes pressing downward on both hips to feel for pelvic stability.

The genitourinary area is inspected for the presence of blood at the urinary meatus. A digital rectal exam is performed. In males, the presence of a high riding prostate or scrotal hematoma indicates trauma to that area, with possible bladder rupture. Urethral catheterization should not be performed in these patients until genitourinary injury is ruled out.

If a digital rectal exam reveals the loss of anal sphincter tone, spinal cord injury should be suspected.

Back

The entire spinal column is palpated without turning the patient and felt for tenderness or deformity. If spinal cord injury has been ruled out and the patient can be turned, the back is inspected. Again, one looks for penetrating injuries or blunt injuries, which might appear as contusions, marks, or abrasion. The flank areas are inspected and palpated for costovertebral angle tenderness suggestive of kidney trauma or infection.

Extremities

The extremities are inspected and palpated for areas of tenderness, pain, crepitus, or deformity. A useful mnemonic is the six Ps of evaluation[5]:

- pain
- puffiness (swelling, edema)
- pallor
- pulselessness
- paresthesia
- paralysis

Skin

The skin is assessed for color, temperature, and moisture as well as turgor. While certain aspects of the secondary survey may seem unrelated to the neurological patient, associated injuries detected on secondary survey can indirectly and adversely affect the neurological system.

Extracranial injuries to the chest, abdomen, spinal cord, and long bones are major causes of hypotension. Hypotension in the neurological patient leads to decreased cerebral perfusion, resulting in cerebral ischemia and secondary infarction. Blood loss from intracranial injuries is rarely significant enough to cause shock. Likewise, the injured brain can mediate multisystem life-threatening complications, such as neurogenic pulmonary edema and cardiac dysrhythmias (see Chapter 11).

THE MINI-NEUROLOGICAL EXAMINATION

Although the mini-neuro exam is an abbreviated form of neurological assessment, it still contains the four basic elements of assessment in any neurological examination. These are:

- level of consciousness/Glasgow Coma Scale
- pupils
- motor/sensory responses
- vital signs

See Chapter 3 for detailed coverage of the neurological examination.

Level of Consciousness

The level of consciousness (LOC) is probably the most sensitive indicator of intracranial pathology. An alteration in LOC, i.e., agitation, or more commonly, decreasing LOC, is usually the first change observed.

Glasgow Coma Scale

Preferable to trying to classify different levels of consciousness with various labels (see Chapter 14) is the implementation of a scoring system known as the Glasgow Coma Scale (GCS; see Table 1–4).[6] The GCS is easy to use, less ambiguous, and has become internationally recognized as an effective tool for objectively communicating assessment data. It consists of three categories of assessment: eye opening, verbal response, and best motor response.

The highest score of 15 reflects an alert individual interacting with his or her environment. The unconscious, unresponsive patient may have a GCS score of 3. Note that the scale ranges from 1 (not 0) to 15, and the minimum score is 3.

Table 1–4 Glasgow Coma Scale[6]

Response	Score
Eyes Open to	
Spontaneous: eyes open (does not imply awareness)	4
Speech: responds to any speech or shout, not necessarily to command	3
Pain: should apply stimulus to limbs, not face	2
Never: (self-explanatory)	1
Best Verbal	
Oriented: aware of self and environment; should be oriented $\times$ 3 (to time, place, person)	5
Confused: attention can be held; responds to questions in conversational manner, but with varying degrees of disorientation and confusion	4
Inappropriate words: intelligible articulation, but no sustained conversation possible; usually shouting or swearing	3
Incomprehensible sounds: moaning and groaning without recognizable words	2
None: (self-explanatory)	1
Best motor	
Obeys commands: (self-explanatory; do not interpret grasp reflexes as response to command)	6
Localizes pain: pain stimulus causes limb to move as to attempt to remove it	5
Flexor withdrawal: withdraws from pain; flexes arms and legs	4
Abnormal flexion: decorticate; flexion of arms, extension of legs and feet (unless SCI [spinal cord injury] present)	3
Extension: decerebrate; extension of arms, legs, feet, with internal rotation of hands and feet	2
None: flaccid; important to rule out SCI	1

Patients with prolonged coma and a GCS score of 3–5 statistically have poor outcomes.

The GCS, in combination with other studies, is a valuable prognostic indicator.[2] Although the GCS is usually reliable and relatively easy to score, there are areas of misunderstanding among nurses and others performing the scoring. Some find it difficult to differentiate between decorticate posturing and withdrawal from painful stimuli. Others find difficulty scoring a 4 for eye opening in deeply comatose, unresponsive patients in whom the eyes remain open. The best advice to give examiners is to be objective and to not "read into" what is observed, just objectively record it. It should be noted that severe hypotension, alcohol, and other depressant drugs may render the GCS ineffective.

One should score the best response of the patient. For example, a patient with lateralizing signs may exhibit extensor posturing on one side of the body, while exhibiting flexor withdrawal on the opposite side. In this instance, this patient would receive a best motor score of 4.

Some patients are almost impossible to score, for example, the patient whose eyes are swollen shut, is restrained, or is intubated. Before applying a label to this patient's level of consciousness, such as alert, lethargic, or obtunded, one should be sure that all members of the medical team agree on the precise meaning of each term used (see Chapter 14).

Pupils

Pupils are checked as part of the mini-neuro exam during the assessment of the eye-opening phase of the GCS. Although a quick check was done during the primary survey, it is now important to look more closely at the pupils. The nurse should check pupils for:

- size (an enlarging pupil without physiologic anisocoria is indicative of midbrain herniation)
- shape (Figure 1–3 demonstrates an oval pupil, which can indicate early third cranial nerve compression seen in early brain herniation syndromes)
- equality (a 1-mm pupillary difference is significant)
- light reflexes (asymmetric constriction to light may indicate brainstem dysfunction)

See Chapter 3 for further descriptions of pupillary abnormalities.

Motor Function

After LOC, GCS, and pupils are assessed, motor responses are evaluated. The nurse assesses for symmetry of movement and strength in all extremities and the

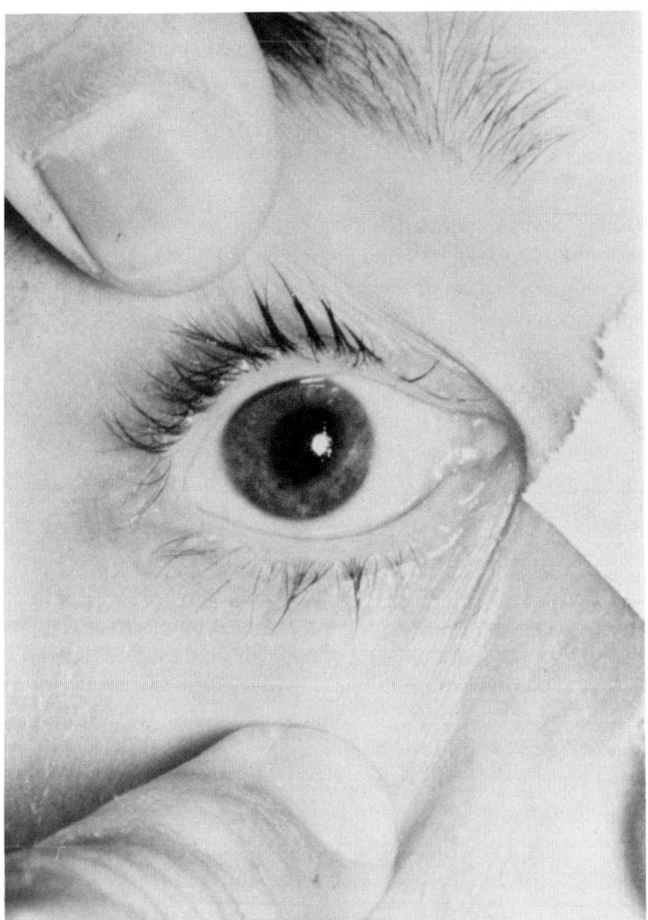

Fig. 1–3—Oval pupil. Early compression of the third cranial nerve can cause the pupil to change from round to oval.

face, comparing right to left, and noting any inequalities. Any abnormal motor movements or ''posturing'' is described (see Chapter 3).

Sensory Responses

A brief sensory examination consists of assessing the patient's ability to sense pain (pinprick) and touch in all four extremities, the trunk, and the face. Any areas of decreased or absent sensation are noted. Frequent follow-up assessments for increasing or decreasing levels of sensation must be performed.

Vital Signs

Another important observation in the neurological patient is the assessment of vital signs.

Respirations

As previously stated, evaluation of the respiratory system is the first priority, with corrections of any deficiencies being carried out during the primary survey.

In the neurological patient there are various changes that may be observed in the rate, rhythm, and depth of respirations (see Chapter 3, Figure 3–8). As ICP rises, there is generally a slowing of the respiratory rate. Respirations may then become irregular in depth and rhythm. Tachypnea or rapid respirations may follow as ICP continues to rise. Unrelieved intracranial hypertension eventually leads to brainstem compression and respiratory arrest.

Chest injury, spinal cord injury, and metabolic and acid-base disorders can also contribute to abnormal respiratory patterns.

Blood Pressure

Blood pressure also yields information regarding the status of the neurological patient. Blood pressure changes to watch for in the presence of intracranial hypertension include an elevating systolic pressure with a widening pulse pressure. Blood pressure changes are considered a late sign in impending brain herniation, however.

On the other hand, hypotension and shock in the head trauma patient are usually due to injury to another area of the body (e.g., chest, abdomen, femur). Although massive facial bleeding, large scalp lacerations, and/or massive head trauma can also produce shock, hypotension is rarely due to brain injury except as a terminal event.

Hypotension caused by spinal (neurogenic) shock can occur with cervical and high thoracic spinal cord injuries. An interruption of sympathetic control of vascular tone occurs and leads to decreased venous return and the peripheral pooling of blood. This results in a relative hypovolemia.[1]

Regardless of the cause, significant hypotension must be treated aggressively to maintain adequate cerebral blood flow.

Pulse

Pulse rates may vary in relation to ICP and various intracranial lesions. Bradycardia is often seen in the following:

- increased ICP
- spinal shock with loss of sympathetic control

Tachycardia can indicate:

- hypovolemia/hemorrhagic shock
- pain or anxiety
- fever
- increased ICP (often a preterminal sign)
- vasodilatory shock[7]

Temperature

This vital sign is frequently forgotten in the emergency setting when attending to critically ill neurological patients. It is important to maintain normothermia in the neurological patient because increased temperature greatly increases oxygen consumption by the brain. The nurse should assess for elevated temperature (hyperthermia) in patients with infections, meningeal irritation, or head trauma with injury to the hypothalamus, the temperature regulating center. Hyperthermia can also result from blood in the CSF as seen in subarachnoid hemorrhage.[7]

Subnormal temperature (hypothermia) can be caused by hypothalamic lesions, spinal shock, CNS depression (including drug overdose), some metabolic disorders such as hypothyroidism, or can be environmentally induced by exposure. The nurse should also remember that the rapid administration of blood products or IV solutions that have not been warmed can also lead to hypothermia.

THE NURSE'S ROLE IN DIAGNOSTIC AND THERAPEUTIC PROCEDURES

Radiological and laboratory studies become critical necessities in the neurological emergency patient. In the unconscious patient this information may provide the only clue to the diagnosis.

Diagnostic Procedures

The nurse's role in diagnostic procedures includes assisting in preparing and positioning the patient, assuring that the ABCs of life support therapy are maintained, observing the patient's response to procedures, performing ongoing physical assessments, and documenting all activities.

Cervical Spine X-rays

Upon arrival in the emergency department, patients with suspected head, neck, or spinal column injury should receive an immediate cross table lateral cervical spine x-ray. Complete immobilization of the spine is carried out prior to obtaining the cervical film. The patient lies in a supine position on the guerney while the x-ray is taken. Those with potential cervical injuries or neck pain should continue in full C-spine immobilization until the full cervical series can be completed and evaluated. A complete cervical series consists of the following views:

- anterior-posterior (AP)
- lateral
- oblique
- odontoid or open mouth (for visualization of C-1 and C-2[8]

The nurse can be helpful during the cross table lateral procedure by assisting the x-ray technician in positioning the patient, as shown in Figure 1–4. The nurse, positioned at the foot of the guerney, clasps both wrists of the patient tightly, and, with gentle, steady traction, pulls the patient's shoulders down. This provides better visualization of all seven cervical vertebrae, particularly C-7. A frequently missed fracture occurs at the C6-7 level, while the most common fracture site is at the level of C5-6.[1]

An alternative patient position that yields similar radiological results is the swimmer's view. The swimmer's view consists of raising the arm of the patient to a 90 degree angle and shooting the x-ray through the axilla. This technique also provides visualization of all seven cervical vertebrae.[8] The swimmer's view may be necessary in the patient with a short, squat neck. The nurse should prepare the patient, if time permits, by explaining the procedure.

During all radiological procedures the nurse must wear a lead apron. Patients of child bearing age should have their pelvic regions shielded as well.

Skull Series

Although skull films are generally overrequested in the emergency department, any patient known to or suspected of having blunt or penetrating trauma to the head will probably receive skull x-rays.[9] Skull x-rays can demonstrate fractures, air-fluid (blood) levels in the sinuses, abnormal intracranial calcifications, facial bone destruction (such as from tumors), location of the brain's midline structures by visualization of the calcified pineal gland (in adults), and widened or prematurely fused sutures (in children).[10]

A complete skull series includes:

- anterior-posterior view
- lateral views
- occipital (Towne) view
- base view
- Water's view (maxillary sinus view)

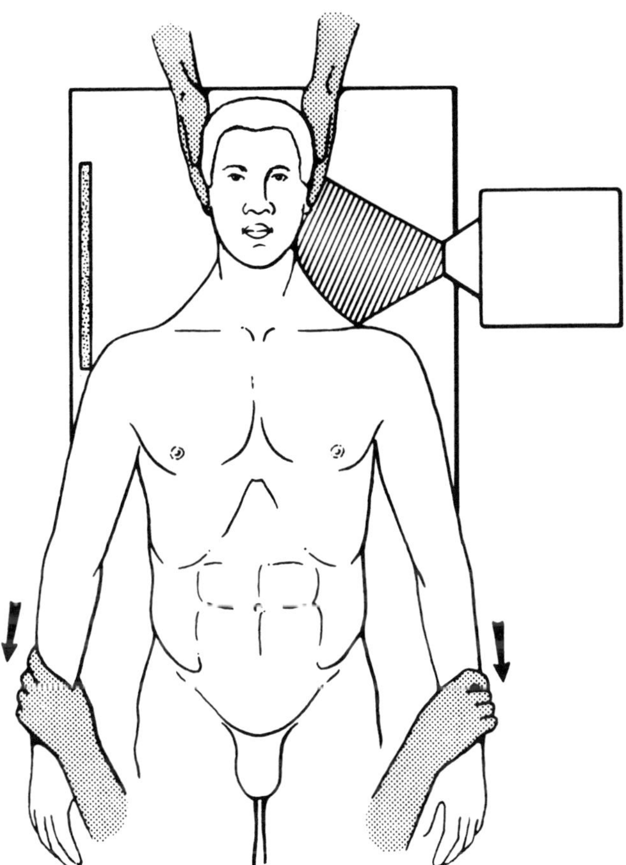

Fig. 1-4—Method of obtaining lateral roentgenogram of the cervical spine with downward traction on the patient's arms to expose all seven cervical vertebrae.
Source: Reprinted from *Emergency Medicine: A Comprehensive Review* (p 624) by TC Kravis and CG Warner (eds), Aspen Systems Corporation, © 1983.

Facial bones, although not part of the skull series, may be ordered if necessary.

With increased utilization of computerized axial tomography scanning (CT scan), skull films may become less routinely taken. This decision, however, will depend on the nature and extent of the neurological illness or injury.

Computerized Axial Tomography

Over the last decade CT scanning has added a new dimension to the field of radiology, particularly in neurological patients. For example, in approximately 12 minutes it is possible to diagnose many intracranial lesions utilizing limited

CT scanning of the head (see Figure 1–5). A CT scan of the head should be obtained in any trauma patient with a suspected skull fracture, neurological deficit, or worsening neurological status. It can make a definitive diagnosis for subdural hematoma, epidural hematoma, intracerebral hematoma, cortical contusion, and cerebral edema.

CT scanning has also had major implications for patients with spinal cord trauma. The CT scan can delineate the anatomy of the spine injury more clearly than simple x-rays and can demonstrate possible spinal canal compromise.[11]

Angiography

Neurological emergency patients will occasionally need emergency angiographic studies. Angiography refers to the radiographic examination of blood vessels made visible by the injection of a contrast agent. Angiography can be helpful when diagnosing vascular disruption, vasospasm, aneurysms, arteriovenous malformations, and other vessel abnormalities. The approach to the intracranial vessels is usually through percutaneous puncture of the carotid artery in the neck or the femoral artery in the groin. These special radiological procedures cannot be performed in unstable patients in whom surgery is the next line of defense. They can, however be additional adjuncts to the diagnosis and subsequent management of the neurological patient.

Adverse hypersensitive reactions to the contrast agent occasionally occur. It the event of an anaphylactic reaction, the procedure must be immediately terminated and treatment of anaphylaxis started at once. Following the procedure the nurse must frequently inspect the puncture site for hematoma formation. The patient should also be assessed for adverse neurological complications caused by vasospasm or emboli resulting from the procedure.

Nuclear Magnetic Resonance Imaging

Nuclear magnetic resonance imaging (NMR or MRI scan) produces detailed images of the body without the use of radiation (Figure 1–6). The patient is placed inside a large tubular shaped machine in which a large magnet generates a strong magnetic field. The hydrogen protons in the body tend to line up with the magnetic field. A radio frequency is applied, then turned off. This causes the protons to ''wobble.'' As the protons then realign with the magnetic field, they emit the absorbed radio frequency signal and these emissions generate the MRI image. It is useful in demonstrating cerebral edema, tumors, blood vessels, hemorrhages, etc. It cannot be used on patients with any ferrous compound prosthesis or surgically implanted clips or hardware. Nonferrous compounds such as surgical stainless steel may be acceptable. It is also contraindicated in patients with pacemakers or metallic heart valves. It is also recommended that it not be used in pregnant women.

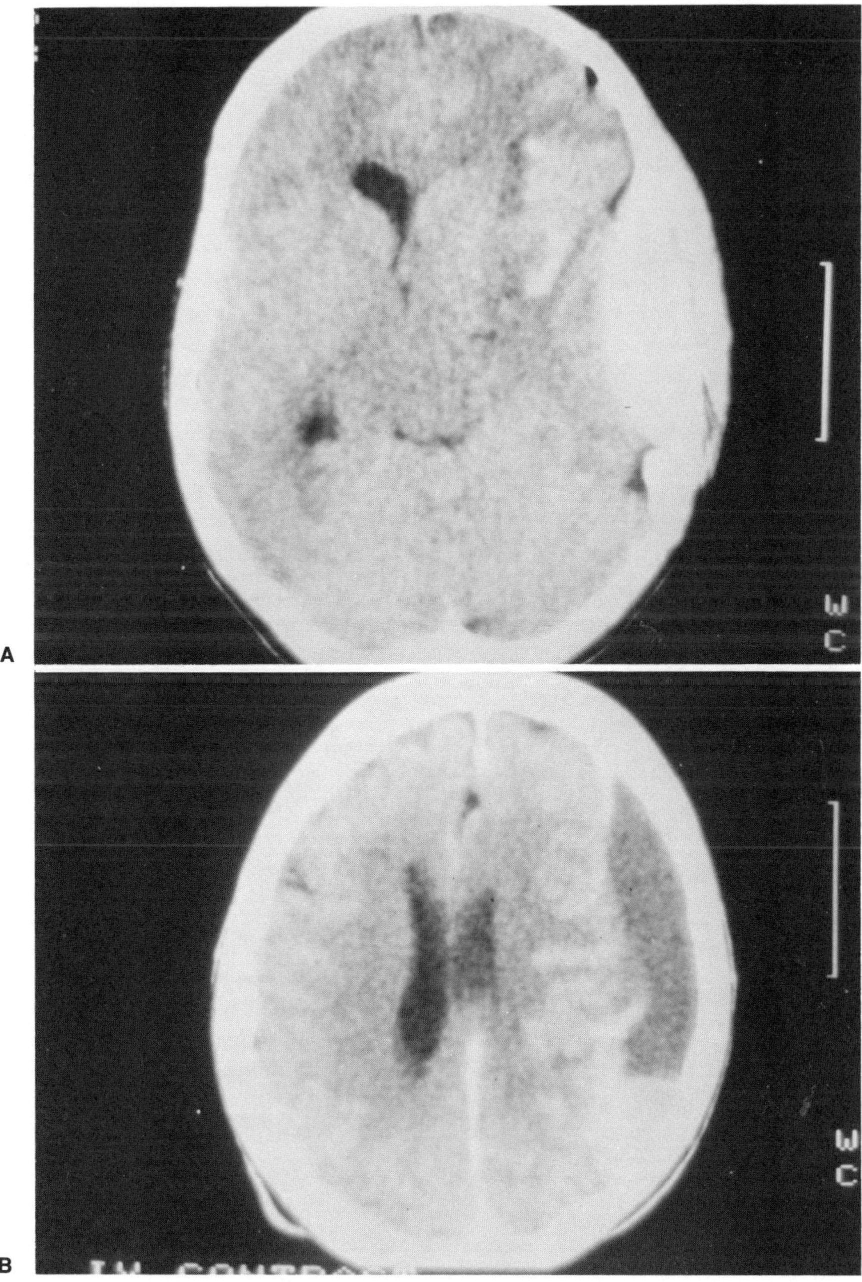

Fig. 1–5—Computerized axial tomography (CT) scans demonstrating (A) an epidural hematoma, and (B) a chronic subdural hematoma.
Source: Courtesy of Grossmont District Hospital, La Mesa, Ca.

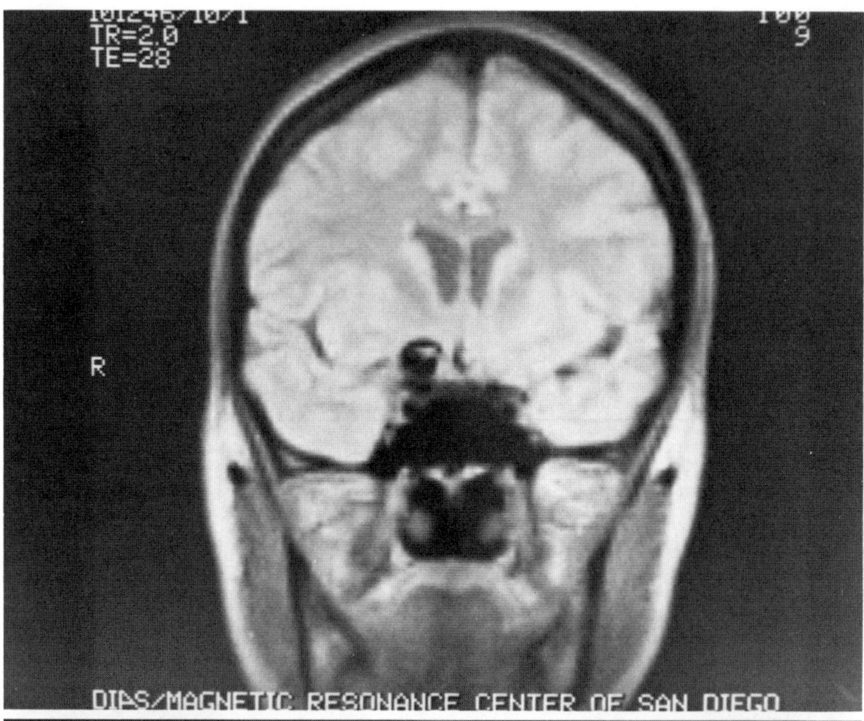

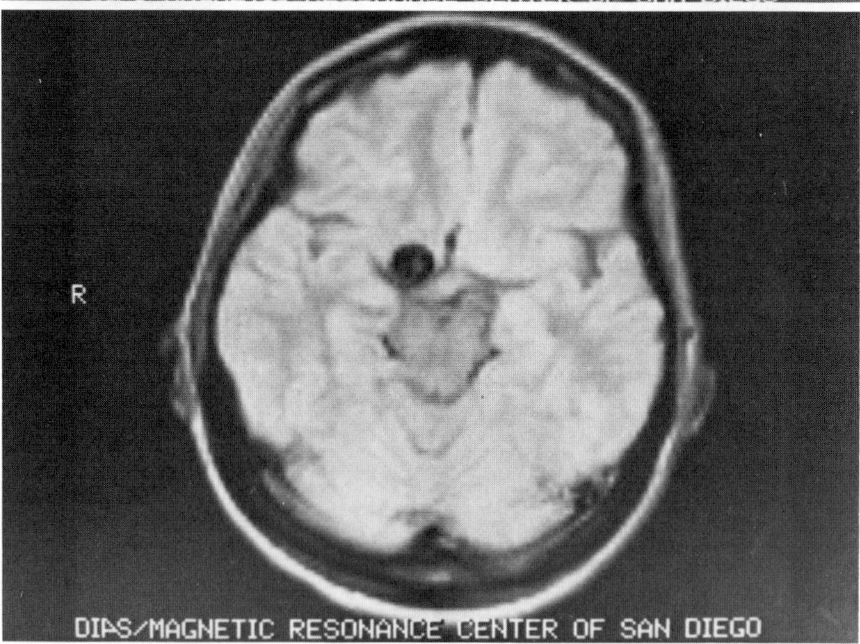

Fig. 1–6—Two nuclear magnetic resonance images of a patient with a right internal carotid artery aneurysm.

Source: Reprinted with permission of the Magnetic Resonance Center of San Diego, San Diego, Ca.

Because the patient is inside the large tubular shaped machine, the nurse has limited access to the patient. The procedure also requires that the patient remain completely still for sometimes up to 45 minutes while the imaging takes place. These factors render MRI scanning less appropriate in acutely ill patients who may be intubated or restless and require constant nursing supervision.

Laboratory

After initial assessment has been performed, the following laboratory data will provide the physician and nurse with valuable information toward obtaining a working diagnosis:

- complete blood count (CBC), including white blood cell (WBC) differential
- urinalysis
- electrolytes (sodium, potassium, chloride, carbon dioxide)
- blood glucose
- blood urea nitrogen (BUN)
- creatinine

This list is obviously not exhaustive but will give the practitioner some baseline data. Many paramedics draw blood specimens prior to administration of drugs in the prehospital phase of care. This is crucial in cases of undiagnosed coma which could be caused by hyper- or hypoglycemia or drug and/or alcohol abuse.

Additional laboratory tests that may be ordered include:

- type and crossmatch
- blood alcohol
- drug or coma panel (for prescription, dangerous, or street drugs)
- blood clotting profile

Cerebrospinal fluid obtained from a lumbar puncture, cisternal puncture, or intraventricular pressure monitoring system may be tested for:

- CSF pressure (done at time obtained)
- gross description of appearance
- cell count
- protein
- culture and sensitivity
- glucose
- electrolytes

- pH
- Wasserman
- other chemical analyses

Therapeutic Procedures

It is the responsibility of the nurse to gather the equipment, prepare the patient, obtain necessary permits, assist with the procedure, and document the events during therapeutic procedures.

Lumbar Puncture

A lumbar puncture (LP) is the insertion of a spinal needle into the lumbar subarachnoid space and withdrawal of CSF for diagnostic and therapeutic purposes.[12] This is a common emergency department procedure in patients suspected of having CNS infections such as meningitis or encephalopathies such as Reye's syndrome. CSF is obtained for laboratory analysis (see Table 1–5) to relieve CSF pressure (although this is done infrequently in the emergency department) and to determine the presence or absence of blood in the CSF. If increased ICP is suspected, an LP can be hazardous. As CSF is removed from the lumbar area of patients with supratentorial lesions and/or increased ICP, the brain may herniate downward.

Equipment. Equipment needed for an LP includes an LP tray or LP set with manometer, sterile gloves, local anesthetic agent, skin prep, and a sterile dressing or bandaid for use at the completion of the procedure.

Preparation. To prepare the patient for the procedure, the nurse opens the LP tray, places the patient in the position as shown in Figure 1–7, and instructs the patient to arch the lower back and to draw the knees up to the abdomen, clasping the knees with the hands.

Procedure. The patient is draped, the skin is prepped with an antiseptic solution, the area is infiltrated with a local anesthetic agent, and the physician then introduces the spinal needle between the L3-4 or L4-5 *inter*space. The needle is advanced until the give of the ligamentum flavum is felt and the needle enters the subarachnoid space. A manometer is attached to the LP needle and an initial CSF pressure reading is obtained. Two to three cubic centimeters of spinal fluid is then withdrawn and placed in test tubes for laboratory analysis.

Spinal fluid should be clear and colorless.[12,13] Blood tinged or bloody spinal fluid may indicate a traumatic tap, cerebral contusion, laceration, or subarachnoid hemorrhage.

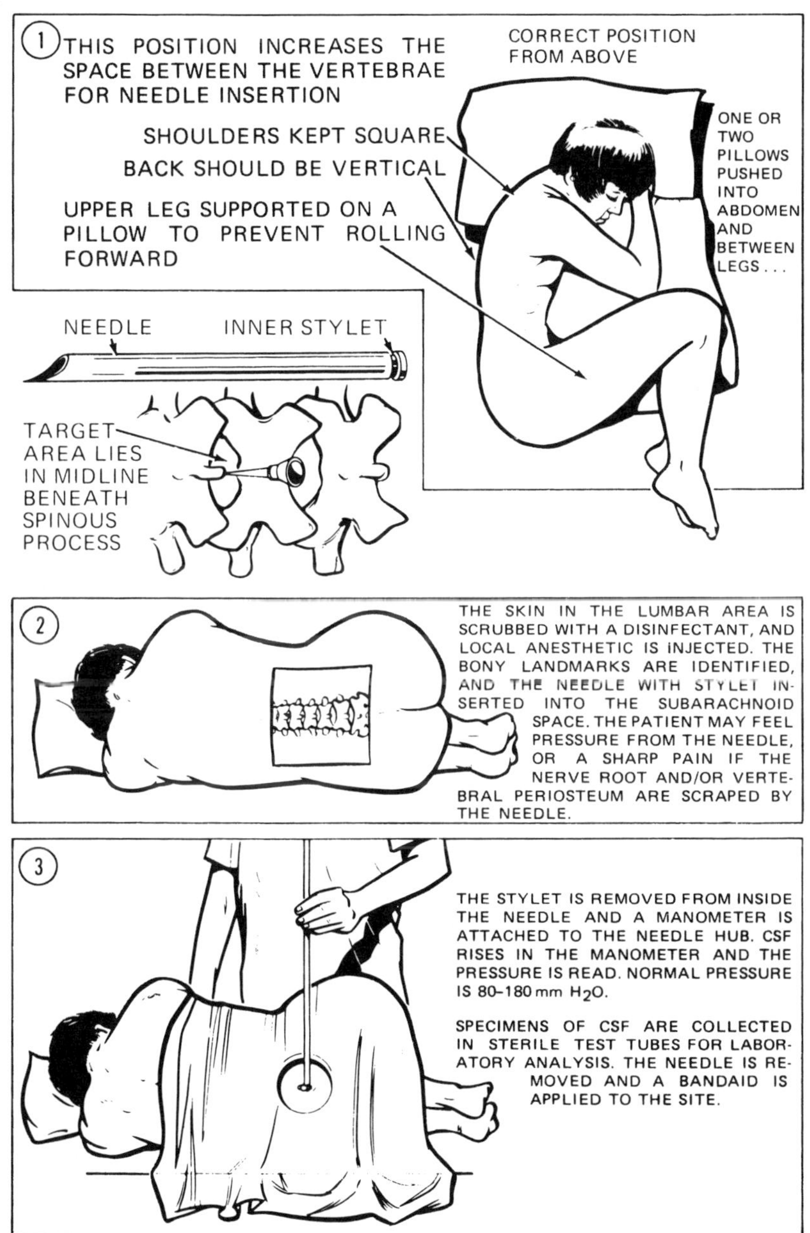

Fig. 1–7—Lumbar puncture procedure.

Source: Reprinted from *Neurological Problems: A Critical Care Nursing Focus* (p 125) by M Snyder and M Jackle with permission of Robert J Brady Company, © 1981.

Table 1–5 Cerebrospinal Fluid[12,13]

Parameters	Normal	Abnormal	Possible cause
Pressure (initial readings)	80–180 mm H_2O	<60 mm	Faulty needle placement Dehydration Spinal block along subarachnoid space Block at foramen magnum
		>200 mm	Muscle tension Abdominal compression Brain tumor Subdural hematoma Brain abcess Brain cyst Cerebral edema (any cause) Internal hydrocephalus Benign intracranial hypertension
Color	Clear, colorless	Cloudy	Increased cell count Increased microorganisms
		Yellow	Xanthochromic (due to RBC pigments) High protein content
		Smoky	Presence of RBCs
Red blood cells	None	Blood-tinged Grossly bloody	Traumatic tap Traumatic tap Subarachnoid hemorrhage
White blood cells	0–6 mm³	>10 mm³ (Cell counts range from below 100 to many thousands depending on causative factor; all are abnormal findings)	Occurs in many conditions: Bacterial infections of meninges Viral infections of meninges Neurosyphilis Tuberculous meningitis Metastatic neoplastic lesions Parasitic infections Acute demyelinating diseases

Table 1–5 continued

Parameters	Normal	Abnormal	Possible cause
			Following introduction of air or blood into subarachnoid space
Protein*	15–45 mg/100 ml (1 percent of serum protein)	<10 mg/100 ml	Little clinical significance
		>60 mg/100 ml	Occurs in many conditions: Complete spinal block Guillain-Barré syndrome Carcinomatosis of meninges Tumors close to pial or ependymal surfaces, or in cerebellopositive angle Acute and chronic meningitis Meningeal hemorrhage Demyelinating disorders Degenerative diseases
Glucose	50–75 mg/100 ml (approximately 60 percent of blood glucose level)	<40 mg/100 ml	Acute bacterial meningitis Tuberculous meningitis Meningeal carcinomatosis
		>100 mg/100 ml	Diabetes
Chloride	700–750 mg/100 ml	<625 mg/100 ml	Hypochloremia Tuberculous meningitis
		>800 mg/100 ml	Not of neurological significance; correlate with blood levels of chloride

*If CSF contains blood this will raise the protein level.

Source: Reprinted from *Advanced Neurological and Neurosurgical Nursing* (p 108) by Ellen B Rudy with permission of the CV Mosby Company, © 1984.

If the physician suspects an obstruction in the spinal subarachnoid space, a test for the Queckenstedt's sign may be performed. This consists of compressing the patient's jugular veins for ten seconds. If no block is present, the CSF pressure will rise.

Aftercare. Aftercare of the patient undergoing LP includes dressing the puncture site and documenting the following: the procedure, including the condition of the patient, lab tests ordered, the time the procedure began and ended, and the results of tests. The patient is sometimes maintained in a prone, supine, or lateral position for six hours as a means of preventing headache. Liberal fluid intake should be encouraged, if not contraindicated. The physician is to be informed of any change in the patient's condition. Supportive care is administered as needed.[14]

Skull Tongs

Skull tongs and traction are used to stabilize and reduce certain fractures and dislocations of the cervical or high thoracic spine (see Figure 1–8). Patients with unstable vertebral fractures with potential for neurological deficit often go to the operating room for surgical stabilization.

Equipment. The equipment needed for skull tongs placement includes skin prepping solution, antiseptic solution, local anesthetic agent, skull tongs (Crutchfield, Gardner-Wells, Trippi-Wells), scalpel, traction apparatus, and weights.

Preparation. The sites for application of the tongs (above the ears and below the temporal ridges for Gardner-Wells tongs) are prepped. There is usually no need to shave the scalp. Some practitioners recommend that an aerosol spray be used prior to skull tong penetration because it coats and adheres the hair to the skin.

Procedure. Once the sites have been identified and prepped, the areas are injected with a local anesthetic. Small stab wounds are made over the sites and the tongs are placed into the skull with the metal face plate facing upward. The spring-loaded points of the tong apparatus are advanced until the 1-mm protrusion indicator with its knob shows that the proper "squeeze" is exerted. As the points are advanced the skin is slightly stretched. This is effective and safe because this method of insertion prevents bleeding and acts as a seal at the point of entry. Once the bone is encountered the spring pin stops. The tongs should be tilted back and forth several times to situate the points. The indicator protrusion should be checked and retightened if necessary. The appropriate weight is applied for traction and stabilization purposes. The weight used will depend on the level of cervical injury. The general rule is five pounds of weight per cervical level involved. For example, a C-6 fracture injury would receive 30 pounds

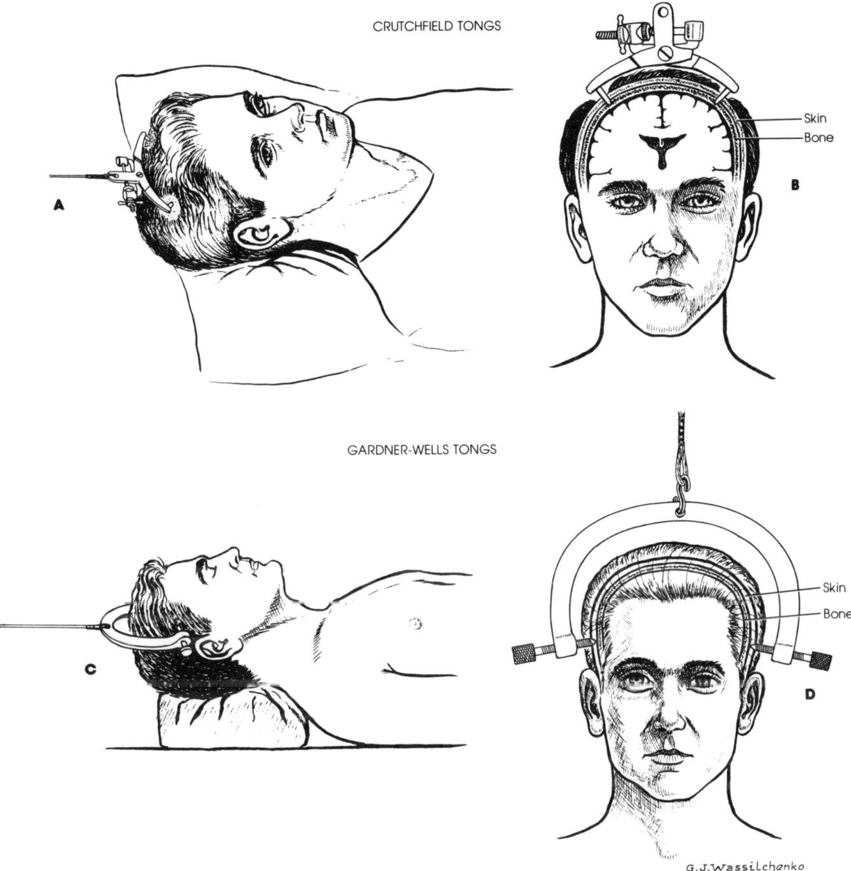

Fig. 1–8—Skull tongs for cervical traction. (A) Supine position. (B) Cross section. (C) Supine position. (D) Cross section.
  Source: Reprinted from *Advanced Neurological and Neurosurgical Nursing* (p 404) by Ellen B Rudy with permission of CV Mosby Company, © 1984.

(6 × 5 = 30) of cervical traction.[5] Sometimes an additional 10 pounds of weight for the head may be added.

Tong placement is contraindicated in infants or where there is Paget's disease of the skull or massive open/comminuted skull fractures.[1]

Aftercare. The patient is usually placed on a turning frame such as a Stryker or Foster frame, or may be placed in a regular hospital bed with a firm mattress and bedboard. Circoelectric beds are used less because of the problem of orthostatic hypotension. The tong sites must be inspected, cleaned, and dressed daily.

Burr Holes

A burr hole is an emergency procedure performed to remove a blood clot from the subdural or epidural space. It is a surgical opening made through the skull using a twist drill.

Equipment. The equipment used for a burr hole procedure includes a twist drill, scalpel, hemostat, suction, retractors, periosteal elevators, prepping solution, and sterile dressings.

Preparation. The decision to evacuate a blood clot from the head is made rapidly. If there is time to perform an adequate prep, the hair should be clipped, then shaved with a sterile razor. The skin is prepped with an antiseptic solution, such as Betadine, and draped with sterile towels. It is then infiltrated with a local anesthetic.

Procedure. The actual procedure for burr hole entrance into the skull begins with a vertical skin incision made one finger breadth in front of the tragus of the ear, and extending 2½ inches cephalad. The depth is extended down to the temporal bone. The incision is retracted and the temporalis muscle pulled away with a periosteal elevator. The incision will bleed considerably since it is at the level of the superficial temporal artery. Use of retractors will help control bleeding and still provide necessary exposure to the clot. Hemostatic control must be maintained and direct pressure with the finger may be used. The burr hole is drilled into the skull through the center of the incision by a simple clockwise rotation of the drill. When penetration of the inner table of the skull occurs, increased resistance is felt. If an epidural hematoma is discovered, it is suctioned with a frazier tip. If no hematoma is discovered, the dura must be incised with a crosshatch X incision. If a subdural hematoma is present, suction should again be applied. Burr hole placement is usually ipsilateral to the dilated pupil or contralateral to the side with the worst motor deficit.[15]

Aftercare. After assisting with the burr hole procedure, the nurse's role includes performing a follow-up neurological assessment, documenting the events, preparing the patient for rapid transport to the operating room or intensive care unit, and providing nursing care enroute.

Monitoring Intracranial Pressure

The emergency department nurse's role in monitoring intracranial pressure is to assemble the equipment, prepare the patient, assist with the procedure, record the events and patient condition, and monitor the patient's care until he or she is transferred to the intensive care unit.

ICP monitoring is not routinely performed in most emergency departments, but may be used occasionally in life threatening situations. Utilization of ICP monitoring depends on the capabilities and resources of the emergency department resuscitation area. If an emergency department has the ability to provide invasive monitoring techniques for therapeutic and diagnostic evaluation, then ICP monitoring can easily be performed. See Chapter 4 for a detailed discussion of ICP monitoring.

PEDIATRIC CONSIDERATIONS

This year in the United States alone 250,000 children will require hospitalization for neurological emergencies.[16] Pediatric neurological emergencies are difficult to manage in even the best of circumstances. Because of inexperience or unfamiliarity with pediatric patients, emergency department nurses frequently experience a sense of anxiety when caring for a critically ill child. To capably and confidently manage the critically ill child the nurse needs an understanding of pediatric concepts and of the unique and individual needs of the pediatric patient, as well as the principles of managing pediatric neurological emergencies. Recognition of when to call in neurological specialists and when to transfer children to other facilities equipped to handle the critically ill pediatric patient is a key issue in reducing morbidity and mortality.[17]

General Differences between Children and Adults

It must be emphasized that children are not little adults. General overall differences between children and adults are:

- pediatric trauma more often involves injury to the head and/or spinal cord (75 percent in children versus 70 percent national average)
- with regard to cerebral insults, the outcome and survival of pediatric patients are statistically better than that of adults
- children have greater resilience but less reserve in their reactions to CNS insult

Anatomical Differences

Some of the most basic anatomical differences between children and adults are:[18]

- the neck in children is short, and if hyperextended, can block the airway
- the child has a larger tongue and smaller mandible
- the infant has a U-shaped epiglottis whereas the adult's is flattened
- the narrower nasal passages in children are easily blocked

- children have a more vascular vertebral column with greater potential for hemorrhage at site of trauma

Physiological Differences

Distinct physiological differences also exist. Among these are:[18]

- a proportionately greater total body surface area in the child
- a greater metabolic rate in children because of a greater per unit weight
- an increased ability of the young child's skull to expand with increasing pressure
- a greater tendency for children to suffer from hypothermia which commonly causes acidosis
- a limited total blood volume in a child, which produces profound shock more rapidly than in an adult

A respiratory arrest with hypoxia is the usual cause of cardiac arrest in the child.

Developmental Differences

- Children tend to ignore symptoms (especially children under two years of age).
- Children are usually unable to describe their neurological symptoms.
- It is difficult to elicit reproducible neurological signs in the child during the performance of the physical examination.[19]

Common Pediatric Neurological Emergencies

The most common pediatric neurological emergencies include seizures, CNS infections, and head trauma. Congenital malformations also account for a very small percentage of pediatric neurological emergencies.

Seizures

Seizures in children are usually the result of febrile episodes. However, other cerebral insults such as head injury and CNS infections can cause seizures. In the absence of a primary seizure disorder, seizures in children are commonly a symptom and not the actual cause of a neurological disorder.

CNS Infections

Infections among the pediatric population include meningitis of various etiologies and encephalopathies such as Reye's syndrome (see Chapter 7).

Head Trauma

Annually in the United States 5 million children sustain some degree of head trauma. Fifty percent of illness and injury in children 1 to 14 years of age is directly related to some traumatic incident. Each year in the United States one-half of the severely injured children will be dead on arrival to emergency departments. Head trauma from child abuse, especially in children under the age of two years, is also a major cause of death and disability.

Head trauma can range from minor superficial head injuries to severe brain injuries. Minor head injuries include forehead contusion, abrasions to the scalp, small localized hematomas, and minor lacerations. Moderate to severe head injuries range from skull fractures and cerebral concussions to severe contusions and lacerations of the brain. Skull fractures can be moderate or severe, depending on their location, size, and involvement of intracranial structures. Three skull fractures frequently encountered in the pediatric patient are linear, basilar, and depressed.

Intracranial bleeding resulting from major head trauma can result in any of the following extra-axial hematomas[17]:

- epidural hematoma
- subdural hematoma
- subarachnoid hemorrhage

Diffuse cerebral edema can occur secondary to severe head trauma. While there may be no skull fracture or bleeding into the epidural or subdural spaces, severe swelling of the brain can cause irreversible neuronal injury leading to death.

Medical and Nursing Management

In the pediatric head trauma patient, rapid medical and/or surgical intervention must occur within the first few hours of injury to avoid permanent disability or death. When a major intracranial bleed occurs, surgical management is often the only alternative. In the presence of brain swelling and cerebral edema, aggressive medical management is needed. Surgical intervention for the placement of ICP monitoring devices is followed by specific medical and nursing management consisting of:

- head positioned midline at a 30 degree elevation to facilitate venous return and reduce ICP
- hyperventilation to $PaCO_2$ of 25–30 mm Hg to vasoconstrict cerebral vessels
- maintenance of cerebral perfusion pressure by control of blood pressure and reduction of ICP

- pharmacological therapy including mannitol, phenytoin, pentobarbital or other barbiturate (see Chapter 5)
- control of seizures (initially with diazepam)
- careful suctioning preceded and followed by hyperoxygenation and hyperventilation, and sometimes preceded by prophylactic intravenous administration of lidocaine[7]

The advancement of techniques such as pediatric intubation and airway management in the prehospital setting are crucial adjuncts to the survival of the pediatric neurological patient. Specialized pediatric centers to care for these patients and programs to combat nonaccidental trauma are goals for the future.

MEDICAL-LEGAL IMPLICATIONS

The nature of emergency care rarely allows for lengthy deliberation in making treatment dispositions. This is especially true in neurological emergencies, where outcomes are so unpredictable.

It is the responsibility of the emergency department nurse to see all patients who present themselves for treatment. Examples of neurological emergencies which by law require immediate attention are severe head injuries and extra-axial hematomas.[20]

Emergency clinicians have been especially prone to potential malpractice litigation primarily because true emergency patients represent high risk clients. Professional negligence occurs when the community standard of care is not observed for the emergency patient.[20]

Important components in preventing or defending against professional negligence claims are:

- consent signing
- charting/documentation
- preservation of evidence

Consent

The patient's informed consent must be obtained before procedures or treatment are rendered. However, in a true emergency, where immediate treatment is necessary to prevent disability and death, consent for treatment is legally implied. The rationale for this practice is that the patient would have given consent had his or her status allowed the informed consent process. Although oral consent is valid, written consent is preferred because it is easier to substantiate. When possible, a consent is signed by the patient for any procedure including an emergency procedure if the patient can physically sign the consent and is under no sedation. To be valid, consent forms must be signed voluntarily unless they are obtained under implied consent.[20] With neurological patients, consents should be obtained for procedures such as:

- CT scan with contrast
- lumbar puncture
- burr holes
- ICP monitoring
- angiography
- MRI scanning

Controversy exists when emergency department nurses are asked by law enforcement officers to draw a blood sample from an arrestee suspected of drunken driving. The written request of the law enforcement officer should be obtained and the blood drawn in the physical presence of the officer. Most states provide that blood can be taken without written consent of the arrestee, including suspected drunken drivers that are unconscious or incapable of giving consent.[4(p45)] Guidelines established by the U.S. Supreme Court in Schmerber v. California (1966) state that blood can be taken from a nonconsenting arrestee provided it is done in a reasonable, medically approved manner, is incident to the person's arrest, and is based on the officer's reasonable belief that the person is intoxicated.[4(p44)] If the appropriate procedures are followed, the nurse/hospital will incur no civil or criminal liability. If a patient violently resists the taking of blood, this may be considered unreasonable taking of blood and the nurse is advised not to do so.

To avoid a legal argument that an alcohol skin prep influenced the test outcome, a cleansing agent other than alcohol should be used. This should also be noted on the laboratory slip.[4(pp44–45)]

Documentation

Another responsibility of the emergency nurse is to provide accurate and complete documentation of the patient's status and all diagnostic and therapeutic procedures performed. This facilitates quality assurance and continuity of patient care, as well as satisfying medical-legal requirements. No longer can nurses count on word-of-mouth reporting at shift change. The standard of care that continues to exist is, "if it is not charted, it's as if it wasn't done."

Meticulous documentation of patient assessment data is vital in identifying subtle changes in level of consciousness, eye opening, verbal response, motor movement, pupillary responses, and sensory changes. These observations can determine the subsequent care the patient receives.

Recording repeated observations on a neurological flow sheet facilitates the comparison of observations, clarifies subtle changes in the patient's condition, and saves nursing time (see Chapter 3, Exhibit 3–1).

Hourly or more frequent charting of patient observations is optimal but often not feasible. Unstable patients may need observations recorded at least every 15 minutes. Some institutions use computer entries and charting to facilitate the documentation of the volume of information that must be recorded. Neurological charting will often include:

- neurological check lists (GCS, pupils, etc.)
- narrative charting (to describe observations)
- graphic charting of vital signs

Terms such as coma, stupor, responsive, obtunded, and lethargic are controversial for communicating findings. It is more accurate and more acceptable to describe in objective, unambiguous detail exactly what the patient can or cannot do. For example, the patient pushes the examiner's hand away with the same hand used when interdigital pressure is applied. This corresponds to a 5 in the motor category of the GCS. This gives the examiner an easy method of comparison with subsequent assessments.

Preservation of Evidence

The preservation of evidence is another important nursing responsibility when caring for patients who may be victims of battery, homicide, suicide, or accident of any suspicious nature. Any patient with an injury that may have been caused by violence or other criminal act that requires further legal investigation must have rapid care and have the appropriate law enforcement agencies notified. The remaining evidence must also be carefully preserved. This evidence includes but is not limited to:

- weapons
- clothing
- material removed from the site of injury (bullet fragments, dirt, grass, etc.)
- other possessions

The following procedures should be adhered to when caring for a patient who may be either a victim or a suspect:

- never cut through clothing unless it is necessary to render care, and when cutting off clothes, cut around the area where the bullet or knife entered

- before wound irrigation, note and document the size, location, and description of the contents of the wound
- save all belongings, but do not place them in plastic bags because of the effects of moisture. Place and seal articles in a clean brown paper bag and label with patient name, date and time, and articles contained within; sign it and give it to the investigating officer, or confine it to a secure area until the arrival of the officer
- take pictures of the injured area whenever possible

It is important that care of the patient never be compromised, but the preservation of evidence can be critical to securing justice and legal recourse for the individual(s) in question.

REFERENCES

1. Collicott PE: *Advanced Trauma Life Support Course*. Chicago, American College of Surgeons, 1984, pp 129–137.
2. Bowers S, Marshall L: Severe head injury: Current treatment and research. *J Neurosurg Nursing* 1980;14:210–219.
3. Lewis F, Oreskovich M: Field care: Do paramedics make a difference? Presented at symposium "Modern Concepts in Trauma Care," Orange County Trauma Society, Anaheim, Ca, May 1984.
4. Budassi SA, Barber JM: *Emergency Nursing, Principles and Practice*. St Louis, Mosby, 1981, pp 151.
5. Barber JM, Budassi SA: *Manual of Emergency Care: Practices and Procedures*. St Louis, Mosby, 1979, pp 226–271.
6. Teasdale G, Jennett B: Assessment of coma and impaired consciousness: A practical scale. *Lancet* 1974;2:81–84.
7. Galada S, Ranieri-Ambrogi D: Monitoring your patient, in *Coping with Neurologic Disorders*. Springhouse, Pa, Intermed Communications, 1982, pp 72–73.
8. Armstrong P, Wastie M: *X-ray Diagnosis*. Boston, Blackwell Scientific, 1981, pp 301–344.
9. The Royal College of Radiologists, England: Patient selection for skull radiography in uncomplicated head injury. *Lancet* 1983;1:115–118.
10. Troupin R: *Diagnostic Radiology in Clinical Medicine*, ed 2. Chicago, Year Book, 1978, pp 143–150.
11. Trunkey D, Lewis F: *Current Therapy of Trauma 1984–1985*. Philadelphia, BC Decker, 1984, pp 47–52.
12. Conway-Rutkowski BL: *Neurological and Neurosurgical Nursing*, ed 8. St Louis, Mosby, 1982.
13. Alpers BJ, Mancall EL: *Essentials of the Neurological Examination*. Philadelphia, Davis, 1971.
14. Brunner L, Suddarth D: *The Lippincott Manual of Nursing Practice*. Philadelphia, Lippincott, 1978, pp 1403–1404.
15. Ruben T: Emergency burr hole, in *UCSD Trauma Management Seminar Manual*. San Diego, Division of Trauma, University of California, 1984, pp 114–115.
16. Bruce DA: Brain injury: Field and emergency management, in *Modern Concepts in Trauma Care Manual*. Orange County, Ca., Orange County Trauma Society, May 1984, pp 103–105.

17. James HE: Head injury in infants, children, and adolescents, in *Intracranial Dynamics Following Head Injuries: Pediatric Intensive Care,* presented at "Modern Concepts in Trauma Care," Orange County Trauma Society, Anaheim, Ca, May 1984.
18. Weibley RE, Holbrook PR: Airway management in the traumatized child. *Topics in Emerg Med* 1982;4:1–7.
19. Rucker R: Monitoring critically ill children. *Topics in Emerg Med* 1981;3:1–5.
20. Mancini M, Gale AT: *Emergency Care and the Law.* Rockville, Md, Aspen Systems, 1981, pp 87–103.

Structure, Function, and Dysfunction of the Nervous System

The nervous system is composed of two divisions: the central nervous system (CNS), which includes the brain and the spinal cord, and the peripheral nervous system, made up of the spinal nerves, the cranial nerves, and the autonomic nervous system. Neural connections between all parts of the nervous system are numerous, multiple, and extremely intricate. The nervous system is responsible not only for regulating itself but also for regulating and coordinating activities of all other body systems. The CNS is also the best protected of all body systems. It is situated almost entirely within bony structures (the skull and vertebrae) and it floats on a waterbed of cerebral spinal fluid (CSF). Further protecting the vitally important neural structures are the meninges and the blood-brain barrier.[1(p16)] All of these factors are discussed in this chapter. Brief reviews of common pathological conditions are included to assist in bringing together a basic understanding of the structure, function, and dysfunction of the nervous system.

SUPPORTING STRUCTURES OF THE CENTRAL NERVOUS SYSTEM

The various supporting structures play an important role in protecting the delicate CNS from trauma and disease. They include the bony structures, meninges, and CSF.

The Skull

The skull (Figures 2–1 and 2–2) is made up of 8 cranial bones, 14 facial bones, and the teeth. The cranium, that part of the skull encasing the brain, is composed of the frontal, occipital, sphenoid, ethmoid, two temporal, and two parietal bones. The bones of the cranium are joined at the suture lines.

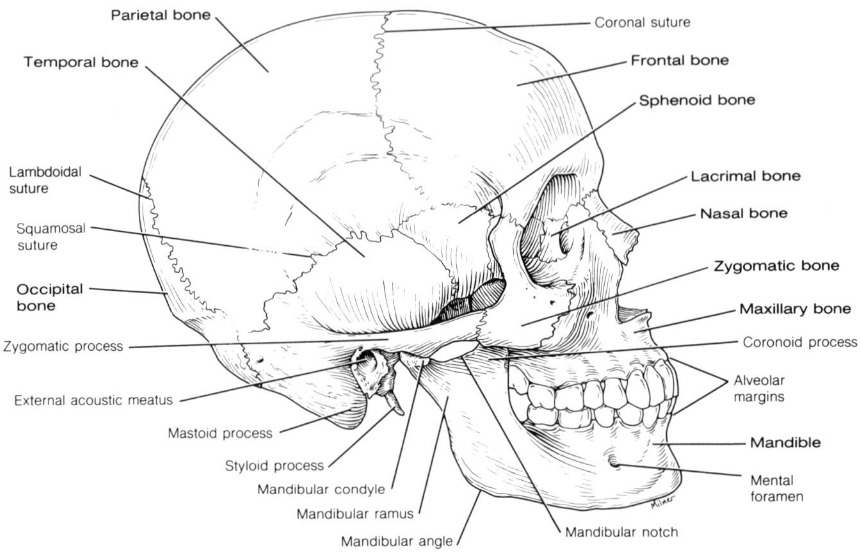

Fig. 2–1—Lateral view of the skull.
Source: Reprinted from *Basic Human Anatomy* (p 101) by Alexander Spence with permission of the Benjamin-Cummings Publishing Company, © 1982.

The base of the skull is thicker and stronger than the roof or walls. The temporal bones are much thinner, especially just superior to each auditory meatus. Viewed from above, the base of the skull contains several depressions or fossae. The frontal lobes of the cerebrum rest in the two anterior fossae; the temporal lobes rest in the middle fossae; and the cerebellum rests in the lower, posterior fossa. The spinal cord passes from the brain through the foramen magnum, an opening in the occipital bone at the base of the skull. The interior of the base of the skull is very irregular, particularly in the area of the sphenoid bone. In head trauma, considerable brain injury can occur as the brain is shaken and forced against these irregular surfaces. The frontal and temporal lobes of the cerebrum are particularly vulnerable to injury because of their location.

Vertebral Column

The flexible vertebral column is composed of 33 vertebrae each stacked one upon the other (Figure 2–3). Seven cervical vertebrae support the muscles of the head and neck. Twelve thoracic vertebrae articulate with the ribs and support the muscles of the chest. Five lumbar vertebrae, the largest and strongest of the vertebral column, support the back muscles. Five sacral vertebrae are fused as the

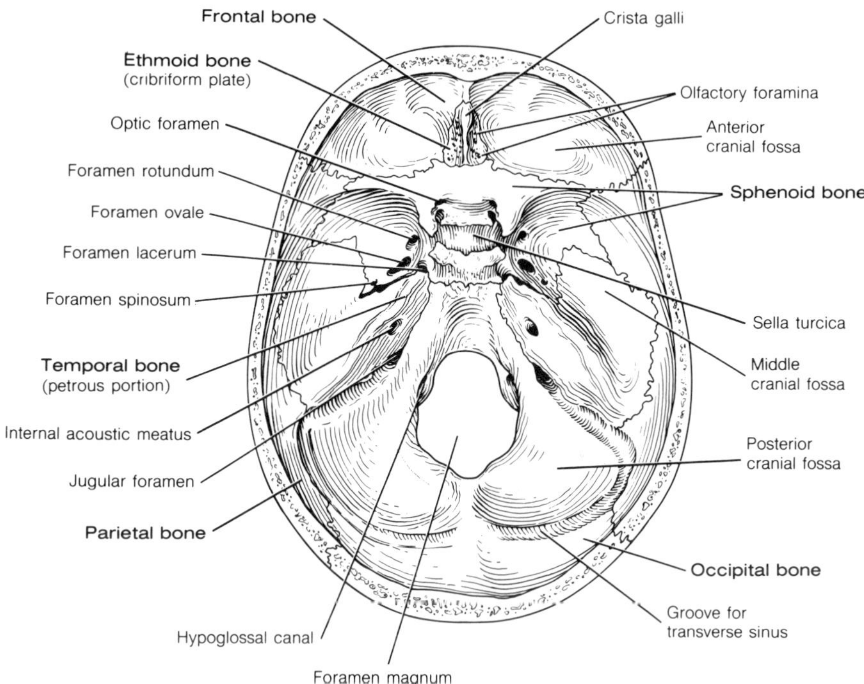

Fig. 2–2—Superior view of the skull with the calvarium removed, showing the floor of the cranial cavity.

Source: Reprinted from *Basic Human Anatomy* (p 102) by Alexander Spence with permission of the Benjamin-Cummings Publishing Company, © 1982.

---

triangular-shaped sacrum. The last four rather rudimentary vertebrae are fused to form the coccyx.

The skull rests on the ring-shaped first cervical vertebra, the atlas (Figure 2–4). The second cervical vertebra, the axis, contains the perpendicular bony projection called the odontoid process which allows the head to rotate. Viewed from above (Figure 2–5), the cervical vertebrae differ structurally from the thoracic and lumbar vertebrae in certain respects. They are smaller and have foramens through the transverse processes for passage of the vertebral arteries. The spinal cord passes through the vertebral foramen.

Ligaments that connect the vertebrae allow for movement of the spinal column (Figure 2–6). Cushioning the movements of the spinal column are the fibrocartilaginous disks located between the verterbral bodies from the second cervical to the sacral vertebrae.

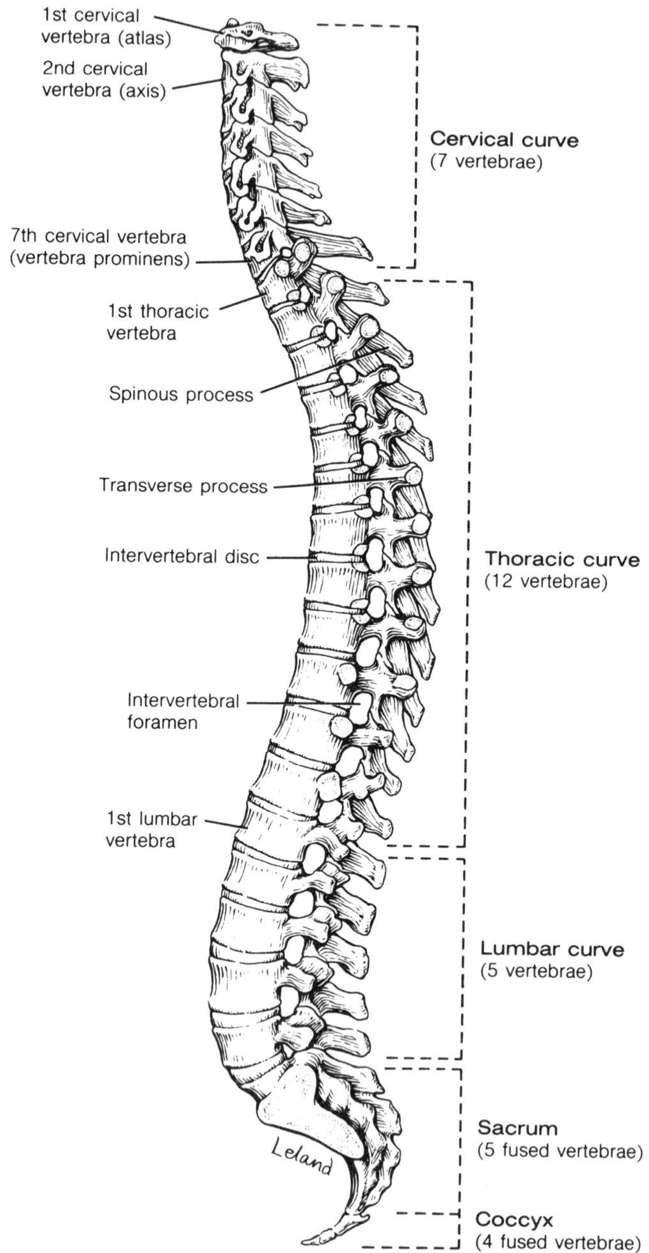

Fig. 2–3—Lateral view of the vertebral column.

Source: Reprinted from *Basic Human Anatomy* (p 115) by Alexander Spence with permission of the Benjamin-Cummings Publishing Company, © 1982.

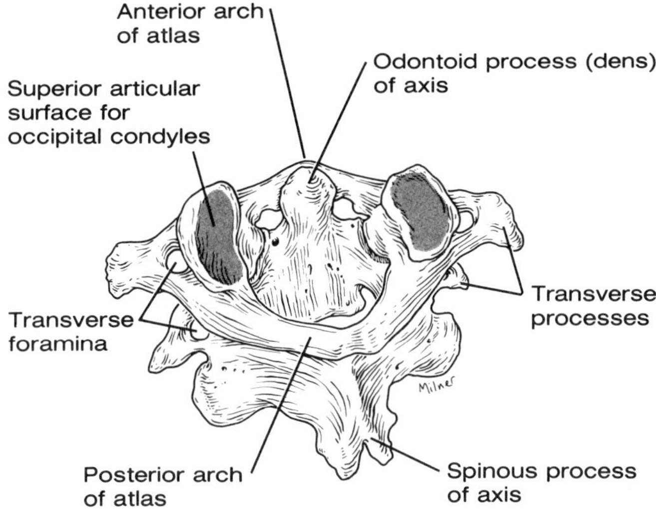

Fig. 2–4—Superior-lateral view showing the articulated first and second cervical vertebrae (the atlas and the axis).
Source: Reprinted from *Basic Human Anatomy* (p 116) by Alexander Spence with permission of the Benjamin-Cummings Publishing Company, © 1982.

Pathophysiological Considerations

Fractures account for probably the greatest number of emergencies related to pathological conditions of the skull and vertebrae.

Skull Fractures

Type and extent of skull fractures not only depend on the velocity, direction, and momentum of the impact object but also vary with the age of the patient. In young children, separation of the sutures may occur. In neonates, the more flexible skull may only be indented, with no actual interruption of the continuity of the bone.[2]

Skull fractures are not always clinically significant and frequently require no emergency treatment. Forces strong enough to cause skull fractures though can also cause injuries to important structures within the skull such as brain tissue, blood vessels, meninges, and cranial nerves. Skull fractures and associated injuries are covered in Chapter 8.

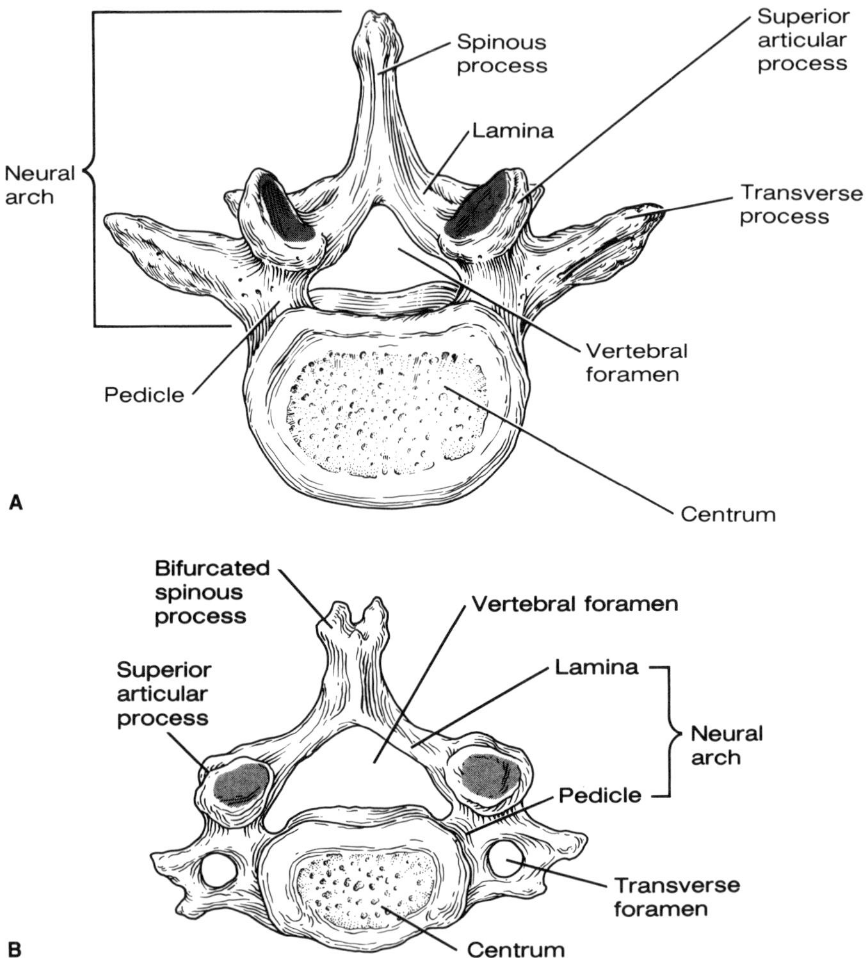

Fig. 2–5—Structural features of typical vertebrae. (A) Thoracic. (B) Cervical.
Source: Reprinted from *Basic Human Anatomy* (p 116) by Alexander Spence with permission of the Benjamin-Cummings Publishing Company, © 1982.

Vertebral Injuries

Vertebral injury refers to trauma only of the bony segment of the vertebral column. The cervical and lumbar regions are the most flexible and thus most vulnerable to injury. The major mechanisms causing vertebral injuries are hyperflexion, hyperextension, vertical compression, and rotation of the spinal column. Persons with preexisting or degenerative diseases of the spine, such as scoliosis, spondylosis, or arthritis, are more vulnerable to vertebral injury.

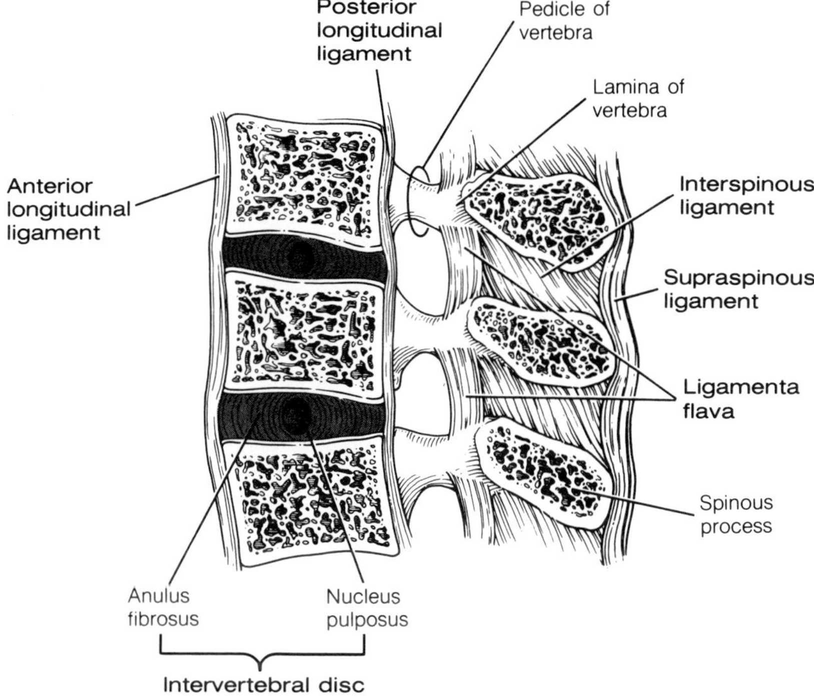

Fig. 2–6—Ligaments of the vertebral column as seen in a median saggital section through two lumbar vertebrae.
Source: Reprinted from *Basic Human Anatomy* (p 158) by Alexander Spence with permission of the Benjamin-Cummings Publishing Company, © 1982.

Injuries to the vertebral column can occur with or without spinal cord injury. Vertebral fractures or partial dislocations do not always cause compression of the spinal cord. The degree of disruption in the alignment of the vertebral column will, of course, influence the degree of spinal cord involvement. Spinal cord injury is covered in detail in Chapter 8.

Herniated Intervertebral Disk

The cervical and lumbar regions are again the most often affected because of the flexibility and stress in these areas. Trauma caused by falls on the back and lifting heavy objects accounts for approximately 50 percent of disk herniations. Other diseases such as osteoarthritis, ankylosing spondylitis, and scoliosis can also predispose a person to disk herniation. Degenerative disk changes commonly occur in middle and later life. An action as simple as sneezing can cause the fibrocartilaginous nucleus pulposus to protrude through the anulus fibrosis, compressing nerve roots against the vertebra (see Figure 2–6).

The Meninges

Further protecting the brain and spinal cord are the meninges. The layers, from the outermost layer inward, are the dura mater, the arachnoid, and the pia mater (Figure 2–7). Although the spinal cord terminates at approximately the level of the first lumbar vertebra, the spinal dura and arachnoid continue further and envelop the cauda equina.

Dura Mater

The dura is a double layered, off-white, glossy, tough, and inelastic membrane. The outer layer of the dura forms the periosteum of the inner skull, while the inner meningeal layer envelopes the brain. Large venous sinuses lie between the layers of the dura. The dura divides the skull into several compartments by forming four major folds, which further serve to support and protect the brain. Clinically, the two most significant are the falx cerebri, which descends vertically between the two cerebral hemispheres, and the tentorium cerebelli, a tentlike double fold of dura that separates the cerebellum from the temporal and occipital lobes resting above (Figure 2–7). The tentorium separates the posterior cranial fossa from the

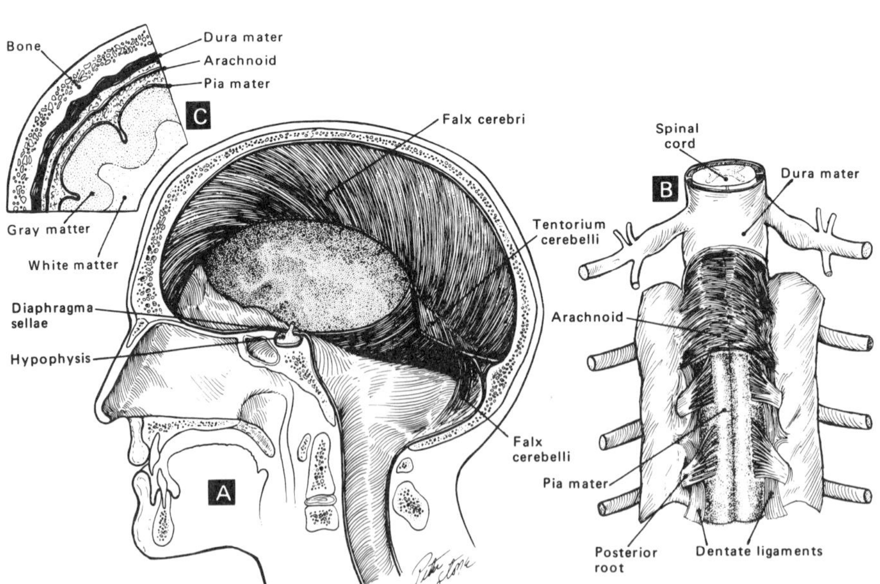

Figure 2–7—Meninges.
Source: Reprinted from *Dynamic Anatomy and Physiology* (p 238) by L Langley, I Telford, and J Christensen with permission of the McGraw-Hill Book Company, © 1974.

rest of the cranial cavity. It serves as an important anatomical landmark for describing lesions as being above the tentorium (supratentorial) or below the tentorium (infratentorial). The upper part of the brainstem, the midbrain, lies partially in a large oval opening in the tentorium, the incisura.

Arachnoid

The arachnoid is the transparent middle layer of meninges that loosely covers the brain and spinal cord. It does not follow the folds and fissures of the brain. Cerebral spinal fluid flows through the spongy subarachnoid space, the space between the arachnoid and the underlying pia mater.

Pia Mater

The innermost layer of meninges, the pia mater, closely covers the entire surface of the brain and spinal cord. It dips down beneath the convolutions of the surface of the brain. By various invaginations, this membrane, rich in minute blood vessels, helps form the choroid plexuses of the lateral, third, and fourth ventricles.[3(p25)]

The pia mater and arachnoid collectively are known as the leptomeninges, distinct from the dura because they are thinner and more delicate.

Pathophysiological Considerations

Three spaces within the meninges are of significance pathologically: the epidural, subdural, and subarachnoid.

The Epidural Space

The epidural or extradural space is a potential space lying between the skull and the outer layer of the dura. Much of the blood supply to the dura arises from the middle meningeal artery, which lies in this epidural space. This artery can be torn in head trauma, especially temporal bone fracture, since this artery lies in a groove in the temporal bone. The bleeding that results is called an epidural hematoma (see Chapter 8).

The Subdural Space

The subdural space separates the inner dura mater from the arachnoid layer. Large venous sinuses lie within the dura and drain venous blood from underlying cerebral veins and from the inner layer of the skull. The blood from the dural sinuses ultimately drains into the jugular veins. Following head trauma, bleeding can occur within this subdural space. It is most often venous in origin and is called subdural hemorrhage or hematoma.

The Subarachnoid Space

The subarachnoid space lies between the arachnoid and the pia mater. Blood vessels of various sizes are found in the arachnoid. Trauma and rupture of cerebral aneurysms or arteriovenous malformations can result in bleeding into the subarachnoid space (see Chapter 9).[3(p25)]

Cerebrospinal Fluid

The CSF cushions the brain and spinal cord, decreasing their effective weight. Whether or not CSF plays a role in metabolism is unknown. Cerebrospinal fluid is a clear, colorless, odorless fluid containing glucose, electrolytes, oxygen, carbon dioxide, and small amounts of protein. The CSF exerts a pressure of 80–100 mm H_2O when collected through a lumbar subarachnoid puncture done with the patient lying in a lateral recumbent position. The pressure of CSF fluctuates normally because of the cardiac cycle and respirations.

Formation

Cerebrospinal fluid is formed in the choroid plexus of the ventricles of the brain (see Figure 2–8). The largest proportion is produced in the lateral ventricles. Small amounts may also be produced by meningeal linings and small blood vessels of the brain. Approximately 20–30 ml of CSF are produced every hour. At any one time there may be about 125–150 ml of CSF present in the ventricular and subarachnoid spaces; 60 percent of this is located in the lumbar subarachnoid space.

Circulation

Cerebrospinal fluid circulates from the lateral ventricles through the interventricular foramen (foramen of Monro) to the third ventricle. From here it traverses the narrow aqueduct of Sylvius to the fourth ventricle. It leaves the fourth ventricle and enters the cisterns via the foramina of Luschka and Magendie. From here the CSF enters the subarachnoid space and bathes the brain and spinal cord.

Absorption

As CSF is continually being produced, it must also be continuously reabsorbed. The entire volume is replaced once every 12–24 hours. A hydrostatic pressure gradient determines the reabsorption of CSF back into the circulatory system. Most of the CSF is reabsorbed into the arachnoid villi, which project from the subarachnoid space into the dural venous sinuses. The largest arachnoid villi, called pacchionian bodies, are located along the superior saggital sinus.[4]

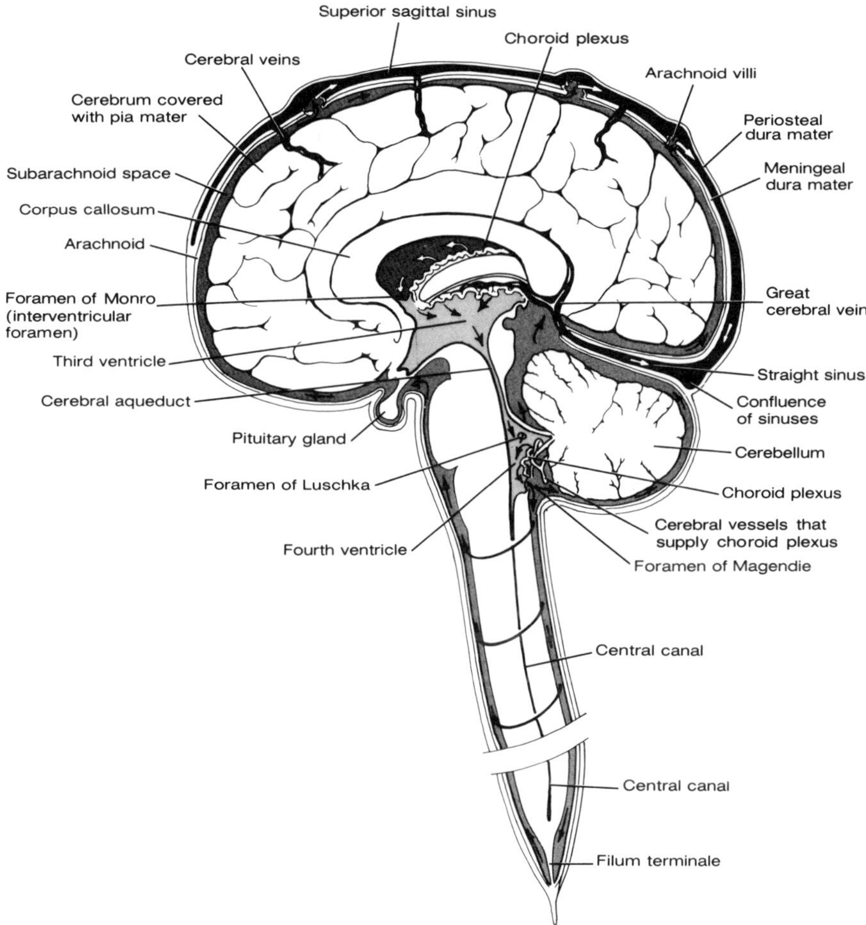

Fig. 2–8—Location of cerebrospinal fluid that surrounds brain and spinal cord. Arrows indicate direction of flow of the fluid.

Source: Reprinted from *Basic Human Anatomy* (p 378) by Alexander Spence with permission of the Benjamin-Cummings Publishing Company, © 1982.

Pathophysiological Considerations

Hydrocephalus, an increased accumulation of CSF in the ventricles of the brain, can result from interference with the normal circulation or reabsorption of CSF. Anomalies, infection, injury, intracranial hemorrhage, or brain tumor may cause hydrocephalus. The symptoms will depend upon the rapidity with which the intracranial pressure rises. If pressure changes occur rapidly, the patient may exhibit rapid deterioration in neurological status. Other patients may develop what is called normal pressure hydrocephalus from any one of the same causes. As ventricular enlargement occurs slowly, there is compression of cerebral tissue, yet lumbar puncture will reveal normal CSF pressure. Neurological changes occur very slowly and are often attributed to the aging process when older patients are involved.[3(p170)]

The pressure of the CSF in the head has been measured directly since the 1950s. The CSF fluid pressure accurately reflects the overall intracranial pressure (ICP). This procedure has proved useful in the assessment and treatment of patients with acute intracranial pathologies. Procedures for monitoring intracranial pressure and nursing implications are discussed in Chapter 4.

VASCULAR SUPPLY TO THE CENTRAL NERVOUS SYSTEM

The brain is a very metabolically active organ. Brain metabolism accounts for approximately 20 percent of the total oxygen consumption of the body.[5(p596)] Most of this oxygen is utilized for the oxidation of glucose, the brain's chief source of energy. Approximately 15 percent of the resting cardiac output is received by the brain.[5(p596)] Since neither glucose nor oxygen can be stored by the brain, a constant flow of blood must be maintained. With cessation of blood flow, the oxygen within the brain is used up within ten seconds, resulting in loss of consciousness.[6] Within two to five minutes, irreversible brain damage can occur.[3(p28)]

Arterial Circulation to the Brain

The brain is supplied with blood via two major pairs of arteries (Figure 2–9). Two internal carotid arteries enter the cranium anteriorly. Two vertebral arteries enter posteriorly, then fuse to become the basilar artery. These arteries then communicate at the base of the brain through the circle of Willis (Figure 2–10), which ensures blood supply to any portion of the brain should one of the four main channels be interrupted. The internal carotid arteries supply the basal ganglia, the upper portion of the diencephalon, and all but the occipital lobes of the cerebrum (Figure 2–11). The vertebral arteries supply blood to the remaining portions of the brain.

Venous Circulation from the Brain

Major venous channels lying in the dura, called sinuses, drain blood from the brain (Figure 2–12). Along the upper portions of the cortex, venous blood drains

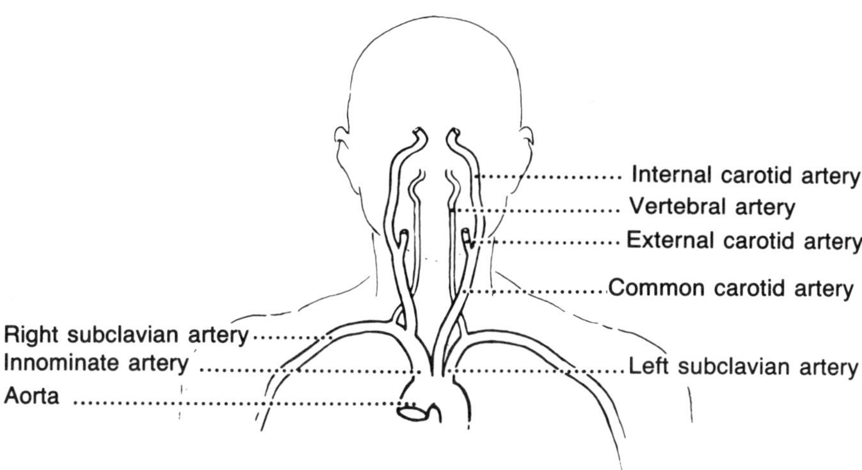

Fig. 2–9—Major arteries supplying the brain.

 Source: Reprinted from *Technique of the Neurologic Examination* ed 3 (p 91) by William DeMyer with permission of the McGraw-Hill Book Company, © 1980.

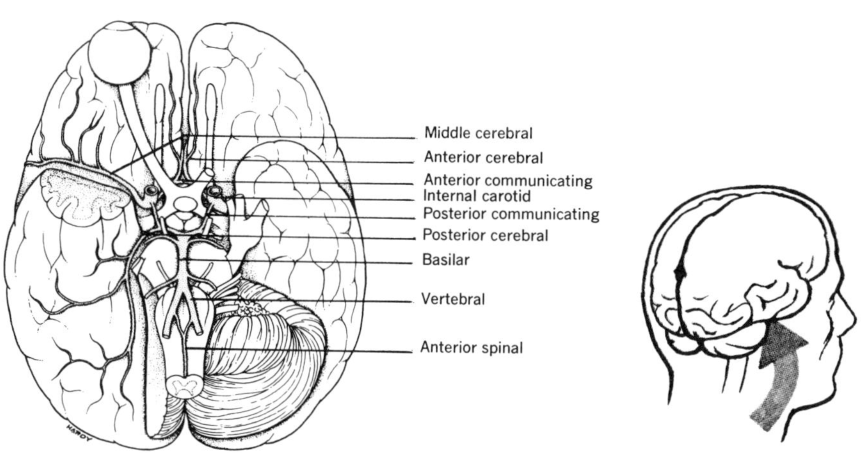

Fig. 2–10—The circle of Willis as seen at the base of the brain that has been removed from the skull.

 Source: Reprinted from *Basic Physiology and Anatomy* ed 4 (p 339) by E Chaffee and I Lytle with permission of the JB Lippincott Company, © 1980.

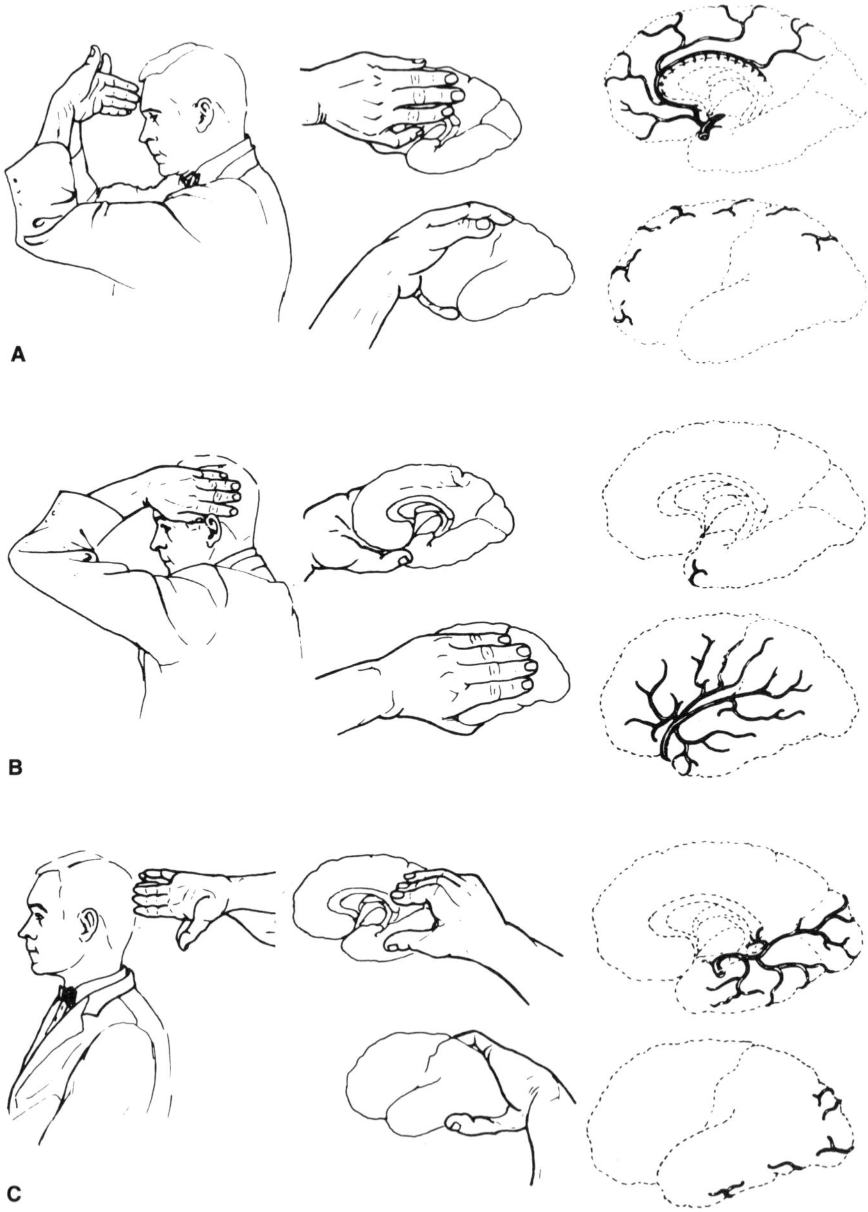

Fig. 2–11—Position of the hands for remembering the irrigation areas of (A) anterior, (B) middle, and (C) posterior cerebral arteries.

Source: Reprinted from *Technique of the Neurologic Examination* ed 3 (p 94) by William DeMeyer with permission of the McGraw-Hill Book Company, © 1980.

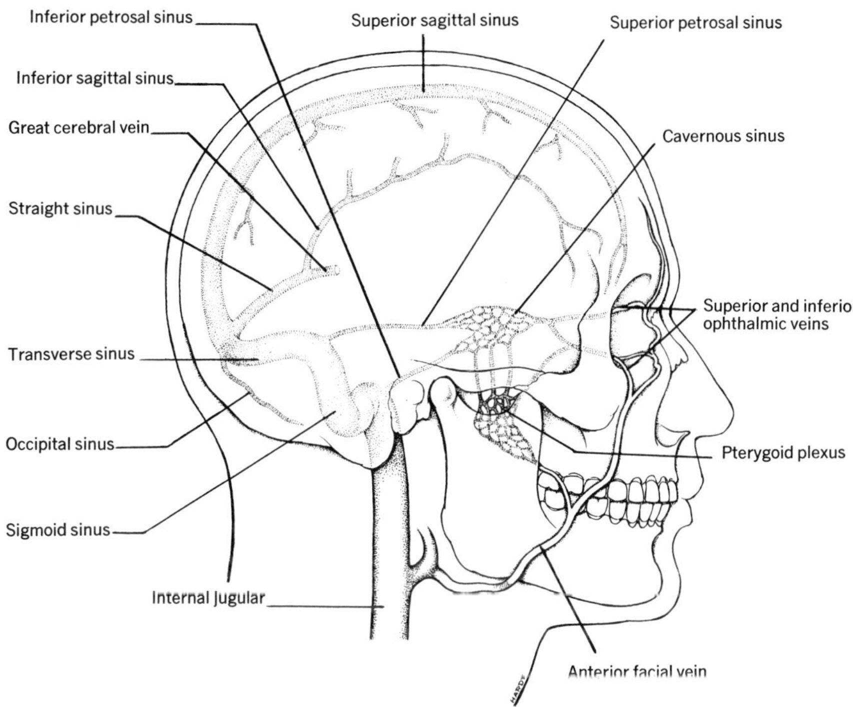

Fig. 2–12—Cranial venous sinuses. Sigmoid portion of transverse sinus continues on as the internal jugular vein.

Source: Reprinted from *Basic Physiology and Anatomy* ed 4 (p 345) by E Chaffee and I Lytle with permission of the JB Lippincott Company, © 1980.

into the superior sagittal sinus. Blood from the medical surfaces of the brain drains into the inferior sagittal sinus. Inferiorly, blood drains into the cavernous sinus. These and other sinuses ultimately empty into the internal jugular veins.

Several factors distinguish the venous system of the brain from venous drainage systems of other parts of the body: (1) the veins have no valves, (2) the venous return does not trace the course of corresponding arteries, and (3) the dural sinuses are unique to cerebral circulation.[3(p29)]

Meningeal Blood Supply

The meninges are richly supplied with blood by the anterior, middle, and posterior meningeal arteries. As previously mentioned, much of the blood supply to the dura arises from the middle meningeal artery, a branch of the external carotid artery.

Blood Supply to the Spinal Cord

The spinal cord receives part of its blood supply from one anterior spinal artery and two posterior spinal arteries, all arising from the vertebral arteries. As these vessels pass down the cord, they receive additional blood at various levels through lateral spinal arteries. Also, small feeder vessels from the deep cervical, intercostal, lumbar, and sacral arteries further ensure adequate blood supply.

Venous drainage comes from various intradural and extradural veins. Multiple communications with veins of the abdomen, thorax, and neck exist to carry blood ultimately back to the vena cavae.[3(p31)]

The Blood-Brain Barrier

A protective barrier exists between circulating blood and the brain and between the blood vessels of the choroid plexus and the CSF. These barriers prevent certain potentially harmful substances from entering the extracellular fluid or the CSF of the brain. Separating cerebral capillaries from neurons are portions of glial astrocytes, supporting cells of the CNS. The barrier created by the close approximation of glial cells and capillary walls is known as the blood-brain barrier. In the ventricles of the brain, epithelial cells of the choroid plexus form the blood-CSF barrier.[3(p31)]

The movement of a substance from the blood to the brain depends on its chemical dissociation, particle size, lipoid solubility, and protein-binding potential. Alterations in systemic pH can produce changes in the permeability of the blood-brain barrier to allow certain substances though.[7(p20)] Water, carbon dioxide, oxygen, and glucose readily cross the blood-brain barrier. The passage of ions such as sodium, potassium and chlorine is slower. Uptake of lipid insoluble molecules is much slower or nonexistent. Consequently, certain drugs necessary for treating CNS infections must be administered directly into the CSF. Passage of substances from the CSF to the brain and to the blood are not hindered by what seems to be a selected ''one-way'' blood-brain and blood-CSF barrier.

These barriers help determine the metabolic level and ionic composition of brain tissue fluids and thus help maintain the homeostatic environment of the neuron, the functional unit of the nervous system.[4]

Pathophysiological Considerations

Brain circulation may be affected by various extracranial and intracranial factors. Extracranial factors affecting cerebral blood flow include systemic blood pressure, cardiovascular function, and blood viscosity. Intracranial factors include cerebral autoregulation, cerebral blood vessels, and intracranial or CSF pressure.[5(p597)]

Decreased Cerebral Blood Flow

Extracranial Factors. Cerebral blood flow depends upon a pressure gradient; therefore, factors that affect systemic blood pressure may indirectly affect cerebral circulation. Shock states, orthostatic hypotension, and some cardiac dysrhythmias can decrease cardiac output and thus impair blood supply to the brain. Increased blood viscosity such as seen in polycythemia may decrease cerebral blood flow by as much as 50 percent.[5(p597)]

Intracranial Factors. The status of cerebral vessels, especially the arterioles, greatly influences blood flow to the brain. Certain vasoconstrictor drugs, decreased arterial $Paco_2$, increased Pao_2, and vascular spasm can all decrease the amount of cerebral blood flow. Likewise, edematous brain tissue can compress the vascular bed, further decreasing cerebral circulation. Anomalous or pathological changes such as cerebral arteriosclerosis can also lead to decreased blood flow and ischemia of certain areas of the brain.

Resistance of blood flow through the brain is further affected by the intracranial pressure. As intracranial pressure rises, moderate to severe restriction of cerebral perfusion can occur.[6]

Physiological mechanisms affecting cerebral blood flow and the dynamics of increased intracranial pressure are discussed in greater detail in Chapter 4.

Increased Cerebral Blood Flow

Extracranial Factors. Significant increases in brain blood flow may occur in hyperdynamic states such as hyperthyroidism. Decreased blood viscosity seen in anemia may increase cerebral blood flow by as much as 30 percent.

Intracranial Factors. Normally, autoregulation of blood flow by the brain maintains a constant cerebral blood flow regardless of fluctuations in systemic arterial blood pressure. This is done through constriction or dilation of the cerebral vessels in response to systemic blood pressure changes. Autoregulation may fail if the mean systolic blood pressure exceeds 150 mm Hg. Cerebral blood flow then increases as a function of increasing arterial blood pressure. Autoregulation may also be lost because of cerebral trauma or various disease processes.

Certain vasodilator drugs or chemicals such as histamine may also increase blood flow to the brain.[6] Carbon dioxide retention as well as severe hypoxemia (Pao_2 less than 50 mm Hg) will also cause cerebral vasodilation, increasing cerebral blood flow.[8(p35)] Vasodilation of cerebral vessels can also result from increased metabolic demands such as those induced by seizures. Vascular anomalies such as hemangioma or arteriovenous malformation can contribute to excessive blood flow in the brain.[6]

Disruption of the Blood-Brain Barrier

A number of factors can cause breakdown of the blood-brain barrier, the result of which is often the formation of cerebral edema. Retention of carbon dioxide (hypercapnia) produces increased vascular permeability. Epileptic seizures also influence the blood-brain barrier, a phenomenon probably also related to carbon dioxide retention. Some toxic agents can cause increased penetration of the blood-brain barrier and thus enter the brain. Many forms of brain injury, including inflammatory processes of the brain and meninges, can cause breakdown of the blood-brain barrier.

The drug mannitol, commonly used to treat cerebral edema, has been shown to promote the breakdown of the blood-brain barrier when serum osmolality levels exceed 310 m Osm/L.[7(p179)]

CELLS OF THE NERVOUS SYSTEM

Billions of neurons make up the functional units of the nervous system while neuroglial cells, ten times more numerous, provide structural support.

Neurons

The basic functional unit of the nervous system is the neuron (Figure 2–13). Neurons are classified in various ways: according to their structure, their location, and their function. Afferent, or sensory, neurons conduct impulses toward the central nervous system. Efferent neurons conduct impulses away from the central nervous system, while internuncial neurons transmit impulses from one neuron to another.

Structure

Each neuron is divided into three major components: (1) the cell body, in which metabolic functions are carried out; (2) dendrites, which are multiple, thin afferent fibers that conduct impulses toward the cell body primarily from other neurons; and (3) the axon, or efferent fiber, which conducts impulses away from the cell body.

Nerve cell bodies are part of the gray matter of the CNS. Nerve cell bodies located outside the CNS are mainly collected into groups called ganglia. Typical examples are the dorsal root ganglia of the spinal nerves (see Figure 2–22), or the chain of ganglia of the sympathetic nervous system that lies anterior to the spinal cord (see Figure 2–26).

Making up much of the white matter of the CNS are the myelinated axons of the neurons. Myelin is a lipoidal, whitish substance that encircles many axons.

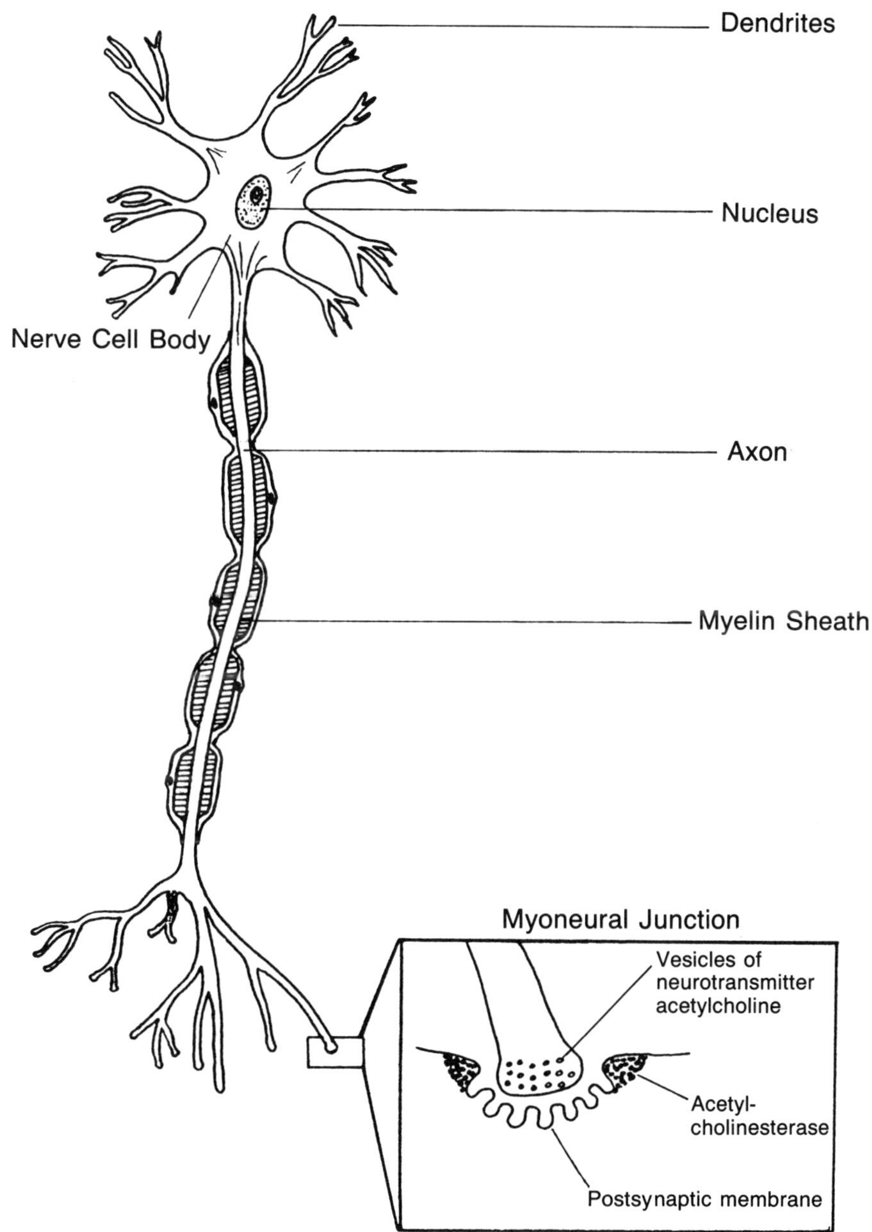

Fig. 2–13—The neuron.

Generally, the axons of larger neurons are myelinated, while those of smaller neurons are unmyelinated. In the CNS, the myelin sheath is laid down by the oligodendrocytes; in the peripheral nervous system the Schwann cells perform this function.[9] Further surrounding the peripheral nerves is the neurilemma, or sheath of Schwann, said to be necessary for axonal regeneration.[3(p14)]

In the peripheral nervous system the neurilemma and myelin sheath have regular interruptions at 1–2 mm intervals known as nodes of Ranvier. Nerve impulses are conducted from node to node as they travel down the axon. In the CNS, nodes of Ranvier occur only at points of bifurcation of a nerve fiber.

Nerve Impulse Transmission

Action Potential of Neurons. At rest a neuron is an electrically charged cell. Because of an unequal distribution of electrolytes on either side of the cell membrane, the inside environment of the neuron has a negative electrical charge in relation to its outside environment. The cell membrane of the neuron is semipermeable and allows passage of these electrolytes between the extracellular and intracellular compartments. When a stimulus of threshold intensity is applied to a neuron, membrane depolarization begins. Sodium ions flow into the cell while potassium ions move out. A stimulus exciting a neuron can arise from within the neuron itself or from a variety of chemical, mechanical, electrical, or thermal means. In larger neurons, transmission is faster. In myelinated nerves this wave of depolarization leaps from one node of Ranvier to the next, speeding the transmission of the nerve impulse. This is known as saltatory conduction. Following depolarization, the cell repolarizes and returns to its resting membrane potential, awaiting the next stimulus.

Synaptic Transmission. The transmission of the nerve impulse from one neuron to the next takes place at a junction known as the synapse. Whereas impulse conduction along a nerve fiber is an electrical process, transmission across a synapse is a chemical process. The terminal projections of the axon of the presynaptic neuron secrete certain neurotransmitter chemicals that are taken up by the dendrites or cell body of the postsynaptic neuron. This neurotransmitter lowers the cell membrane potential of the receiving neuron, renewing the spread of the wave of electrical depolarization.

Each neuron in the nervous system, of which there are billions, secretes one neurotransmitter. Neurotransmitters can be classified as excitatory or inhibitory. An excitatory neurotransmitter causes the membrane of the postsynaptic neuron to depolarize. Acetylcholine, norepinephrine, dopamine, and serotonin are all excitatory neurotransmitters. Inhibitory neurotransmitters cause ionic permeability changes in the postsynaptic membrane, causing the cell membrane to depolarize less easily. The result is membrane stabilization or hyperpolarization. Gamma-aminobutyric acid (GABA) is an inhibitory neurotransmitter.[4(pp194–196)]

Neuromuscular Transmission. The transmission of a nerve impulse to a muscle takes place across the myoneural junction. When the action potential of the neuron reaches the terminal end of the axon, vesicles in these motor end plates release acetylcholine into the synaptic cleft (see Figure 2–13). The acetylcholine then attaches to receptor sites on the receiving muscle membrane increasing its permeability to sodium and potassium. An action potential results, spreading in both directions along the muscle fiber. Combined with the temporary release of calcium ions into the muscle fibers, a muscle contraction results.

To prevent repetitive muscle stimulation, acetylcholinesterase, an enzyme found in the muscle fibers, inactivates the acetylcholine by hydrolyzing it to choline and acetic acid. The muscle fibers repolarize and are then ready for the next impulse.

Neuroglia

The glial cells (neuroglia) provide structural support, protection, and nutrition for the neurons (Figure 2–14). Making up the interstitial elements of the CNS, neuroglia are ten times more numerous than neurons. Included in the neuroglia are (1) oligodendrocytes, which produce the myelin sheaths of the axons in the CNS; (2) astrocytes, large star-shaped cells, which provide nourishment for neurons (many astrocytes are in contact with blood vessels in the CNS and are thought to be involved in the formation of the blood-brain barrier); (3) ependymal cells, which line the ventricles and choroid plexuses and contribute to the production of CSF; and (4) microglia, which are the phagocytic cells of the CNS.[9]

Pathophysiological Considerations

Neuronal Degeneration

Nerve cell bodies shrink and eventually dissolve as a natural process of aging. Degenerative changes in neurons can also occur because of trauma and various disease processes.

If a nerve cell body is destroyed, axonal degeneration begins within a matter of hours. The myelin sheath breaks down and is ultimately removed by phagocytic cells. In the CNS, limited true regeneration of cells occurs, and lost neurons are replaced by glial or supporting cells. In peripheral nerves, degeneration occurs as described, but the innervated end organs, such as muscles or glands, will also degenerate or show functional changes. Regeneration of some peripheral neurons may occur, although there may be abnormalities in nerve distribution and thus persistent functional abnormalities.[10(pp897–898)]

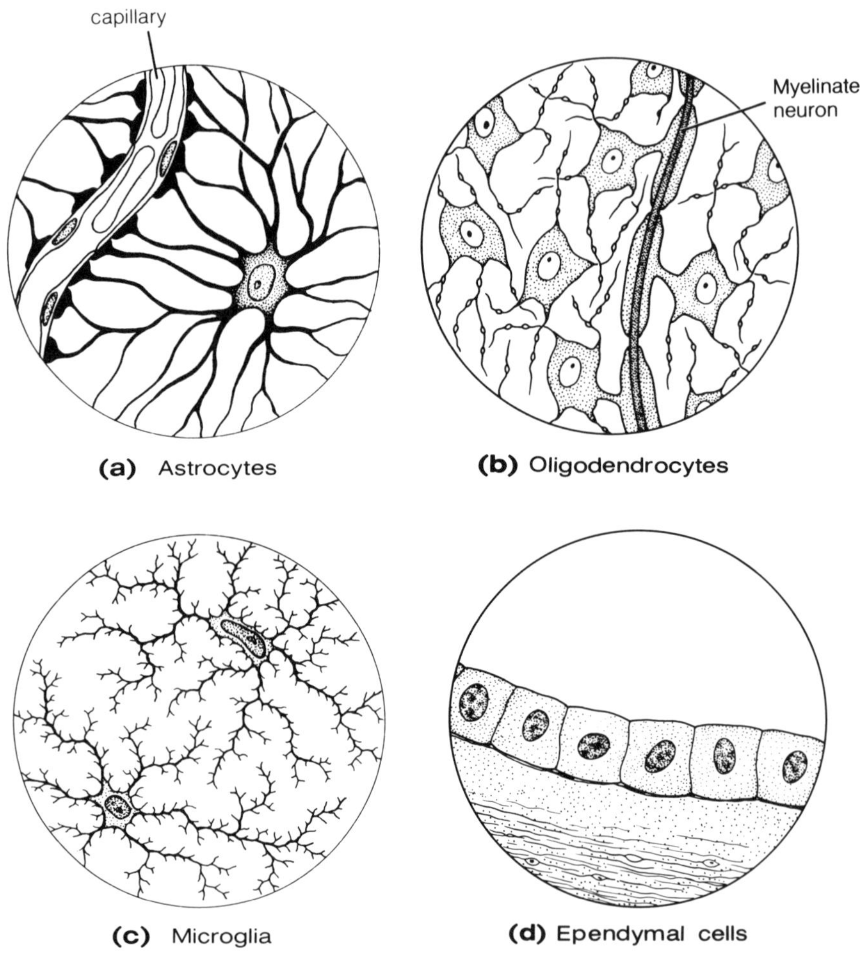

Fig. 2–14—Types of neuroglial cells.
Source: Reprinted from *Basic Human Anatomy* (p 355) by Alexander Spence with permission of the Benjamin-Cummings Publishing Company, © 1982.

Demyelinating Disease

Demyelinating diseases affecting axons ultimately interrupt or retard nerve impulse transmission. For example, multiple sclerosis is a demyelinating disease characterized by scattered sclerotic lesions of the white matter of the brain and spinal cord. Although characterized by remissions, progressive degeneration of myelin occurs and symptoms become progressively worse and permanent. Guillain-Barré syndrome represents a reversible demyelinating disease caused by edema and inflammation of the nerve roots. As the edema and inflammation resolve, remyelination occurs. In most cases nerve impulse transmission returns to normal.[4(pp238–239)]

Disorders of Neuromuscular Transmission

Myasthenia gravis is a disease of impaired neuromuscular transmission characterized by progressive fatigability and weakness of certain voluntary muscles. Its exact cause is unknown, but some feel that there is a deficiency in the amount of acetylcholine in the nerve endings. Recent evidence points toward a disorder in the muscle receptor sites. It is thought that myasthenia gravis may involve an immunological block of acetylcholine receptors at the myoneural junction. Syptoms are usually relieved by rest and the administration of anticholinesterase agents (see Chapter 11).[5(pp618–620)]

Neuroglial Cell Disorders

A primary disorder of neuroglial cells is tumor formation. Gliomas account for approximately 40 to 50 percent of all brain tumors. They may arise from astrocytcs, oligodcndrocytcs, or cpcndymal cclls. Most, but not all, astrocytomas arc benign, while ependymomas tend to be malignant. Gliomas affect the brain by invasion and infiltration. Signs and symptoms, which vary with tumor location, size, and speed of growth, are usually related to six areas of pathophysiology: (1) cerebral edema, (2) increased intracranial pressure, (3) focal neurological deficit, (4) seizure activity, (5) endocrine imbalance, and (6) CSF obstruction.[3(p330)]

THE BRAIN

In the evolution of the CNS, the spinal cord was functionally developed before the brain. Being the last developed, the brain became the most complicated and highly developed component of the CNS. The brain must integrate all incoming information from the senses and initiate the body's reactions. In addition, it may also store this information for future use. The brain is divided into three major areas: the cerebrum, the brain stem, and the cerebellum (Figure 2–15).

The Cerebrum

Sometimes referred to as the telencephalon, the cerebrum is the most highly developed and complex structure in the nervous system. It accounts for humans' sophisticated intellectual abilities. Within the cerebrum lie the basal ganglia and the limbic system. Located deep within the cerebrum and just above the brainstem is the diencephalon or ''between brain'' containing the thalamus and the hypothalamus.

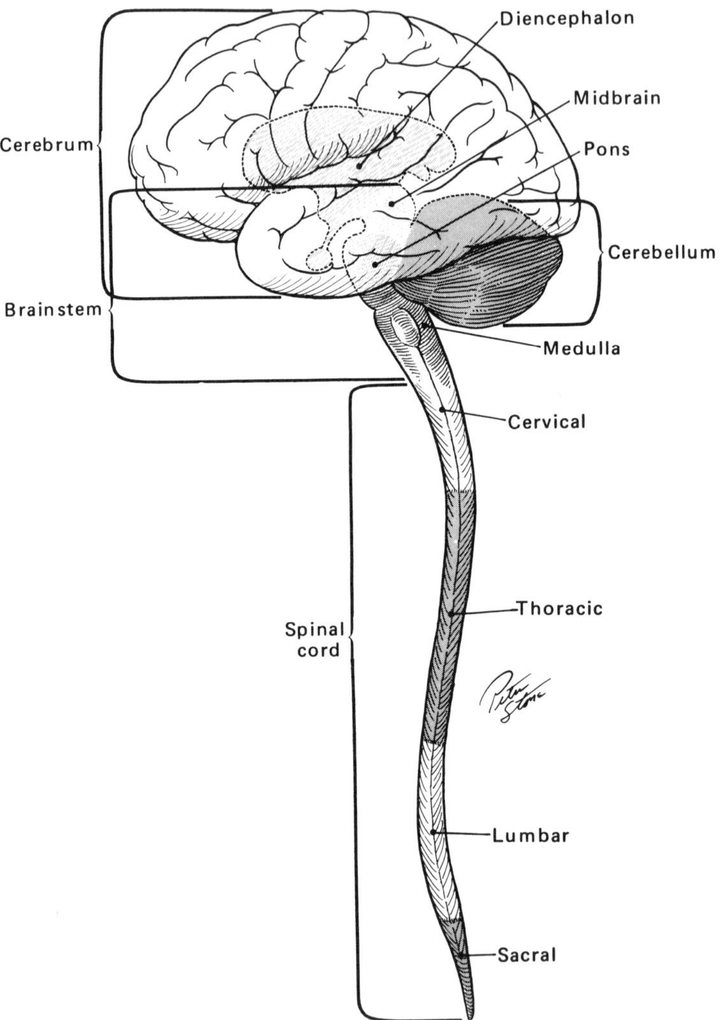

Fig. 2–15—Lateral view of the central nervous system.
Source: Reprinted from *Dynamic Anatomy and Physiology* ed 4 (p 228) by
L Langley, I Telford, and J. Christensen with permission of the McGraw-Hill Book
Company, © 1974.

The surfaces of the cerebral cortex contain many grooves known as fissures or
sulci. Those portions of brain lying between these fissures are called convolutions
or gyri.

The cerebrum is subdivided into two cerebral hemispheres. These hemispheres
are incompletely separated by the longitudinal fissure. The falx cerebri, an

extension of the dura mater, projects into this fissure. This fissure is traversed by a broad band of nerve fibers, the corpus callosum, which makes possible the transfer of information between the two hemispheres (Figure 2–16).

In most people, one cerebral hemisphere is more highly developed and becomes, functionally, the dominant hemisphere. Ninety percent of the population is believed to be left hemisphere dominant. Regardless of the handedness, the left hemisphere is also dominant for the function of speech in 90 percent of the population.[11]

Each cerebral hemisphere is further subdivided into four lobes: frontal, parietal, temporal, and occipital. Each lobe rests approximately beneath its similarly named bone of the skull. Separating each frontal lobe from the parietal lobe is a central sulcus or fissure of Rolando. The parietal lobe is separated posteriorly from the occipital lobe by an indistinct parieto-occipital sulcus. Each temporal lobe is separated from the frontal and parietal lobes by a deep lateral fissure of Sylvius.

Very discrete areas can be identified within the four lobes, which perform specific functions such as control of certain motor activity or the processing of certain sensory information (Figure 2–17). It should be kept in mind, though, that no area of the brain functions alone. Extensive association tracts connect various

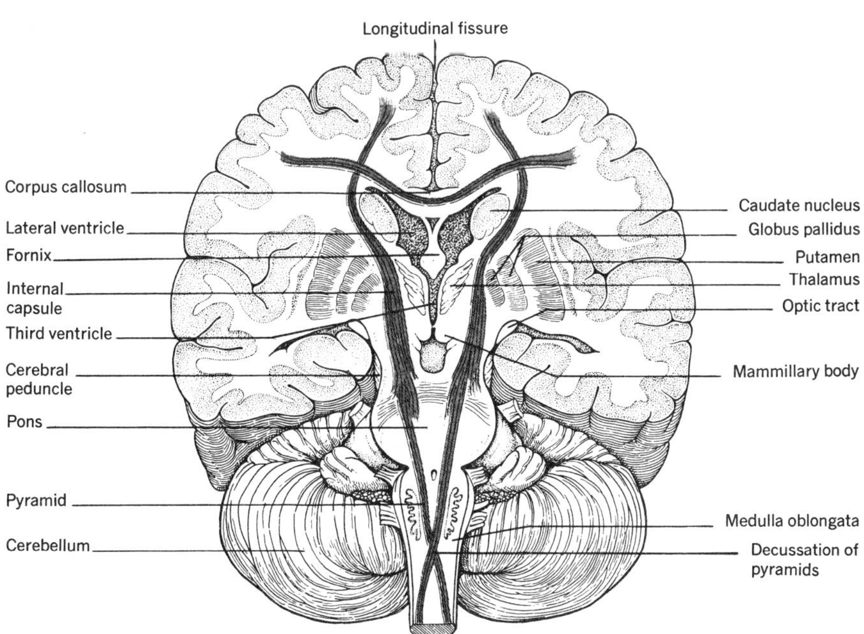

Fig. 2–16—Oblique coronal section through cerebrum and brainstem.
Source: Reprinted from *Basic Physiology and Anatomy* ed 4 (p 204) by E Chaffee and I Lytle with permission of the JB Lippincott Company, © 1980.

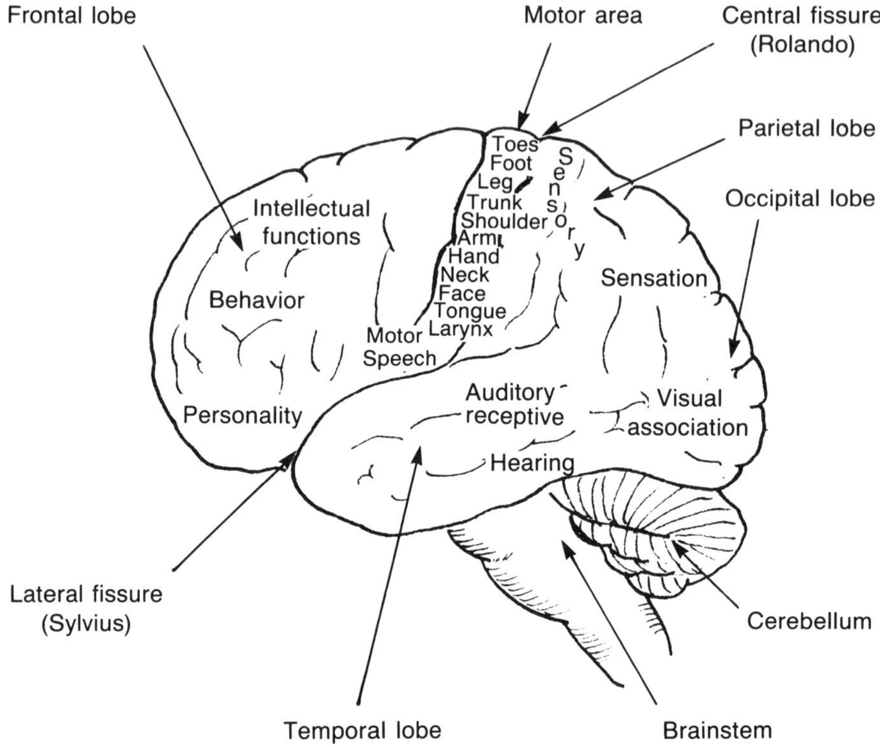

Fig. 2–17—Functional areas of the cerebrum.

areas of the cerebral cortex within the same hemisphere, so that any function attributed to a specific cortical area probably involves several cortical areas.[9]

Frontal Lobes

Higher intellectual activities and attributes such as personality, behavior, learning, abstract thinking, problem solving, and social, moral, and ethical values are among the characteristics of humans that arise from the sophisticated, highly developed frontal lobes.[11]

The motor cortex, lying anterior to the central fissure, is the origin of most voluntary movement. Nerve fibers originating in the motor cortex terminate in the spinal cord and make up what is called the corticospinal (pyramidal) tract. Most of these fibers from the motor cortex cross over or decussate at the level of the medulla (Figure 2–16). Hence, the left cerebral motor cortex controls movement of the right side of the body while the right cerebral motor cortex controls movement of the left side of the body.[1(pp96–97)] Different regions along the motor cortex regulate movement in different parts of the body. Those parts controlling skilled movements that require fine dexterity have a much larger area of representation.

Motor association areas lying anterior to the motor cortex are connected to several cranial nerves and correlate many motor activities. Each premotor cortex contains a center that controls coordinated eye movements and turning of the head.

A language area (Broca's area) lies at the inferior frontal gyrus. This area is believed to affect the production of both written and spoken language, and is sometimes referred to as the motor speech area. It is located in the left cerebral hemisphere in 90 percent of the population.[11]

Parietal Lobes

The parietal lobes are concerned mainly with the receiving of sensations. A sensory cortex located immediately posterior to the central sulcus parallels the same functional areas located along the adjacent motor cortex. The sensory cortex receives fibers via the thalamus that convey cutaneous as well as deep sensations arising from the opposite side of the body, with the exception of the special senses of sight, smell, hearing, and taste. Although the sensory cortex analyzes only gross aspects of sensation, it communicates through the thalamus with sensory association areas, also located in the parietal lobe, which analyze the specific characteristics of sensory input.[3(p36)]

The parietal lobes also interpret size, shape (stereognosis), weight, texture, and consistency of objects and distinguish between two simultaneous skin contacts (two-point discrimination).[11] Touch, position sense (proprioception), pressure, and vibration are also identified here. The parietal lobes are essential for a person's awareness of body parts and their orientation in space.

Temporal Lobes

The temporal lobes interpret the senses of hearing, taste, and smell. The temporal lobe of the dominant hemisphere is important in the whole complex of language related behavior, including the ability to understand the meaning of words and symbols. This auditory association area located in the superior temporal gyrus is known as Wernicke's area (Figure 2–17). At the junction where the temporal, parietal, and occipital lobes meet lies the interpretive area. It integrates somatic, auditory, and visual association areas and plays a major role in cerebration. Memory that requires more than one sensory modality is stored in part in this region. Great impairment of intellectual ability can result from destruction of this area.[3(p36)] Visual fibers of the optic radiations travel through the temporal lobes enroute to their termination in the occipital lobes (see Figure 2–28).

Occipital Lobes

The medial surfaces of the occipital lobes contain the primary receptive areas for vision. Visual association areas nearby allow a person to recognize or identify objects seen.

Basal Ganglia

Located deep within the white matter of the cerebrum lie several masses of gray matter (cell bodies) known collectively as the basal ganglia (Figure 2–16). These are identified as the caudate nucleus, the amygdaloid nucleus, the lentiform nucleus, which is subdivided into the globus pallidus and the putamen, and the claustrum. The basal ganglia are involved in skeletal muscle motor function and make up part of the extrapyramidal system. They exert an inhibiting or regulating effect on motor function, suppressing muscle tone and smoothing out muscle movements, especially those of the hands and lower extremities.

A band of white matter located between the basal ganglia and the thalamus is called the internal capsule. Major motor and sensory tracts passing to and from the cerebral cortex make up the internal capsule.[9]

Limbic System

Anatomically, the limbic system, or limbic lobe as it is sometimes called, consists of certain cortical and subcortical structures that form the border of the lateral ventricles on the medial surface of each cerebral hemisphere. The limbic system has many connections with the thalamus and hypothalamus and is concerned with primitive behaviors such as biological rhythms, sexual behavior, emotions of rage and fear, instincts, and self-preservation. Sometimes referred to as the "visceral brain," these emotional responses are expressed through endocrine, visceral, and somatic reactions (see Figure 2–18).[3(pp36–37)]

The hippocampus, structurally a medial part of the temporal lobe, is part of the limbic system. It is thought to be concerned with the formation of recent memory.[6] The anterior portion of the hippocampal gyrus curves in the form of a hook and is known as the uncus. This area lies just above the tentorium and immediately adjacent to the incisura.

Diencephalon

The diencephalon is divided into four regions: the thalamus, hypothalamus, subthalamus, and epithalamus. The thalamus and hypothalamus are the most important diencephalic structures.

Thalamus. The thalamus is made up of two large oval masses of gray matter that form part of the lateral walls of the third ventricle (Figure 2–16). The thalamus

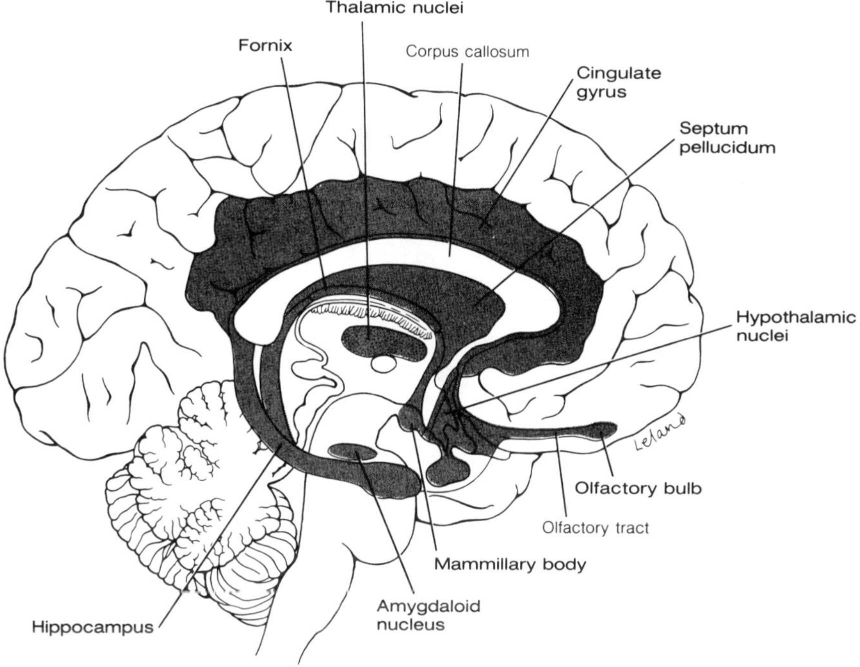

Fig. 2–18—Structures that constitute the limbic system.
Source: Reprinted from *Basic Human Anatomy* (p 373) by Alexander Spence with permission of the Benjamin-Cummings Publishing Company, © 1982.

---

is the vital integrating center of the brain. It acts as a final relay station for incoming sensory impulses prior to their termination in the cerebral cortex. All sensory pathways (except for the olfactory pathways) have direct afferent and efferent connections with the thalamus. In addition to its sensory role, the thalamus is involved with the limbic system and with the reticular activating system.

Hypothalamus. As the name implies, the hypothalamus lies below the thalamus, where it forms part of the walls and floor of the third ventricle (Figure 2–19). Like the thalamus, it is composed of several nuclei, each of which has specific functions. The mammillary bodies function as relay stations for olfactory neurons. They also relay limbic data from the cortex to the thalamus. The pituitary stalk connects the hypothalamus to the pituitary gland. The optic chiasm, located just above the pituitary gland, is the point at which some of the neurons of the optic nerves cross.

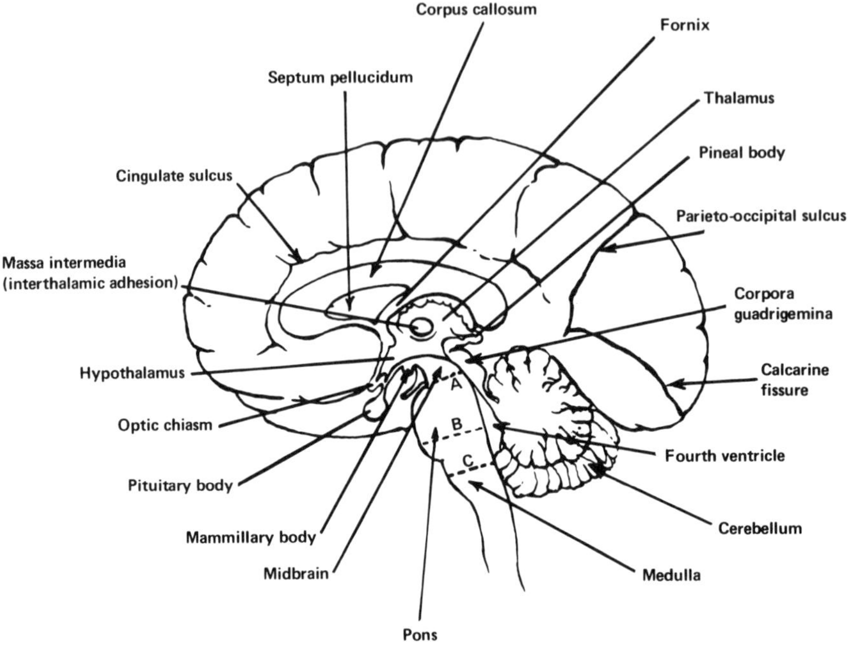

Fig. 2–19—Midsaggital section through the brain.
   Source: Reprinted from *Correlative Neuroanatomy and Functional Neurology* ed 18 (p 26) by Joseph Chusid with permission of Lange Medical Publications, © 1982.

The hypothalamus controls much of the activity of the autonomic nervous system. Some hypothalamic nuclei regulate sympathetic activity, while others control parasympathetic functions. The hypothalamus is involved in regulating body temperature, water balance, appetite, gastrointestinal activity, sexual activity, and emotions of fear and rage.[9] It is thought to play a role in the sleep-wakefulness cycle.[3(p38)] The hypothalamus also regulates the release of the hormones of the pituitary gland (Table 2–1).

Subthalamus. Located below the thalamus, the subthalamus is closely related to the basal ganglia in function.[3(p38)]

Epithalamus. Located posteriorly, the epithalamus forms a thin roof over the third ventricle. It contains the pineal body (epiphysis), which is thought to play a role in retarding sexual maturation and mediate some of the endocrine and metabolic effects of light.[9] Normally calcified in the audit, the pineal is an important radiologic landmark for locating the brain's midline structures.

Table 2–1 Hormone Secretions of the Pituitary Gland (Hypophysis)

Hormone	Target Organs	Actions
Anterior Lobe (Adenohypophysis)		
Adrenocorticotrophic (ACTH)	Adrenal cortex	Stimulates secretion of glucocorticoids and mineralcorticoids that protect against stress and influence metabolism of carbohydrates, proteins, fats, sodium, and potassium
Thyroid-stimulating (TSH)	Thyroid gland	Stimulates secretion of thyroxine that influences rate of many chemical reactions in the body
Follicle-stimulating (FSH)	Testes	Stimulates growth of gonads and reproductive activities
Luteinizing (LH)	Ovaries	
Growth (GH)	Muscles, bone, cartilage	Promotes tissue synthesis and body growth; affects carbohydrate and fat metabolism
Prolactin	Mammary alveolar cells	Stimulates milk production and secretion
Posterior Lobe (Neurohypophysis)		
Antidiuretic (ADH)	Kidneys	Promotes reabsorption of water from urine forming structures of kidneys, thereby controlling water content of body; mild circulatory pressor effect
Oxytocin	Uterus	Stimulates contraction of uterus
	Breast	Stimulates release of milk

Brainstem

The brainstem is the second major subdivision of the brain. It extends from the cerebral hemispheres to the foramen magnum at the base of the skull, where it merges with the spinal cord. The brainstem also connects with the cerebellum. Within the brainstem are the nuclei of ten of the cranial nerves. These cells lie principally in the dorsal portion. The ventral part of the brainstem contains the ascending and descending pathways that connect the cerebrum with the spinal cord.

Within the brainstem is an interlacing network of nerve fibers known as the reticular formation. These fibers extend from the lower brainstem up into the diencephalon. Motor and sensory neurons scattered throughout the CNS provide information concerning muscle activity. The reticular formation provides impulses to the muscles to support the body against gravity.[3(p40)]

Selected sensory impulses ascending through the reticular formation are relayed to the cerebral cortex and activate it (Figure 2–20). This activating or arousal system is involved in maintaining wakefulness. It is referred to as the reticular activating system (RAS). Injury to the RAS can cause coma. Anatomically, the brainstem can be subdivided into three major regions: the midbrain, the pons, and the medulla (Figure 2–19).

Midbrain

The midbrain makes up the upper portion of the brainstem and lies between the diencephalon and the pons. The nuclei of cranial nerves III and IV are located in the midbrain. Through numerous specific nuclei, the midbrain functions as a relay station. It coordinates impulses between the cerebellum and the cerebral hemispheres. It also contains relay centers (tectal regions) for auditory and visual reflexes.

Pons

The pons (bridge) lies between the midbrain and the medulla. The nuclei of cranial nerves V through VIII are located in the pons. Transverse tracts in the pons connect with the cerebellum. Longitudinal tracts pass through the pons as well, connecting the cerebrum with lower levels of the nervous system. Certain pontine centers influence the pattern and rate of respirations.

Medulla

The medulla extends from the pons to the foramen magnum where it becomes continuous with the spinal cord. The nuclei of cranial nerves IX through XII are located in the medulla.

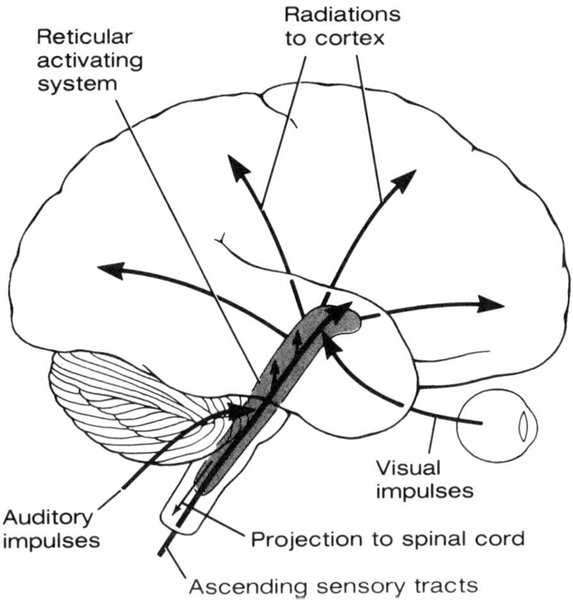

Fig. 2–20—Reticular formation. Arrows indicate input to and output from the reticular activating system.
    Source: Reprinted from *Basic Human Anatomy* (p 377) by Alexander Spence with permission of the Benjamin-Cummings Publishing Company, © 1982.

Also located in the medulla are neurons that are involved in the control of a variety of vital functions such as respiration, heart rate, dilation and constriction of blood vessels, coughing, swallowing, and vomiting.[9]

On the ventral surface of the medulla are two large columns of nerve fiber tracts call the pyramids. The pyramids contain the corticospinal tracts that extend from the motor cortex down through the spinal cord. Some of these motor tracts cross from one pyramid to another, referred to as the ''decussation of the pyramids.''

The Cerebellum

The cerebellum lies in the posterior fossa and is separated from the cerebrum by the tentorium cerebelli. The cerebellum connects with the brainstem via three paired cerebellar peduncles. Two lateral cerebellar hemispheres are connected by a structure called the vermis. Like the cerebrum, the cerebellum contains an outer cortex of gray matter, or nerve cell bodies, surrounding the inner white matter, composed of pathways connecting the cerebellum with other parts of the CNS.

Of major importance is the cerebellum's coordination of muscle activity on the basis of certain sensory information. It is believed that almost all sensory input is relayed through the cerebellum. In response to sensory input, motor impulses are then sent from the cerebellum to the cerebrum and the spinal cord, resulting in muscle synergy and the maintenance of equilibrium and balance. Unlike the cerebrum, cerebellar control is ipsilateral. The right side of the cerebellum influences the right side of the body, and the left side of the cerebellum influences the left side of the body.[1(pp105–106)]

Pathophysiological Considerations

Because of the complexity of the brain structures, a multitude of abnormalities can result from trauma, neoplasms, infectious and inflammatory disorders, or other disease processes. Brain dysfunctions can be very serious because of the very limited ability of neurons within the CNS to adequately regenerate once they have been damaged.

Signs and symptoms may vary from a mixture of motor, sensory, speech, cognitive, and intellectual disorders to seizures, coma, and death. A description of common cerebral hemispheric disorders is covered in detail in Chapter 9.

Dysfunctions of the Basal Ganglia

Since the basal ganglia are primarily concerned with supressing or smoothing out muscle function, lesions in the basal ganglia generally result in spastic movements. Dyskinesias, or abnormal involuntary movements seen with basal ganglia disorders, are often referred to as extrapyramidal signs. These may include tremors, writhing, flinging of extremities, or more graceful choreiform movements.

Dysfunctions of the Limbic System

Because the limbic system is thought to be the seat of emotional experience and expression, damage to this area of the brain may induce a multitude of signs and symptoms. Restlessness and hyperactivity are common.

Seizures that originate in the temporal lobe are sometimes referred to as psychomotor or limbic seizures and reflect an emotional component. There may be hallucinations, illusions, bizarre or violent behavior, and memory disturbances.[1(pp538–539)]

Complex brain mechanisms for memory storage and retrieval are affected by damage to structures in the limbic system. Infarctions of hippocampal areas retard recent memory. Thalamic lesions impair the formation of new memory as the ability of the thalamus to give the "print" order for new memory is affected. A severe brain contusion may cause various degrees of retrograde amnesia. Amnesia can also result from electroconvulsive therapy (ECT), chronic alcoholism (Korsakoff's syndrome), and Alzheimer's disease, a form of dementia caused by brain atrophy.[12]

Dysfunctions of Diencephalic Structures

Lesions of the thalamus cause contralateral anesthesia. Sometimes, certain sensations return, but they may be exaggerated. Tactile and thermal stimuli that were once not unpleasant may become very uncomfortable. Spontaneous intractable pain may occur with thalamic lesions. Emotional instability with outbursts of laughter or crying may occur with vascular lesions that affect diencephalic structures.[13]

Lesions of the hypothalamus can result in diverse autonomic disturbances. One such manifestation of sympathetic disruption at the hypothalamic level is the appearance of very small reactive pupils. With unilateral hypothalamic damage, only the pupil on that same side will appear small. This may be an early sign of transtentorial herniation.

In addition, hypothalamic lesions may cause disorders of water balance, sugar and fat metabolism, and temperature regulation. Like the thalamus, the hypothalamus is part of the limbic system. Emotional disorders may result from lesions in this region.[13]

Dysfunctions of the Brainstem

Since all motor and sensory tracts of the CNS must traverse the brainstem, complex mixtures of motor and sensory deficits may be seen with lesions of the brainstem. Cranial nerve, respiratory, and autonomic nervous sytem dysfunctions can also occur. Trauma, tumor, infarction, or hemorrhage in the brainstem can also result in coma if the reticular activating system is affected.[9]

Expanding lesions in the supratentorial or infratentorial structures of the brain can result in the displacement of brain structures, leading to compression of the brainstem. Various brain herniation syndromes are discussed in more detail in Chapter 4.

Dysfunctions of the Cerebellum

Lesions of the cerebellum or its pathways produce disturbances of gait, posture, and equilibrium. Rapid, orderly movement is not possible, and jerky movements or tremors may be seen when the patient reaches for a given object. Unable to stop movement at a particular place, the patient may stop short of a given object or reach beyond it (past pointing). Eye muscles may be affected leading to jerky eye movements (nystagmus). Speech may be slurred or halting and broken.

SPINAL CORD

The spinal cord is essentially an extension of nerve tracts of the brain. Its primary purpose is to carry messages to and from the brain. It also serves as a center for reflexes not necessarily requiring input from higher centers in the brain. It is continuous with the medulla at its rostral end and is enclosed within the vertebral column. Like the brain, it is also surrounded by CSF and meninges. A central canal extends from the fourth ventricle through the length of cord. It is lined with ependymal cells and also contains CSF.

Occupying the upper two-thirds of the vertebral canal, the spinal cord extends from the foramen magnum to the level of the first or second lumbar vertebra and is approximately 42–45 cm long in the adult (Figure 2–21). A thin filament of pia mater called the filum terminale extends from the lower spinal cord, the conus medullaris, to the coccyx.

Thirty-one pairs of spinal nerves emerge from the spinal cord. Each level of spinal cord giving rise to a spinal nerve is called a "spinal segment." There are eight pairs of cervical spinal nerves, twelve thoracic, five lumbar, five sacral, and one coccygeal. The first pair of cervical spinal nerves leaves the cord above the C-1 vertebra, while C-2 through C-7 spinal nerves leave through the intervertebral foramina above each corresponding vertebra. The C-8 spinal nerves leave the cord below the C-7 vertebra. All spinal nerves from T-1 down leave the cord by way of the foramina immediately below the corresponding vertebrae.

Two prominent enlargements appear in the spinal cord where innervation of the upper and lower extremities takes place. The cervical enlargement gives rise to spinal nerves that form the brachial plexus and supply the arms. The lumbar enlargement gives rise to the nerves forming the lumbar plexus and supplies the legs.

Because the vertebral column grows at a faster rate than the spinal column, the spinal nerves from the lumbar area down must descend from their point of origin to their respective vertebral foramina. These spinal nerves develop long roots that resemble the shape of a horse's tail and are known as the cauda equina.

Each spinal nerve contains a dorsal root that conveys sensory information into the spinal cord, and a ventral root that conveys motor impulses out from the spinal cord (Figure 2–22). These two nerve roots join just outside the cord to form the spinal nerve. After leaving the spinal cord, each spinal nerve divides into several branches making up the peripheral nerves.

Gray Matter

The spinal cord contains an H-shaped central gray matter made up of nerve cell bodies and nonmyelinated nerve fibers. The anterior (ventral) horn of the gray matter contains the cell bodies of motor nerves whose axons leave the cord and

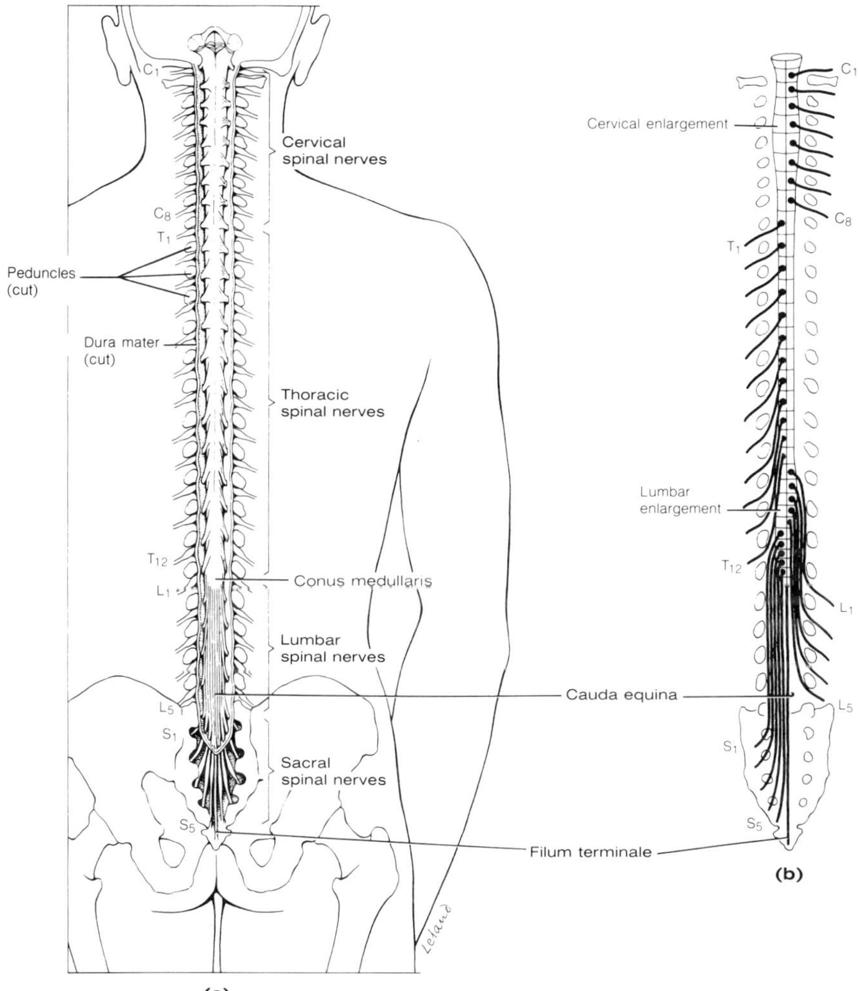

Fig. 2–21—Spinal nerves as they leave the spinal cord and pass between the vertebrae.
Source: Reprinted from *Basic Human Anatomy* (p 416) by Alexander Spence
with permission of the Benjamin-Cummings Publishing Company, © 1982.

supply voluntary striated muscle. The posterior (dorsal) horns contain axons of
sensory nerves and internuncial (connecting) neurons. In the thoracic and upper
lumbar regions, the spinal cord has a pair of lateral horns or columns of gray matter
that give rise to the preganglionic fibers of visceral motor (autonomic) nerves.[9]

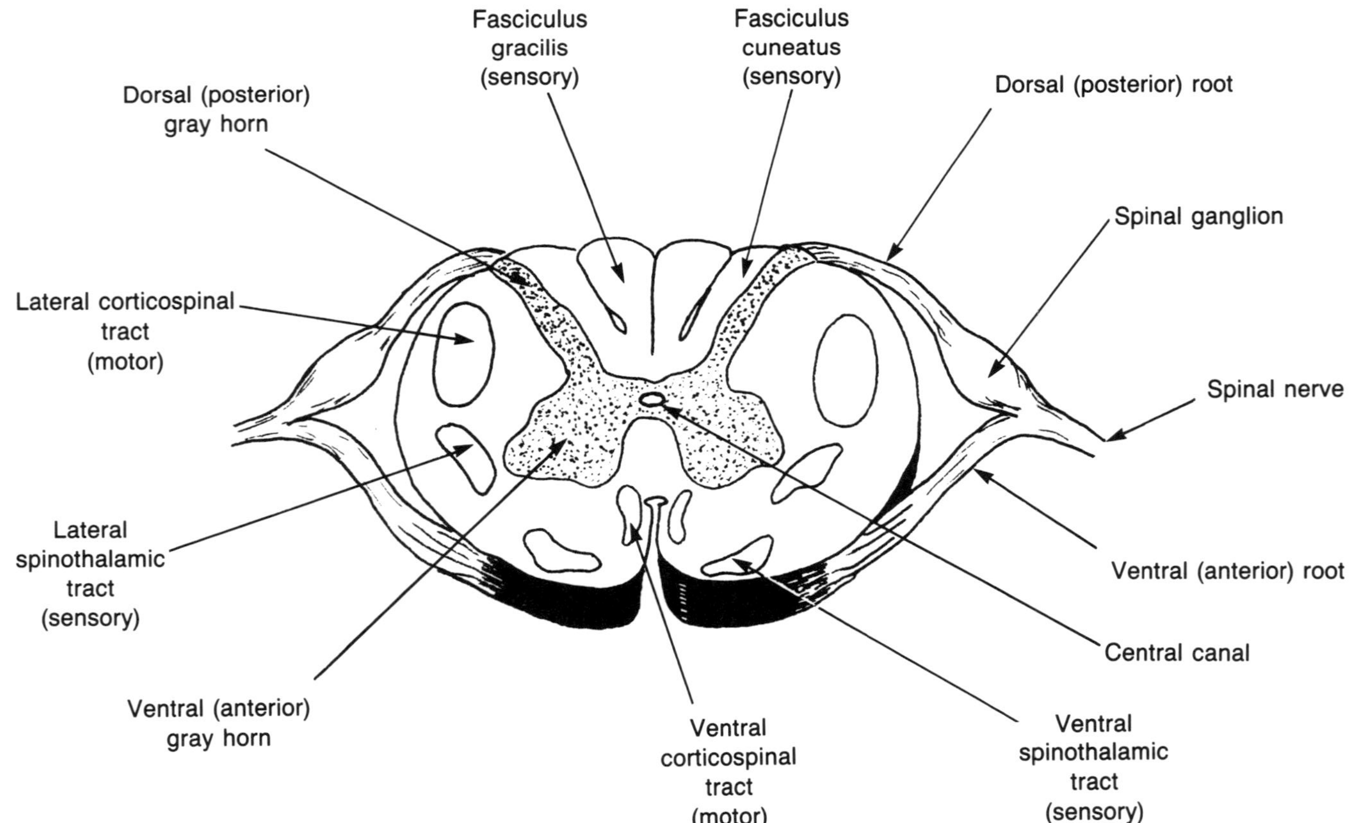

Fig. 2–22—Cross section of the spinal cord.

White Matter

The white matter of the spinal cord surrounds the gray matter. It is composed of axons, most of which are myelinated, that convey messages between various levels of the spinal cord and between the brain and the spinal cord. Although not visibly discernible, these nerve fibers can be divided into bundles making up pathways or tracts that carry information. Some tracts are ascending, or sensory, carrying impulses to the brain. Other tracts are descending, or motor, carrying impulses from the brain.[9]

The Sensory System

The ascending spinal tracts carry sensory information from peripheral sensory receptors to various centers in the brain. Sensory tracts generally contain three neurons (Figure 2–23). Dendrites of the first sensory neuron extend from the peripheral receptor to its cell body, which is located in a dorsal root ganglion. Its axon then travels into the dorsal horn of the spinal cord where it synapses with the dendrites of the second sensory neuron. The cell bodies of these second level sensory neurons are located in the dorsal gray horn of the spinal cord or in the brain stem. The axon of this second neuron terminates in the thalamus. The third sensory neuron of the tract conveys the impulse from the thalamus to the appropriate area of the parietal cerebral cortex where the perception of sensation occurs.

Almost all ascending tracts cross to the other side of the CNS. Some cross at or a few segments above entry level into the cord, or within the medulla. Sensory information from the right side of the body is subsequently interpreted by the left cerebral cortex and vice versa.[9] Major ascending sensory spinal tracts of clinical significance include the fasciculus gracilis, fasciculus cuneatus, spinothalamic, and spinocerebellar.

Fasciculus Gracilis and Fasciculus Cuneatus

Sensory fibers in the fasciculus gracilis and fasciculus cuneatus convey muscle position and movement sensation (proprioception), vibratory sense, and two-point discrimination. They enter the dorsal portion of the spinal cord and ascend in the posterior columns. The crossover of these tracts to the other side of the CNS takes place in the medulla.

Spinothalamic Tracts

The lateral spinothalamic tract conveys pain and temperature sensation. The anterior spinothalamic tract carries the sensations of light touch and pressure. Fibers from both of these tracts cross over in the cord before they ascend on the opposite (contralateral) side.

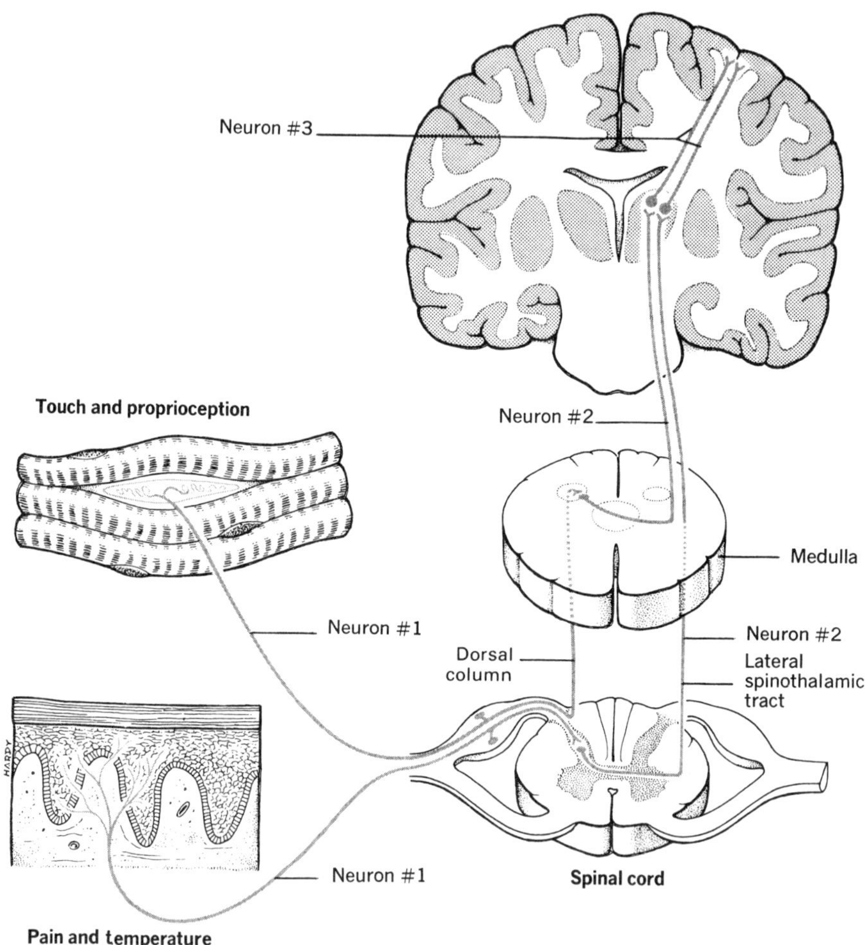

Fig. 2–23—Decussation (crossing) of ascending tracts.
Source: Reprinted from *Basic Physiology and Anatomy* ed 4 (p 242) by E Chaffee and I Lytle with permission of the JB Lippincott Company, © 1980.

Spinocerebellar Tracts

Dorsal and ventral spinocerebellar tracts convey unconscious proprioception from neuromuscular receptors to the cerebellum. The dorsal tracts do not cross over before ascending to the cerebellum while the ventral tracts cross in the cord.

The Motor System

The motor system consists of upper motor neurons and lower motor neurons. Upper motor neurons, which are totally contained within the CNS, descend from the cerebral cortex, cerebellum, or basal ganglia and synapse with lower motor neurons in the brain stem (cranial nerves) and with lower motor neurons originating in the anterior horns of the gray matter of the spinal cord (Figure 2–24). There are two types of descending (motor) tracts, the pyramidal and the extrapyramidal.

Pyramidal Tracts

The pyramidal tracts are also called the corticospinal tracts. They carry impulses for voluntary skeletal muscle movement. These tracts originate in the pyramidal cells of the cerebral cortex and descend through the internal capsule, midbrain, pons, and medulla, where 90 percent of the tracts cross over to the opposite side before descending the entire length of the cord as the lateral corticospinal tracts. The remaining 10 percent descend uncrossed as the ventral or anterior corticospinal tracts. Crossover of these fibers occurs a few spinal segments above their termination in the cervical and thoracic cord.[9]

Extrapyramidal Tracts

Numerous extrapyramidal tracts exist, but they will not be discussed in individual detail. These tracts may originate from various regions of the cortex, from subcortical structures, such as the basal ganglia, and from the brain stem. There is considerable overlap between the actions of some of these tracts and the pyramidal (corticospinal) tracts. While the pyramidal tracts convey impulses to initiate voluntary muscle movement, some extrapyramidal tracts exert inhibitory influences that modify muscular contractions. Consequently, these extrapyramidal tracts unconsciously influence balance and posture.[9] Some extrapyramidal tracts influence respiration, circulation, and sweating, while others influence certain sensory cranial nerves, thereby mediating audio and visual reflexes. Still other tracts mediate voluntary control of motor cranial nerves.

Spinal Reflex Arc

A reflex is a stereotyped response, mediated by the nervous system, to a stimulus of sufficient magnitude.[3(p50)] Not all sensory impulses carried into the spinal cord need to enter one of the ascending tracts to be carried to the brain. Some sensory neurons synapse directly or through internuncial neurons with motor neurons in the anterior horn of the gray matter at the same level in the spinal cord. Other neurons travel up or down only a few segments of the cord before synapsing

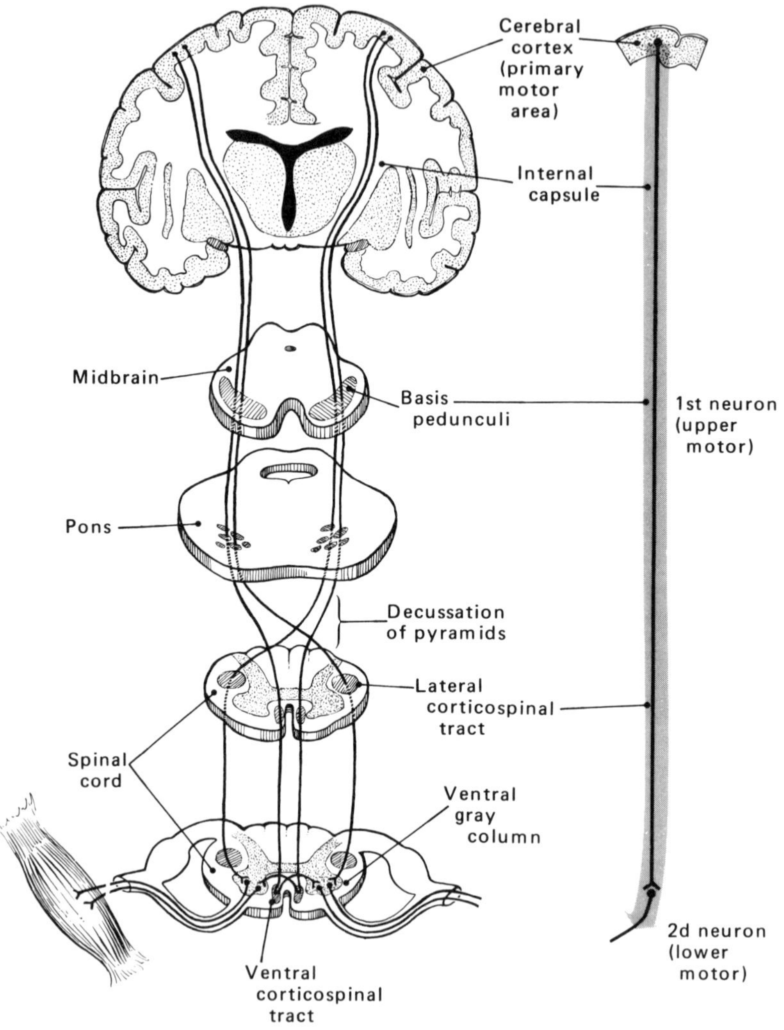

Fig. 2–24—Pyramidal motor pathways; the corticospinal tracts.
Source: Reprinted from *Dynamic Anatomy and Physiology* (p 286) by L Langley, I Telford, and J Christensen with permission of the McGraw-Hill Book Company, © 1974.

with a motor neuron. These neural pathways making up this direct communication of sensory to motor neurons are called spinal reflex arcs. They do not require conscious thought, although at the same time the stimulus may also be carried to the brain where we become aware of it. The event may then be committed to memory. This all happens, though, after the reflex action mediated by the spinal cord has taken place. For instance, one may quickly pull a hand away from contact with a hot object before becoming aware of a burning sensation (Figure 2–25).[9] Descending upper motor neurons such as those of the corticospinal tracts do exert an inhibitory or modulating influence on certain spinal reflexes.

Muscle Stretch Reflexes

A muscle stretch reflex is monosynaptic, meaning the afferent or sensory nerve synapses directly with the efferent or motor nerve without an internuncial neuron (Figure 2–25). When a muscle is stretched by striking a tendon, the nerve impulses that are generated travel via a sensory nerve to the spinal cord. Here the sensory nerve synapses with a motor nerve that carries the impulse to the muscle. Acetylcholine is released at the motor end plate causing the muscle to contract, resisting the stretch.

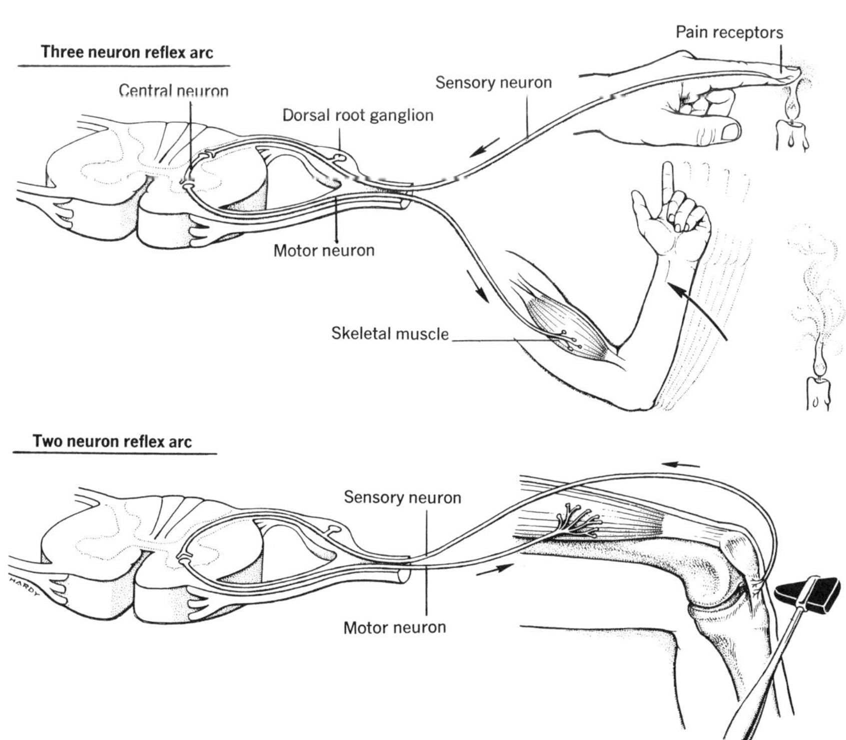

Fig. 2–25—*Above,* flexor reflex; *below,* stretch reflex.
Source: Reprinted from *Basic Physiology and Anatomy* ed 4 (p 240) by E Chaffee and I Lytle with permission of the JB Lippincott Company, © 1980.

The knee jerk reflex involves contraction of the quadriceps muscle and extension of the lower leg in response to tapping the patellar tendon.[9] Concurrently from higher centers in the CNS come the modulating controls over these deep tendon reflexes. Without this inhibiting or modulating control, muscle tone is increased, leading to hyperactive reflexes and spasticity.

Flexor Reflexes

Flexor reflexes, also known as withdrawal reflexes, are protective reflexes that involve several spinal segments (intersegmental). As in the previous example, if a finger touches a hot object, the arm immediately flexes and pulls the hand away. Simultaneously, motor neurons supplying extensor muscles are inhibited.[9]

Cutaneous Reflexes

Cutaneous reflexes are superficial reflexes that involve the contraction of groups of muscles in response to stimulation of the skin. In the abdominal reflex, the skin of the abdominal quadrants is stroked. The normal response is contraction of superficial abdominal muscles, leading to a twitching of the umbilicus toward the quadrant being stimulated.[14]

Pathological Reflexes

Pathological reflexes are seen in neurological diseases. Destruction or depression of the corticospinal or other upper motor neuron tracts releases their inhibition of spinal reflexes and results in hyperactive reflexes. The Babinski reflex represents a pathological superficial plantar reflex, although it is known to occur normally in infants.[14]

In addition to the Babinski reflex, the Hoffman's sign also indicates pyramidal tract disease. A positive sign (flexion and adduction of the thumb) occurs when the terminal phalanx of the middle finger is pressed or snapped.[3(p86)] Lower motor neuron lesions result in absent reflexes for those parts of the body supplied by that spinal segment.

Pathophysiological Considerations

While acute spinal cord dysfunction can occur as a result of such disease processes as disk protrusion, tumors, infections, or ruptured vascular malformations, the emergency department nurse is most likely to encounter patients who have sustained traumatic spinal cord injury. Typically, the patient is a young man under age 30, injured during a motor vehicle accident, a fall, or a sporting activity such as diving or skiing.[5(p629)] While there may or may not be vertebral fracture, severe spinal cord injuries result from forces that cause severe hyperflexion, hyperextension, or rotation of the spinal column. The spinal cord may be concussed, compressed, stretched, or contused. Cord laceration can occur from bony vertebral fragments and from penetrating injuries. Interruption of blood supply to the cord from bony angulations can further enhance the severity of cord injury.

Spinal cord injury can be classified by level of injury and by degree of cord involvement (see Chapter 8). Most spinal cord injuries occur in the lower cervical or lumbar regions where relatively mobile segments of the vertebral column meet relatively fixed portions.[5(p629)] Signs and symptoms can vary from minimal motor and sensory impairment to complete paralysis, sensory loss, and spinal shock.

THE PERIPHERAL NERVOUS SYSTEM

The peripheral nervous system includes all neurons other than those in the CNS. It is composed of cranial nerves that emerge from the base of the brain, spinal nerves that originate in the spinal cord, and the autonomic nervous system (Figure 2–26).

A peripheral nerve trunk contains many nerve fibers wrapped within a sheath. Nerve fibers can be classified as sensory or afferent, motor or efferent, or autonomic (efferent in function). Afferent nerves may be somatic, carrying sensations from the body wall, or visceral, carrying sensations from the internal organs. Efferent nerves are also somatic or visceral. Somatic efferent nerves carry voluntary motor impulses to skeletal muscle. Visceral motor neurons are involuntary and comprise the autonomic nervous system. They transmit visceral motor impulses to cardiac and smooth muscles and to glands.

The Cranial Nerves

There are 12 pairs of cranial nerves (CN) arising from the brain. Nerves I (olfactory) and II (optic) are actually nerve fiber tracts rather than true nerves. With the exception of part of the fibers of CN XI arising from the upper cervical cord, CNs III through XII emerge from the brain stem (Figure 2–27). Cranial nerves are classified as sensory, motor, or autonomic. Some nerves such as CN V have both motor and sensory fibers (Table 2–2).

Cranial Nerve I (Olfactory)

The olfactory nerves are the organs for the sense of smell. Hairlike filaments in the mucous membranes over the upper part of the nasal septum enter the skull through the midline portion of the frontal fossa, the cribiform plate. These filaments terminate in the olfactory bulbs. From each bulb, fibers go along the base of the brain to each side of the optic chiasm, where they enter the brain and reach the medial sides of the temporal lobes of the cerebral cortex.[11]

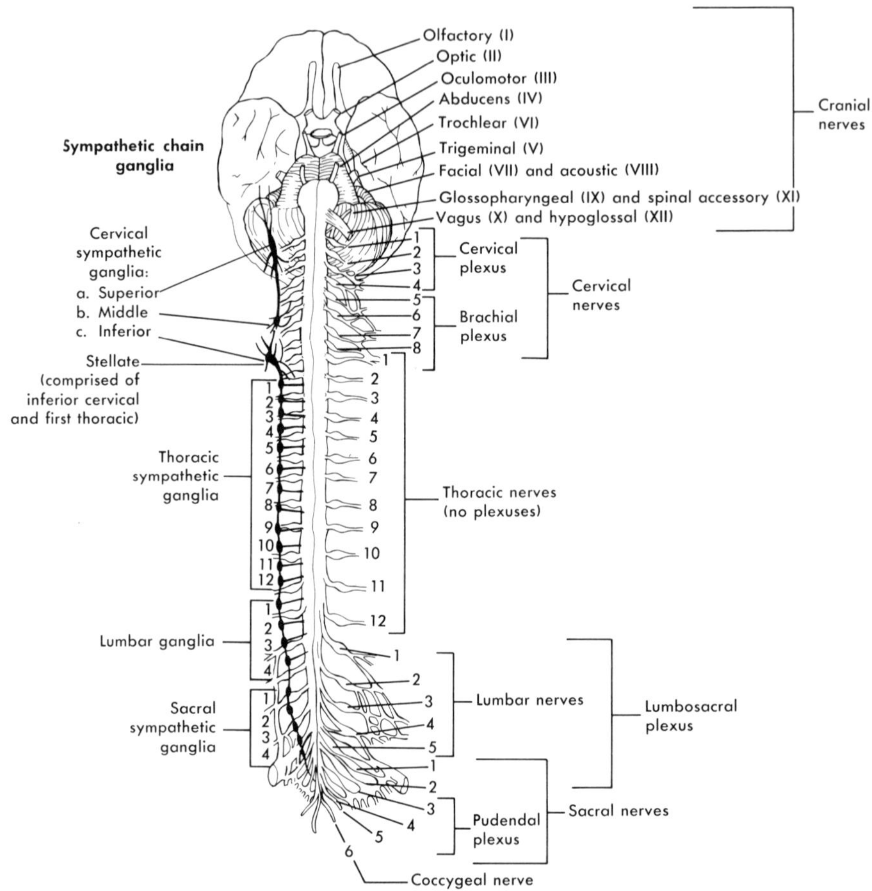

Fig. 2–26—Anterior view of brain and spinal cord. *Right,* spinal nerves; *left,* sympathetic chain. *Source:* Reprinted from *Carini and Owens' Neurological and Neurosurgical Nursing* ed 8 (p 85) by Barbara Conway-Rutkowski with permission of the CV Mosby Company, © 1982.

Cranial Nerve II (Optic)

The optic nerves serve the sense of vision. Nerve fibers arising from the inner layer of the retina join to form each optic nerve, which proceed posteriorly to enter the cranial cavity via the optic foramen. Shortly after entering the cranium, the two optic nerves meet at the optic chiasm just anterior to the pituitary gland. Nerve fibers from the medial half of each retina cross to the opposite side while fibers

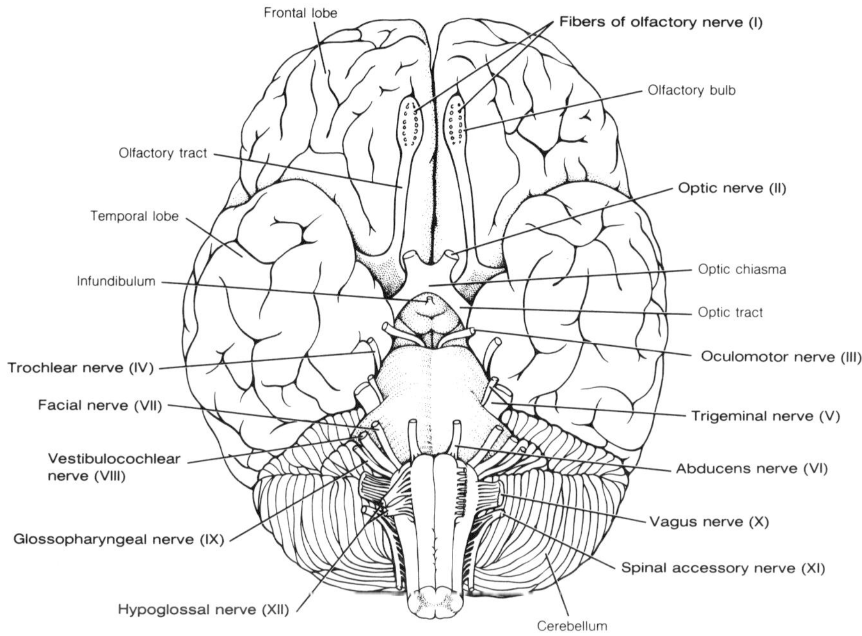

Fig. 2–27—Ventral surface of brain showing the cranial nerves.
Source: Reprinted from *Basic Human Anatomy* (p 404) by Alexander Spence with permission of the Benjamin-Cummings Publishing Company, © 1982.

---

from the lateral half of each retina do not cross (Figure 2–28). These fibers all pass back through the brain as the optic tracts, terminating in the lateral geniculate of the thalamus. From the geniculate bodies, optic radiations fan back to the optic cortex and visual association areas of the occipital lobes. Thus, each optic tract and optic radiation carry some fibers from each eye. Also from the optic tracts come pathways to the midbrain, which when connected to the third cranial nerve, mediate the pupillary light reflex.

Cranial Nerve III (Oculomotor)

The oculomotor nerves arise from the midbrain and innervate four of the six muscles responsible for movement of the eyeballs. They control motion of the eyeballs up, in, and down. In addition, the oculomotor nerves innervate the muscles that raise the eyelids and the muscles of the iris that constrict the pupils in response to light and accommodation. The oculomotor nerves are both motor and autonomic.

Table 2–2 Cranial Nerves

Cranial Nerve	Point of Origin	Structures Innervated	Function	Dysfunction
I Olfactory (sensory)	Olfactory mucous membranes	Same	Sense of smell	Anosmia (unilateral or bilateral loss of sense of smell)
II Optic (sensory)	Retina of eye	Same	Sense of vision	Visual field defects
III Oculomotor (motor, autonomic)	Midbrain	Superior, medial, inferior rectus, oblique, levator superioris, ciliary muscles, sphincter of iris	Moves eye up, down, in; raises eyelid; constricts pupil	Loss of ability to adduct eye; loss of pupillary constriction; diplopia; ptosis
IV Trochlear (motor)	Midbrain	Superior oblique muscle	Moves eye down and out	Slight impairment of downward gaze
V Trigeminal (sensory motor)	Pons	Skin and mucous membranes of head; teeth; muscles of mastication	Sensations from head, face, nasal, and oral cavities; mastication	Sensory loss in one or all divisions; weakness of jaw muscles; tic douloureux; herpes zoster
VI Abducens (motor)	Lower pons	Lateral rectus muscle	Rotates eyeball outward	Loss of ability to turn eye laterally (abduct)

VII Facial (motor, sensory, autonomic)	Cerebellar-pontine angle	Muscles of face and scalp; taste buds ant. ⅔ of tongue	Muscles of facial expression; close eyelids; sense of taste; secretion by salivary and lacrimal glands	Weakness of all muscles on same side of face,* eyelid does not close; loss of taste ant. ⅔ of tongue
VIII Acoustic (sensory)	Pons and medulla	Structures of inner ear	Hearing (auditory branch); equilibrium (vestibular branch)	Hearing loss, tinnitus; vertigo, nausea, vomiting, nystagmus
IX Glossopharyngeal (motor, sensory, autonomic)	Medulla	Pharynx; taste buds post. ⅓ of tongue; carotid sinus and body	Motor and sensory control of pharynx; secretion by parotid glands; sense of taste; afferent limb of circulatory and respiratory reflexes	Impaired sensation over palate and pharynx; loss of sense of taste posterior ⅓ of tongue
X Vagus (motor, sensory, autonomic)	Medulla	Organs of thoracic and abdominal cavities; larynx, pharynx, and palate	Pharyngeal and laryngeal movement and sensation; motor to walls of bronchi; constrictor to coronaries; visceral activities; active in cardiac, circulatory, and respiratory reflexes	Disturbances of swallowing and phonation; decreased gag reflex; hoarseness; palate and uvula deviate away from side of lesion

Table 2–2 continued

Cranial Nerve	Point of Origin	Structures Innervated	Function	Dysfunction
XI Spinal accessory (motor)	Lower medulla to upper cervical cord	Sternocleidomastoid and trapezius muscles	Allows turning of head and shrugging of shoulders; some muscle control of larynx and pharynx	Flatness of neck on affected side; weakness of head turning; dropped shoulder; weakness in shrugging shoulder; difficulty raising arm above horizontal plane
XII Hypoglossal (motor)	Medulla	Muscles of tongue	Movement of tongue	Atrophy of tongue on affected side; deviation of tongue to affected side; fasciculations (fine muscle twitching) of tongue

*The portions of the facial nerve that supply the upper facial muscles receive fibers from the motor strips of each cerebral cortex via the corticobulbar tracts. Therefore, a lesion in either cerebral cortex affecting CN VII upper motor neuron tracts will cause weakness of the lower facial muscles on the opposite side, but will spare the muscles of the forehead (called central facial weakness). A lower motor neuron (facial nerve) lesion will cause weakness of the entire face on the same side as the lesion.

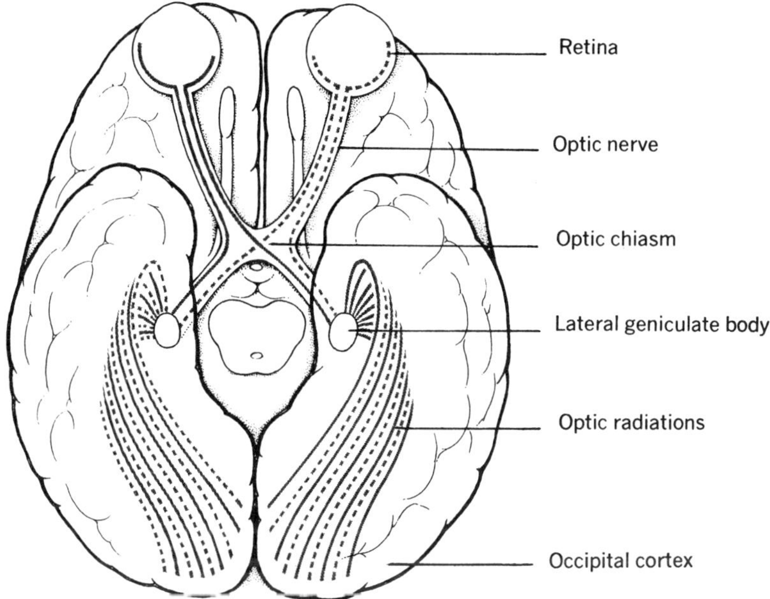

Fig. 2–28—Optic pathways. Note crossing of fibers from medial half of each retina.
Source: Reprinted from *Basic Physiology and Anatomy* ed 4 (p 274) by
E Chaffee and I Lytle with permission of the JB Lippincott Company, © 1980.

Cranial Nerve IV (Trochlear)

Arising from the midbrain, immediately posterior to the oculomotor nuclei, the trochlear nerves supply the superior oblique muscles that rotate the eyeballs down and outward. Unlike CN III and CN VI, CN IV decussates before emerging.

Cranial Nerve V (Trigeminal)

The trigeminal nerves arise from the pons. Three sensory branches, the ophthalmic, maxillary, and mandibular, convey the sensations of pain, temperature, and touch from the supratentorial cavity, meninges, the entire face and scalp, the corneas, the paranasal sinuses, and the nasal and oral cavities. The motor components of the trigeminal nerves innervate the muscles of mastication.

Cranial Nerve VI (Abducens)

The abducens nerves arise from the anterior portion of the lower pons and innervate the lateral rectus muscles of the eyes. This allows each eye to look laterally.

Cranial Nerve VII (Facial)

The facial nerves arise from the lower border of the pons, at the cerebellar-pontine angle. After dividing into several branches, the facial nerves supply the muscles of the face and scalp. The sensory component of the facial nerves innervates the taste buds of the anterior two-thirds of the tongue. CN VII also innervates certain salivary and lacrimal glands.

Cranial Nerve VIII (Acoustic)

Each acoustic nerve has two separate divisions, both sensory and both innervating the inner ear. They join to form each single nerve trunk that enters just below the pons. The cochlear division transmits the sense of hearing from the organ of Corti. The vestibular division's receptors are in the region of the semicircular canals and influence balance and maintenance of body position.

Cranial Nerve IX (Glossopharyngeal)

The glossopharyngeal nerves arise from the medulla and carry motor, sensory, and autonomic impulses. Having five branches, each nerve innervates the tongue and the pharynx. Sensory impulses convey the sense of taste from the posterior third of the tongue, sensation from the mucous membranes of the pharynx and tonsils, and pressure from the carotid sinus and carotid body. Motor fibers supply the muscles of the pharynx. Parasympathetic fibers travel to the parotid salivary glands.

Cranial Nerve X (Vagus)

The vagus nerves arise from the medulla and branch into several segments. They carry motor impulses to and sensory impulses from the pharynx and palate. In addition, they have widespread parasympathetic distribution to the organs of the thoracic and abdominal cavities. Sensation is also conveyed from the heart, lungs, and viscera of the gastrointestinal (GI) tract. The vagus nerves are the only cranial nerves whose distribution is not restricted to the head and neck.[9]

Cranial Nerve XI (Spinal Accessory)

The spinal accessory nerves arise from the lower medulla and upper cervical spinal cord. They supply the sternocleidomastoid and upper trapezius muscles and allow for the turning of the head and shrugging of shoulders. A few of the most cephalad fibers intermix with vagus fibers to supply the muscles of the larynx and pharynx.[9]

Cranial Nerve XII (Hypoglossal)

The hypoglossal nerves arise from the medulla and innervate the muscles of the tongue. They influence normal speech and the ability to swallow.[3(p58)]

Pathophysiological Considerations

Common terminology used in peripheral nerve disorders includes neuritis and neuralgia. Neuritis means inflammation of a nerve, but many neuritis conditions are actually degenerative and inflammatory. Bell's palsy is a term used to describe paralysis of the facial muscles caused by an inflammation of the facial nerve (CN VII) on the affected side.

Neuralgia refers to spasms of severe pain along the path of a peripheral nerve. Trigeminal neuralgia (tic douloureux) is characterized by attacks of excruciating pain along the course of the maxillary and mandibular divisions of the trigeminal nerve (CN V).

Herpes zoster (shingles) is a viral infection of the dorsal root ganglia of the spinal nerves. The disease is characterized by pain and vesicular lesions along the path of a peripheral sensory nerve.

Lesions affecting the peripheral nervous system may be due to congenital defects, neoplasms, trauma, or inflammation. There is interruption in the conductivity of the nerve resulting in neurologic impairment that may be manifested as motor loss, sensory changes, or trophic changes. Motor loss may include muscle weakness or paralysis. Sensory involvement may include pain and paresthesias (numbness, tingling, crawling sensations). These symptoms usually indicate partial or irritative lesions. More complete lesions may cause analgesia or anesthesia in a body part supplied by the affected sensory nerve. Nutritional and metabolic activities that are partially under neurological control may be impaired, leading to trophic changes in those tissues supplied by the affected nerves. In the extremities, early trophic changes include dry, warm, and flushed skin. Within a few weeks, the skin becomes cold and cyanotic, with loss of hair, brittleness of nails, ulcerations, and slow wound healing.[6(p76)] Peripheral nerves do have some ability to regenerate (see Figure 2–29).

Dysfunctions involving the cranial nerves are listed in Table 2–3. The oculomotor nerve (CN III) is of major clinical significance. Abnormal pupillary dilation occurs with interruption of this parasympathetic nerve. This can occur as a result of midbrain lesions, compression of the midbrain by brain shifts (herniation), or by lesions occurring peripherally on the oculomotor nerve.

When abnormal pupillary constriction is noted, it may be due to interruption of sympathetic innervation to the pupils occurring at the hypothalamic, brainstem, or upper thoracic cord levels, or in the ascending sympathetic fibers in the neck or head.

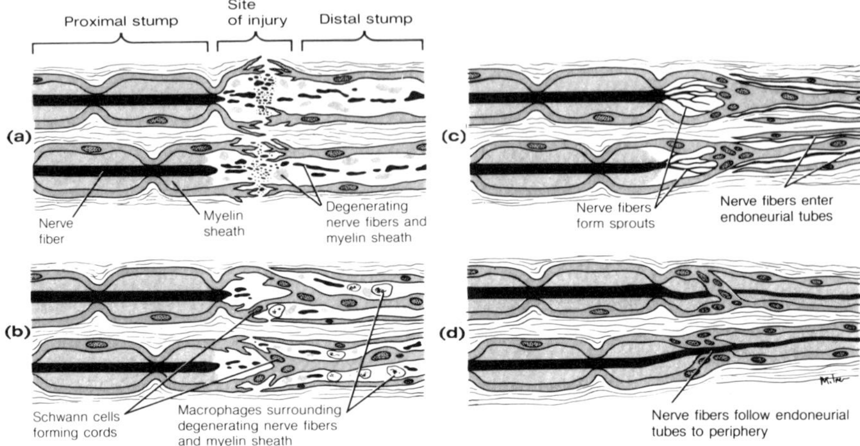

Fig. 2–29—Regeneration of peripheral nerve. (a) Nerve fibers degenerate distal (and a short distance proximal) to site of injury. (b) Schwann cells become active, forming cords within endoneurial tube. (c) Nerve fibers then form sprouts that grow into the endoneurial tube alongside Schwann cell cords. (d) Nerve fibers follow Schwann cell cords. Schwann cells then wrap around the nerve fibers, forming a myelin sheath around new fiber sprouts.

Source: Reprinted from *Basic Human Anatomy* (p 425) by Alexander Spence with permission of the Benjamin-Cummings Publishing Company, © 1982.

The Autonomic Nervous System

The autonomic, or automatic, nervous system is composed of visceral motor, or efferent, neurons. The autonomic nervous system regulates the activity of cardiac muscle, smooth (involuntary) muscle, and the glands of the body. Many neurons of the autonomic nervous system travel in the spinal nerves and certain cranial nerves, so it is an integral part of the nervous system as a whole. Two major subdivisions comprise the autonomic nervous system: the sympathetic and the parasympathetic. Generally these divisions have opposing functions, and for this reason the autonomic nervous system maintains a relatively stable internal body environment.

The Sympathetic Division

Also known as the thoracolumbar division, the sympathetic division has cell bodies of the preganglionic neurons located in the lateral horns of the gray matter of the spinal cord from the first thoracic through the second lumbar segments. These fibers leave the cord with motor fibers of the ventral roots. A short distance

Table 2–3 Effects of the Autonomic Nervous System

Organ or Function	Sympathetic Effects	Parasympathetic Effects
Heart		
Rate	Increased	Decreased
Force of contraction	Increased	Decreased
Blood vessels		
In heart	Dilation	Constriction
In skeletal muscle	Dilation	No innervation
In skin	Constriction	No innervation
In viscera	Constriction	Dilation
In external genitalia	Constriction	Dilation
Blood pressure	Increased	Decreased
Lungs		
Bronchioles	Dilation	Constriction
Respiratory rate	Increased	Decreased
Gastrointestinal tract		
Peristalsis	Decreased	Increased
Secretions	No direct effect	Increased
Liver	Increased conversion of glycogen to glucose	No innervation
Glands		
Salivary	Thick, viscous secretions	Thin, watery secretions
Sweat	Increased secretion	No innervation
Adrenal medulla	Secretion of epinephrine and norepinephrine	No innervation
Bladder		
Muscles of bladder wall	Relaxation	Contraction
Sphincters	Contraction	Relaxation
Pupil of eye	Dilation	Constriction
Pilomotor muscles of skin	Contraction (gooseflesh)	No innervation

Source: Adapted from *Basic Physiology and Anatomy* ed 4 (p 254) by E Chaffee and I Lytle with permission of the JB Lippincott Company, © 1980.

---

from the spinal cord these short preganglionic fibers synapse with postganglionic fibers along a chain of ganglia located on either side just anterior to the spinal cord. Long postganglionic fibers then travel out to the effector organs (see Figure 2–30).

The sympathetic division functions with a mass effect and prepares the individual to meet an emergency through the liberation of norepinephrine from the postganglionic neurons. It is therefore known as the "adrenergic" division. There are exceptions in the sympathetic division where norepinephrine is not the neurotransmitter. Acetylcholine is the neurotransmitter at all preganglionic nerve endings in both the sympathetic and parasympathetic divisions. Acetylcholine is also secreted by the sympathetic postganglionic neurons to the sweat glands and

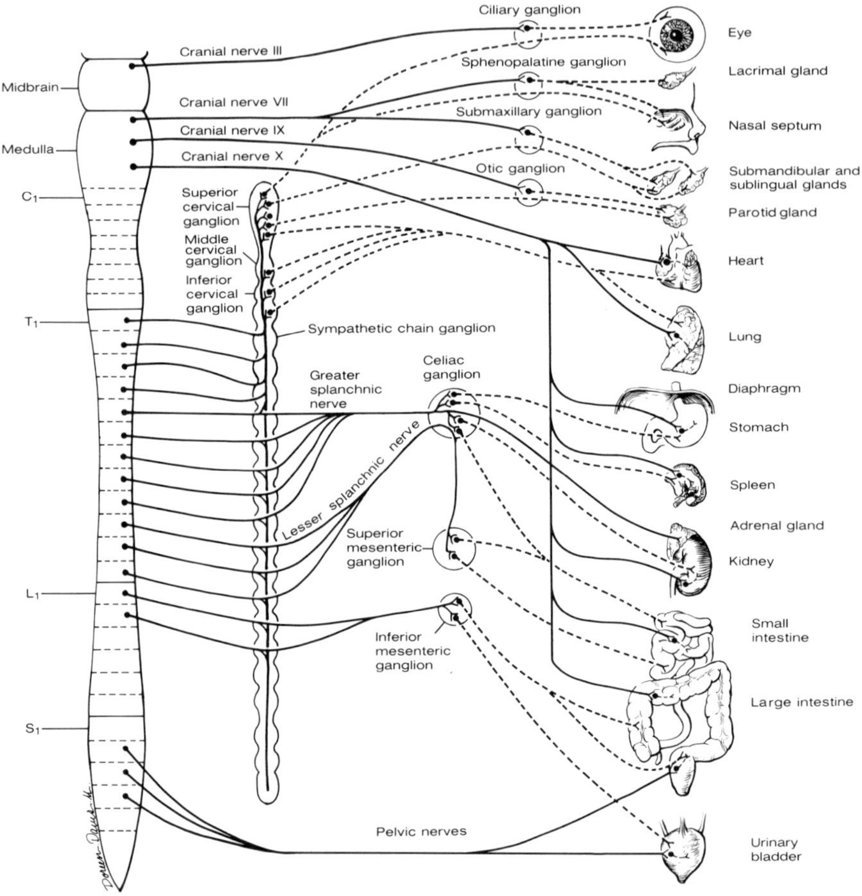

Fig. 2–30—Autonomic nervous system. Solid lines indicate preganglionic nerve fibers; dotted lines indicate postganglionic nerve fibers. Note that the parasympathetic fibers exit from the brainstem and sacral spine and the sympathetic fibers exit from the thoracolumbar spine.

Source: Reprinted from *Basic Human Anatomy* (p 432) by Alexander Spence with permission of the Benjamin-Cummings Publishing Company, © 1982.

the vasodilator neurons to skeletal muscle blood vessels. The adrenal medulla, unlike other viscera, is innervated directly by preganglionic fibers. The postganglionic neurons are located in the adrenal medulla and contain no axons. These neurons secrete epinephrine and norepinephrine directly into the bloodstream.[6(p141)] The effects of sympathetic stimulation are summarized in Table 2–3.

The Parasympathetic Division

Also known as the craniosacral division, the parasympathetic division has its preganglionic cell bodies located with the brain stem and the gray matter of the sacral spinal cord. These long preganglionic neurons synapse with short postganglionic neurons in ganglia located peripherally. Acetylcholine is released from the postganglionic neurons, and for this reason the parasympathetic division is known as the ''cholinergic'' division.

The parasympathetic division functions more selectively, tending to conserve bodily resources and playing a more dominant role when the individual is at rest.[11]

The frontal cortex influences the reactions of the autonomic nervous system through connections to the hypothalamus. Neurons from the hypothalamus descend through the brainstem and spinal cord, synapsing with preganglionic neurons of the autonomic nervous system. In this way the frontal lobes and the hypothalamus influence cardiovascular reactions, GI motility, respirations, peripheral vascular control, sweating, and the secretion of various hormones.[11]

Pharmacologically, the two divisions of the autonomic nervous system differ in their selective reactions to certain drugs. Some drugs such as adrenalin, amphetamines, cocaine, ephedrine, and phenylephrine stimulate the sympathetic division. Other drugs such as beta blockers (e.g., propanolol) selectively block certain sympathetic receptors, thus reducing selective sympathetic responses such as cardiac contractility.

Other drugs known to stimulate the parasympathetic division include Tensilon, neostigmine, physostigmine, metacholine, and pilocarpine. Some work by blocking the action of acetylcholinesterase, the enzyme that breaks down acetylcholine. Atropine and its derivatives depress parasympathetic activity by competing with acetylcholine for receptor sites. Curare and related drugs completely block the action of acetycholine, leading to muscle paralysis.

Although the autonomic nervous system is thought to function below the level of consciousness, research has shown that some conscious control of autonomic functions is possible through the process popularly known as biofeedback. Through electronic instruments, patients can monitor some impulses in the autonomic nervous system. With this conscious awareness of the autonomic nervous system, some people learn to control the responses of their autonomic nervous system. Some individuals are able to lower their blood pressure, slow their heart rate, increase circulation through their limbs, relieve migraine headaches, and control epileptic seizures.[9]

Pathophysiological Considerations

While autonomic dysfunctions can encompass a wide range of conditions, from peripheral vascular manifestations to sexual dysfunctions, only those conditions presenting or indicating a potential threat to life are discussed.

Spinal Shock

Spinal shock (see Chapter 8) includes the loss of vasomotor tone because of the sudden interruption of sympathetic outflow from the spinal cord. It may be due to transection of or severe injury to the spinal cord, or from excessive spinal anesthetic.[6(p144)] It is characterized by bradycardia, vasodilation with hypotension, warm flushed skin below the level of injury, and loss of body temperature. Flaccid paralysis, flaccid sphincters, and absent reflexes are also evident.

Autonomic Hyperreflexia

Also known as autonomic dysreflexia, autonomic hyperreflexia occurs during the rehabilitation or long-term phases of spinal cord injury but represents a very serious emergency. It is a mass reflex representing an exaggerated autonomic response to stimuli that occurs in patients with spinal cord injuries above the T-6 level. Any stimulation into the lower spinal cord such as bladder distention or irritation, bowel distention, or skin lesions trigger hyperactivity of sympathetic neurons. Clinical manifestations consist of severe paroxysmal hypertension, throbbing headache, blurred vision, sweating and/or flushing above the level of injury, pilomotor spasm with goose pimples, chills, nasal stuffiness, nausea, and restlessness.[3(p273)] The high blood pressure is sensed by pressure receptors in the carotid sinus and aorta, which causes a reflex slowing of the heart rate via the vagus nerve. The severe hypertension may result in cerebral hemorrhage or left ventricular failure with pulmonary edema if the condition is not promptly treated. Treatment consists of finding and removing the offending cause and reducing the blood pressure. Rapid acting antihypertensive drugs such as diazoxide may be needed.[15(p693)]

Paralytic Ileus

Paralytic ileus caused by autonomic dysfunction of the bowel may constitute a medical emergency. The patient may exhibit abdominal distention and rigidity, vomiting, and diminished or absent bowel sounds. Pain may not be experienced if there is impaired sensation from the viscera or if the sensorium is altered. This loss of GI peristalsis and bowel tone may result from overstimulation of the sympathetic system or understimulation of the parasympathetic system. The dangers include vomiting with aspiration, hypovolemia due to the third spacing of body fluids into the distended bowel, and bowel necrosis or rupture leading to sepsis.[1(pp271–273)]

Cardiorespiratory Abnormalities

In studies of severe head injury patients, Jennett and Teasdale reported the frequency of autonomic abnormalities occurring within the first week following injury.[16(pp145–146)] Periodic respiration (such as Cheyne-Stokes) occurred in 28 percent of the patients; respiratory rates greater than 30 breaths per minute occurred in 33 percent; pulse rates greater than 120 beats per minute occurred in 34 percent; blood pressure above 160 mm Hg occurred in 22 percent; and temperatures above 39° C were reported in 23 percent. In addition, electrocardiogram (ECG) abnormalities, in particular S-T segment depression, were frequently observed. They reported infrequent observations of bradycardia.

Pulmonary Insufficiency. Pulmonary insufficiency can occur in patients with intracranial hypertension. Intense sympathetic stimulation can alter surfactants leading to decreased pulmonary compliance and atelectasis.[8(p81)] Hypoxemia results from ventilation/perfusion (V/Q) mismatch in which underventilated alveoli continue to be perfused. Excessive rates of blood flow through normal alveolar-capillary units can also lead to V/Q mismatch.[17(p87)]

Neurogenic Pulmonary Edema. Intense sympathetic stimulation causes increased peripheral and pulmonary vascular resistance. Severe peripheral vasoconstriction can result in a sudden shift of blood from the peripheral to the more compliant pulmonary circulation. Pulmonary arterial, venous, and capillary wedge pressures rise. Fluid leaks from the distended capillaries into the pulmonary interstitium and alveoli resulting in pulmonary edema.[18]

REFERENCES

1. Taylor JW, Ballenger S: *Neurological Dysfunctions and Nursing Intervention.* New York, McGraw-Hill, 1980.

2. Budassi SA, Barber JM: *Emergency Nursing: Principles and Practice.* St. Louis, Mosby, 1981.

3. Hickey JV: *The Clinical Practice of Neurological and Neurosurgical Nursing.* Philadelphia, Lippincott, 1981.

4. Nikas DL: The nervous system, in Borg N, Nikas DL, Stark J, et al (eds): *Core Curriculum for Critical Care Nursing,* ed 2. Philadelphia, WB Saunders, 1981.

5. Price SA, Wilson LM: *Pathophysiology: Clinical Concepts of Disease Processes.* New York, McGraw-Hill, 1978.

6. Chusid JG: *Correlative Neuroanatomy and Functional Neurology,* ed 15. Los Altos, Calif, Lange Medical Publications, 1973.

7. Howe JR: *Patient Care in Neurosurgery.* Boston, Little, Brown, 1977.

8. Nikas DL: *The Critically Ill Neurosurgical Patient.* New York, Churchill Livingstone, 1982.

9. Spence AP: *Basic Human Anatomy.* Menlo Park, Ca, Benjamin-Cummings Publishing, 1982, pp 337–440.

10. Gray H: *Gray's Anatomy of the Human Body,* ed 29, Goss CM (ed). Philadelphia, Lea & Febiger, 1973.

11. Conway, BL: *Carini and Owen's Neurological and Neurosurgical Nursing,* ed 7. St Louis, Mosby, 1978, pp 45–70.

12. Herbert W: Remembrance of things partly. *Science News* 1983;124:378–381.

13. O'Brien MT, Pallett PJ: *Total Care of the Stroke Patient.* Boston, Little, Brown, 1980, pp 19–66.

14. DeMyer W: *Techniques of the Neurological Examination,* ed 3. New York, McGraw-Hill, 1980, pp 225–226.

15. Mitchell PH: Neurological Disorders, in Kinney MR, Dear CB, Packa DR, et al (eds): *AACN's Clinical Reference for Critical Care Nursing.* New York, McGraw-Hill, 1981, p 15.

16. Jennett G, Teasdale G: *Management of Head Injuries.* Philadelphia, FA Davis, 1981, pp 145–146.

17. Shapiro BA, Harrison RA, Walton JR: *Clinical Application of Blood Gases,* ed 3. Chicago, Year Book, 1982.

18. Loughnan PM, Brown TC, Edis B, et al: Neurogenic pulmonary oedema in man: Aetiology and management with vasodilators based on haemodynamic studies. *Anaesth Intensive Care* 1980;8:65–71.

Chapter 3

Assessment of the Neurological Patient

A comprehensive neurological examination is usually performed by a physician, nurse practitioner, or physician's assistant. It is beyond the scope of this book to present the details of performing such an examination. In an emergency situation a more practical approach to nursing assessment of the neurological patient is indicated.

When presented with an emergency neurological patient, the nurse's responsibilities include the performance of a baseline neurological assessment followed by periodic ongoing neurological assessments.

BASELINE NEUROLOGICAL ASSESSMENT

The baseline neurological assessment includes obtaining a neurological history and assessing function of the following areas: cerebral, cranial nerves, motor, sensory, cerebellar, reflexes, and vital signs. Abnormalities noted may direct the examiner to expand the scope of the neurological examination or seek assistance if unfamiliar with the performance of a comprehensive neurological examination.

Health History

The patient's history may be the most important determinant in identifying the nature of the neurological disorder. The nurse should ask questions designed to uncover neurological problems using layman's terms in questioning the patient about symptoms. The patient is asked to describe symptoms. It may be advantageous to have a relative or friend present who can confirm a patient's responses to questions. When a patient is unable to provide historical information, a family member should be interviewed.

In addition to vital statistics such as age, occupation, education, and usual activities of daily living, the patient is asked to list or describe any chronic or past health problems, major surgeries, or major injuries, and to list all current prescription and nonprescription medications being taken. The nervous system can be affected by such chronic disorders as diabetes mellitus, anemia, cancer, hypertension, and bowel, bladder, and sexual dysfunctions.[1]

It is important to determine if there has been a recent infection that could be affecting the nervous system such as meningitis, encephalitis, abscessed teeth, sinusitis, middle ear infection, or severe acne.[2]

Rudy[3] suggests that specific questions relating to the neurological history should include the following areas:

Headaches

The patient is asked to describe the character, frequency, location, onset, duration, and accompanying symptoms associated with headaches. He or she is asked if light in the eyes causes increased headache (photophobia). Photophobia may occur with meningitis. Ask the patient what medications or techniques, if any, provide relief from headaches.

Pain in Back or Lower Extremities

The patient is asked to describe the character, frequency, location, onset, duration, precipitating causes of back or lower extremity pain, and if the pain radiates, to where.

Vertigo or Syncope

Inquiry is made about preceding symptoms such as feelings of weakness, dimming of vision, nausea and vomiting, or sweating. The patient is asked if he or she experiences any buzzing or ringing in the ears (tinnitus). It should be determined if syncope occurs with exertion, with specific head movement, or during defecation. Statements from a witness may be extremely helpful.[4]

Convulsive Seizures

The nurse obtains a description of any motor activity observed, where it started, if it spread, and how long it lasted. It should be determined if the convulsive seizure was preceded by an aura, and if so, the patient is asked to describe it. The nurse tries to determine if unconsciousness followed the seizure and for how long, how often seizures occur, and if any provoking mechanism can be identified. The patient should be assessed for any injuries that may have occurred as a result of the seizure.

Paralysis, Paresthesia, or Neuralgia

The patient is asked for a description, location, and onset of any paralysis, paresthesias, or neuralgias.

Visual Difficulties

The patient is asked to describe any areas of blindness, blurred vision, double vision, or loss of eye movements.

Muscle Weakness or Unusual Muscle Activity

The patient is questioned about any facial weakness such as drooping eyelid, cheek, or corner of the mouth, and is asked for a description of any reported weakness or unusual motor activity in any extremity.

Difficulty Swallowing or Drooling

The patient is asked if there has been any difficulty in swallowing (dysphagia) and if it is painful or painless. It should be determined if it is accompanied by regurgitation through the nose, by difficulty handling saliva, or drooling.

Difficulty with Head or Neck Movements

The patient is asked to describe any limitation in head or neck movement and if it is associated with pain.

Memory and Orientation

The nurse tries to obtain a description of any amnesic episodes, and to determine if long-term or short-term memory is affected.

Problems with Gait or Balance

The nurse asks the patient or a family member to describe any noticed abnormality in gait or balance and when it began.

Additional historical information is needed if neurological trauma is suspected.

Mechanism of Injury

Information should be obtained from the patient, witnesses, or prehospital medical personnel about the mechanism of injury. The extent of injury the brain might incur depends on the type of trauma as well as the amount of force applied to the head at the time of impact. If head injury occurred from a motor vehicle accident, knowledge of any broken car windshield, dashboard, or steering wheel provides clues to the potential for associated spinal cord or multisystem injuries. It is helpful to find out the speed of travel at the time of impact, if the patient was wearing a seat belt, and whether or not the patient was thrown from the vehicle. It should be determined when the accident occurred, what the patient was doing prior to the accident, and whether or not there was evidence of alcohol or drug ingestion. It is important to know if the patient was ever unconscious, and if so, if it was immediate with the injury or associated with a lucid interval.

Physical Examination

A neurological assessment begins with the first encounter between the nurse and the patient. The nurse makes note of the appearance of the patient in relation to general health, attire, grooming, manner, behavior, posture, gait, voice, and communication abilities.[1]

Before an accurate assessment can be performed, the patient must be aroused to maximal level of functioning. It is important to record what form of stimulation is needed to elicit arousal. Does the patient respond to voice, such as to name, and follow commands, or is it necessary to shout or provide tactile stimulation such as gentle shaking? If these fail to arouse the patient, then painful stimuli should be applied. Stimuli such as sternal rubs are inappropriate and leave bruises. Preferable stimuli include firm, painful pressure applied to the base of the fingernails by using your own fingernail or the blunt end of a pencil or other firm object, or supraorbital pressure.

Cerebral Function

Assessment of cerebral function includes determining the patient's level of consciousness, cognitive functions, and speech abilities.

Conversation with the patient while obtaining the history gives clues to the patient's thought content, memory (both recent and distant), attention and concentration, attitude, mood, and speech abilities. It may be determined from the family if there has been any change in the patient's mental status.

Level of Consciousness. A change in the level of consciousness is one of the first signs of neurological deterioration and increasing intracranial pressure. Plum and Posner have defined consciousness as the awareness of one's self and environment.[5] Consciousness depends on an intact reticular activating system in the brainstem, which accounts for a person's wakefulness and arousal. For a person to be fully alert and oriented there must also be intact cerebral hemispheres, which account for the content of the consciousness or the sum of the mental functions.[5]

Unfortunately, the assessment of level of consciousness can be quite subjective. See Chapter 14 for definitions of various states of altered consciousness. To avoid using what may be controversial terminology, it is best to describe the patient in terms of behaviors or responses to stimuli. The Glasgow Coma Scale is a more objective assessment tool that encompasses various indicators of cerebral function (see Chapter 1). Composed of three areas—assessment of eye opening, best verbal response, and best motor response—the Glasgow Coma Scale consists of a numerical rating scale for each area. Based on the total score, certain deductions can be made concerning the level of consciousness, the seriousness of the patient's condition, and the need for specialized care. A score of 15 reflects an alert and oriented individual, while a score of 8 denotes coma. Thus a score of 8 or less reflects serious neurological impairment requiring vigorous intervention.[6]

Orientation. The assessment of orientation tests cognitive function. Intracranial pathology affecting the frontal lobes, temporal lobes, or hippocampal gyri may induce memory loss and disorientation.

Three areas to be tested are orientation to time, place, and person. The patient is asked questions such as what month it is, what day of the week it is, the date and the year. If the patient is disoriented, determine if the patient knows whether it is day or night. The patient is asked to recall any recent past or upcoming holiday. Orientation to time is usually lost before orientation to place or person. Testing orientation to place is done by asking the patient's present location, city, state, and home address. Asking patients to state their own name and the names of close family members tests orientation to person.

Memory. Both recent and distant memory are tested. The patient is asked to state the circumstances surrounding admission to the hospital and to recall how he or she was brought to the hospital and by whom.

Distant memory is tested by asking questions concerning the patient's place of birth and date, schooling, marriage age, names and ages of any children, etc.[7(p65)] Recent memory may be more severely disturbed than distant memory. The patient may also have temporary difficulty formulating new memory and might repeatedly ask "Where am I?" or "What happened?" Attempts to reorient the patient are made by consistently responding to these questions with brief explanations.

Speech. While assessing the patient's ability to communicate, the nurse makes note of the clarity and flow of speech as well as thought content and perceptions.

Disorders of communication are complex and can involve pathology in various areas of the brain. For this reason only simple tests of the patient's abilities to understand spoken words and express oneself verbally are performed. If abnormalities are noted in either, then the abilities of the patient to understand written words and to express oneself in writing are tested.[7(p67)]

Testing understanding of spoken words can be accomplished by issuing simple commands such as "Close your eyes." Increase the difficulty of the commands if simple commands are followed appropriately.

If the patient fails to communicate verbally or follow verbal commands, understanding of written words is tested by writing simple commands and observing the patient's responses. The ability of the patient to express ideas verbally has already been tested during the assessment of orientation and memory.

To test expression in writing, the patient is asked to write his or her address on a piece of paper. The inability to express oneself in writing is called agraphia.

Cranial Nerves

Testing of all 12 cranial nerves (CNs) is undertaken unless the chief complaint indicates that immediate medical intervention is needed. See Table 3–1 for techniques in testing the cranial nerves.

Hemispheric lesions often affect CN II, CN V, and CN VII. Assessing pupillary responses to light and eye movements tests CN III, CN IV, and CN VI, while assessing the gag reflex tests CN IX and CN X.[3]

Dysfunctions of certain cranial nerves have serious clinical implications for nursing. Disorders of CN III may indicate an expanding intracranial lesion with brain herniation. Loss of the corneal reflex because of dysfunctions of CN V and CN VII calls for nursing measures to prevent corneal damage. Disorders of CN IX and CN X can lead to airway and aspiration problems calling for critical nursing interventions.

Assessing Pupils. Pupils are assessed for their size, shape, equality, and light reflexes. Normally the pupils are round and equal in size, measuring approximately 2–6 mm, although 17 percent of the population has pupillary inequality of up to 2 mm difference.[7(p73)] If pupillary abnormalities are noted, it should be determined, if possible, whether or not the patient normally has pupillary inequality, has ever sustained an eye injury or had eye surgery, is blind in one eye, or wears a prosthesis.

The shape or regularity of the pupils are inspected. Any torn edges, obvious marks, scars, or abrasions across the cornea are noted. An ovoid shaped pupil can be an early warning sign of a pupil that will go on to become dilated and fixed due to midbrain compression.

Evaluating pupillary reactions to light is a vital component of both baseline and ongoing neurological assessments.

Normal pupillary reaction to light implies an intact optic nerve (CN II-sensory) and oculomotor nerve (CN III; see Figure 3–1). Pupillary constriction to light should be described as normal (brisk), sluggish, or fixed (nonreactive). Injury or compression of the oculomotor nerve anywhere along its course results in a fixed, dilated pupil. When due to brain herniation, pupillary dilation is usually seen on the same side as the expanding lesion. An alert patient with a fixed dilated pupil probably has a peripheral third cranial nerve injury and not compression of the brainstem. Common abnormalities of pupils are depicted in Figure 3–1.

Table 3–1 Assessment of Cranial Nerve Function

Cranial Nerve	Function	Test
I Olfactory	S: Smell	Have patient identify familiar odors, such as coffee, cloves, mint
II Optic	S: Visual fields	These fields of vision can be grossly evaluated by having the patient cover one eye, look straight ahead, and identify when he sees a penlight or wiggling finger. The examiner tests each visual field and then has the patient cover the other eye and repeats the test.
	Visual acuity	Use Snellen eye chart or ask the patient to read normal printed material
II Oculomotor	M: Pupil constriction	With penlight check for pupil constriction in each eye and consensual constriction in opposite eye
	Accommodation	Check pupil constriction as finger is moved from 3 feet to a few inches from the eyes. Pupils dilate for distance, constrict for close vision
	Movement of eye muscle (superior rectus, inferior oblique, inferior rectus, medial rectus); eye moves nasally, up and nasally, up and lateral, and down and in with extorsion	Extraocular eye movements (EOM). Three cranial nerves (III, IV, and VI) innervate the muscles of the eye and have control over coordinated eye movements. Weakness or paralysis of eye muscles is evaluated by having the patient follow the examiner's finger to the six cardinal directions of gaze while holding the head still. Each of these eye movements is controlled by a particular cranial nerve. To test, have patient move eye nasally, up and out, up and in, and down and out.
	Eyelid opening	Check for ptosis by evaluating position of eyelid in relation to rim of pupil
IV Trochlear	M: Movement of eye muscle (superior oblique); eye moves down and out with intorsion	EOM. Strongest primary action is adduction, so test by having patient move eye in and down
V Trigeminal	M: Jaw muscles and muscles of mastication	Have patient open and close jaw tightly; feel for muscle contraction
	Ophthalmic: forehead, cornea Maxillary: cheek Mandibular: jaw, mucous membrane of mouth	Have patient identify sharp and dull sensations by pinprick on each area with eyes closed. If pain sensation is lost, test temperature sensation. Test corneal reflex with cotton wisp if defect is suspected

Table 3–1 continued

Cranial Nerve	Function	Test
VI Abducens	M: Movement of eye muscle (lateral rectus); lateral movement of eyes	EOM. Test by having patient move eye laterally
VII Facial	M: Movement of muscles of face and scalp, eyelid closing	Have patient frown, smile, puff cheeks, close eyes tightly and resist opening
	S: Taste anterior two-thirds of tongue	Often deferred unless neurological problem. Have patient identify familiar taste—sugar, coffee, salt—on anterior part of tongue
VIII Acoustic	S: Cochlear: hearing	Can be grossly evaluated by having patient repeat a whispered word or identify watch ticking. Some also use the Weber and Rinne tests to evaluate hearing. Weber test: Strike the tuning fork (preferably one with 1024 cycles per second frequency), hold it by the stem, and place on patient's forehead or top of skull at midline. Ask where the patient hears the sound. Sounds should be heard equally well in each ear; a distinct lateralization is abnormal. Rinne test: Strike the tuning fork and place the base of it on the mastoid process of the skull, behind the ear. Ask the patient to signal when sound is no longer heard, then quickly place the vibrating fork near the external ear canal and ask if the patient can hear it. In normal individuals the sound will be heard longer through air conduction than bone conduction (AC > BC)
	Vestibular: equilibrium	Romberg test. (See description of test under cerebellar function)
IX Glossopharyngeal	S: Taste posterior half of tongue	Usually deferred unless neurological problem. Patient is asked to close eyes and identify familiar tastes, such as salt or sugar, on back portion of tongue
	Pain, touch, and temperature in pharynx and throat	
	M: Muscles of pharynx	Test these two nerves together by testing gag reflex, swallowing, and phonation. Ask patient to say "ah." Watch for symmetry of soft palate, gross deviation of uvula
X Vagus	M: Muscles of pharynx and larynx	
	S: Sensation in larynx, trachea, lungs, esophagus	

Table 3–1 continued

Cranial Nerve	Function	Test
	Slows heart, contracts bronchial muscles, and produces other involuntary activity	
XI Spinal accessory	M: Muscles of neck (Sternocleidomastoid) and upper shoulders (trapezius)	Have patient turn head to each side against resistance of examiner's hand. Ask patient to shrug shoulders upward against resistance of examiner's hand
XII Hypoglossal	M: Tongue movement	Have patient protrude tongue; note tremors or deviation. Have patient push tongue against cheeks

Source: Reprinted from *Advanced Neurological and Neurosurgical Nursing* (pp 72–74) by Ellen B Rudy with permission of CV Mosby Company, © 1984.

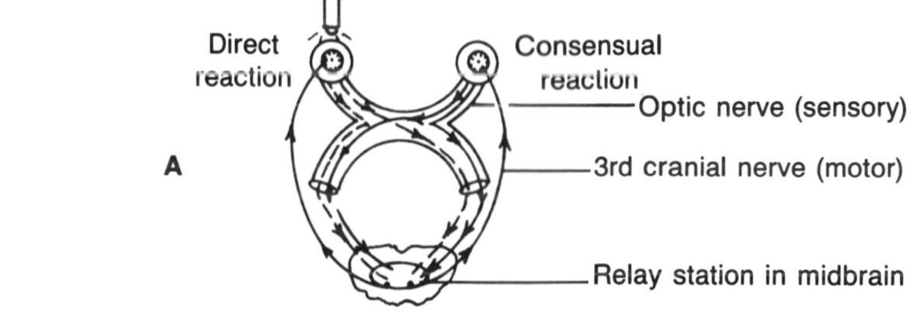

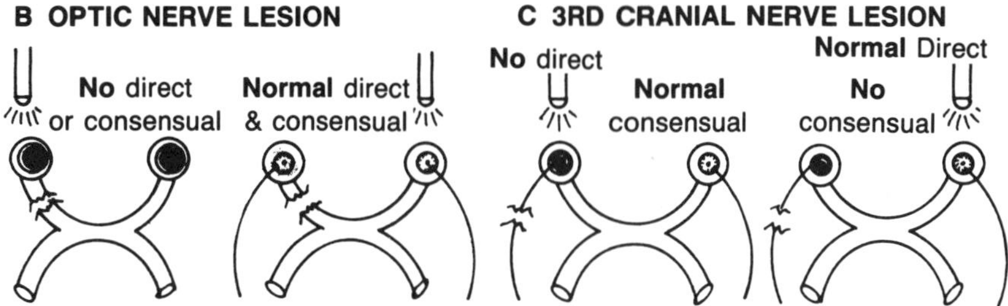

Fig. 3–1—Pupillary light reflex. (A) Normal reflex pathways and reaction of pupils to light shone into the left eye. (B) Responses to light shown into the left and right eyes in the presence of left optic nerve lesion. (C) Responses to light shown into the left and right eyes in presence of left oculomotor nerve lesion.

Source: Adapted from *Management of Head Injuries* (p 68) by Bryan Jennett and Graham Teasdale with permission of the FA Davis Company, © 1981.

It is best to examine the pupils in subdued light when possible. The examiner begins first by observing for ptosis of an eyelid (CN III also controls the ability to open the eyelid). Both eyelids are lifted simultaneously and observed for size, shape, and equality of the pupils. Pupil size is recorded in millimeters. Using a penlight, the beam of light is brought in from the side; the pupil being tested should constrict immediately. This is called the direct light reflex. Similar constriction should occur in the pupil of the opposite eye; this is known as the consensual light reflex. To assure that the consensual light reflex is not an accidental direct light reflex, the light is blocked from entering the opposite pupil by placing an opened hand over the bridge of the patient's nose. This process is repeated in the opposite eye. If one pupil is unreactive to direct light, yet reacts consensually, one should suspect an optic nerve lesion in that eye (Figure 3–2).

It is important to distinguish between an optic nerve or oculomotor nerve lesion as the cause of an unreactive pupil. An optic nerve lesion is not a sign of impending

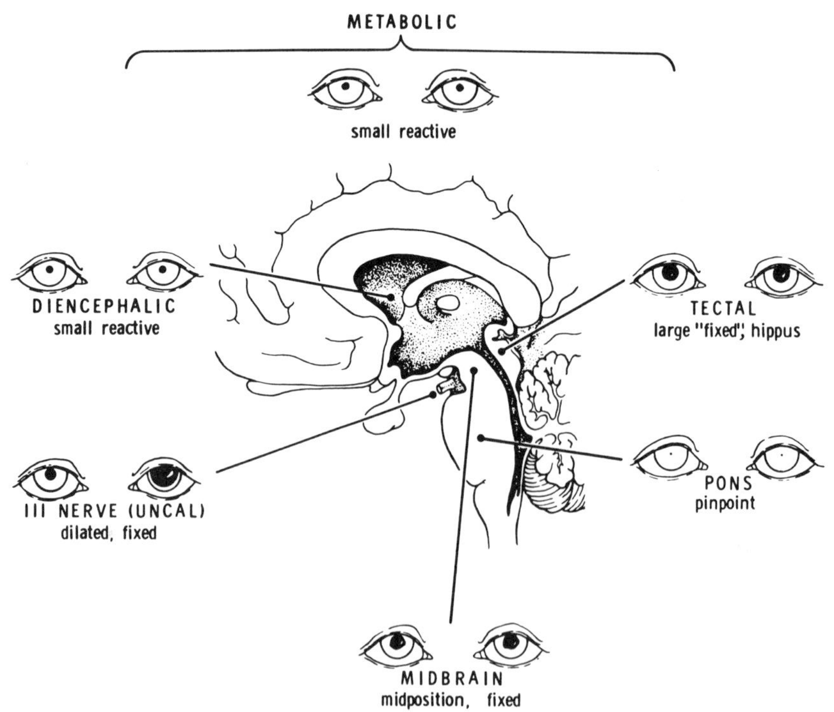

Fig. 3–2—Pupils in comatose patients.
Source: Reprinted from *Diagnosis of Stupor and Coma*, ed 3 (p 46) by Fred Plum and Jerome Posner with permission of the FA Davis Company, © 1980.

brain herniation and is not a neurosurgical emergency while an oculomotor nerve lesion may be. Pupillary signs must be interpreted with other neurological findings to determine their clinical significance. A sudden ''blown'' dilated and fixed pupil that was previously found to be normal constitutes a neurosurgical emergency. It is important to rule out the possibility that the patient received any cycloplegics, e.g., homatropine.

Assessing Eye Movements. While observing pupillary signs, the examiner notes any abnormal eye movements such as nystagmus (rhythmic jerking movements of the eyes). Nystagmus can be caused by various CNS pathologies including lesions of the brainstem or cerebellum, but it is most often caused by drugs such as barbiturates or tranquilizers.

Awake and cooperative patients are instructed to follow the examiner's finger or penlight with their eyes. The eyes should move conjugately (together), up, down, and laterally to both sides. Any defect in the range of movement of one or both eyes is recorded. Inability of an eye to move medially or laterally indicates dysfunction of the eye muscles controlled by CN III and CN VI, respectively. In a patient who previously exhibited normal eye movements, the appearance of limited mobility of one or both eyes may indicate neurological deterioration.

Eyes are often seen deviated toward the side of a destructive hemispheral brain lesion, and away from the side of an irritable focus such as a seizure focus. Pontine brainstem lesions may produce eye deviation toward a paralyzed arm and leg.[5(p60)]

In comatose patients, eye movements are often absent and the eyes assume a prolonged forward stare. Sometimes the eyes will move slowly from side to side. Eye movements can be assessed in the unconscious patient by means of the oculocephalic reflex (doll's eyes phenomenon). This maneuver should not be attempted until all possibility of cervical spine injury has been ruled out. To assess the oculocephalic reflex, the patient's eyelids are held open and the head is briskly rotated from side to side. When the head is rotated, the eyes should move in the direction opposite to the head movement. If the head is rotated to the right, the eyes appear to move to the left. This is the normal response and doll's eyes are said to be present. When the oculocephalic reflex is absent, the eyes do not move but follow the direction of passive head rotation (see Chapter 4, Figure 4–3). Loss of the oculocephalic reflex indicates a brainstem lesion at the midbrain-pontine level.[7(p116)] It can also indicate a poor prognosis.

Vertical eye movements are also tested by briskly flexing and extending the patient's neck. A normal response is upward deviation of the eyes on neck flexion, and downward deviation of the eyes on neck extension.

Like the oculocephalic reflex, the oculovestibular reflex (ice water calorics) also tests the integrity of those brainstem areas conducting impulses from the vestibular nuclei to the abducens nuclei in the pons and the oculomotor nuclei in the midbrain.

To perform the oculovestibular reflex, the patient is positioned with the head elevated 30 degrees to bring the semicircular canals to a vertical plane. The ear is examined with an otoscope to ensure an intact tympanic membrane. The external ear canal is slowly irrigated with 30–50 cc of ice water. If the brainstem is intact, the stimulus is conducted from the vestibular branch of CN VIII to CN VI and CN III. In the awake patient, horizontal nystagmus occurs with the eyes moving slowly toward the irrigated ear and rapidly jerking (fast component) away from it. Simultaneous irrigation of both canals causes fast component nystagmus to occur downward. Warm-water irrigation causes fast component nystagmus to move toward the irrigated ear, whereas bilateral warm-water irrigation causes fast component nystagmus upward.[7(p104)] The eyes are observed for a minute or more before deciding there is no response. Protect the airway in case the patient vomits.

Diffuse cerebral lesions causing unconsciousness may abolish the jerking nystagmus, with tonic eye deviation toward the cold being noted.

In obtunded or lightly comatose patients there may be a slow drift of the eyes to the irrigated ear with a quick return to midline. Five minutes should elapse before undertaking testing in the opposite ear.[5(p56)]

The absence of oculovestibular reflexes in comatose patients does not always imply absent brainstem function. Preexisting vestibular disease and various agents such as ototoxic drugs (gentamycin, etc.), phenytoin, barbiturates, tricyclic antidepressants, and neuromuscular blockers (pancuronium, succinylcholine) are all capable of blocking the oculovestibular reflex in comatose patients.[5(p62)]

Motor Function

Assessment of motor function includes observing muscle size and testing muscle strength, symmetry, and appropriateness of movement. Techniques used to evaluate motor function will vary depending on the patient's level of consciousness. Although motor dysfunctions can occur independently of changes in level of consciousness, when changes occur in the patient's motor function and in the level of consciousness, increasing intracranial pressure should be suspected.

Motor deficits may be due to pressure or damage to the motor cortex of the frontal lobes, or anywhere along the descending motor tracts. Cerebral or brainstem compression of motor tracts will cause weakness or paralysis of muscles on the opposite (contralateral) side of the body. Only a few simple tests of motor strength are needed to establish a baseline for comparison to subsequent ongoing assessments.

The Conscious Patient. When the conscious patient is able to cooperate and follow commands, muscle strength can be graded on a numerical scale (see Table 3–2). This provides objectivity to the examination and allows for comparison of symmetry of strength between muscle groups on both sides of the body.

Table 3–2 Muscle Strength Scale

Scale	Muscle Function
5	Normal muscle strength against full resistance
4	Full range of motion against mild resistance
3	Full range of motion against gravity only; cannot tolerate any resistance
2	Some movement, but limited; not able to lift extremity against gravity
1	Visible or palpable muscle contraction, but no movement of extremity
0	Complete paralysis: important to rule out spinal cord injury

Keep in mind that normal strength varies from person to person and is influenced by age, sex, occupation, and physical conditioning.

The motor exam begins by testing to level 3 (full range of motion against gravity with no resistance applied). If successful, the major muscle groups are then tested against resistance applied by the examiner.

The upper extremities are tested by asking the patient to grasp and squeeze the examiner's index and middle fingers. The strength and equality of the patient's grips are noted. The grips should be strong, firm, and equal, although a right handed individual may exhibit a slightly stronger right-hand grip which is not considered abnormal. The patient is asked to extend both arms with the palms turned upward and hold that position with eyes closed. A weaker arm may be observed to drift downward and pronate. The patient is then asked to pull each arm up off the mattress against resistance, and then flex each forearm against resistance. The strength of all responses are graded using the numerical scale. For example if the patient is unable to make a complete fist with one hand, but movement of fingers is noted, a score of 2 is given. If no movement is noted in any muscle test, the examiner places one hand over the muscle group being tested to palpate for muscle contraction that may not be visible. Muscle contraction or twitching with no movement of the extremity is given a score of 1. A score of zero implies no movement or muscle contraction.

In testing the lower extremities, the patient is asked to lift each leg off the mattress against resistance. If this exercise is painful for the patient, an alternative maneuver can be performed to test the strength of the quadriceps muscles. The patient is asked to extend the lower leg against resistance while the examiner holds the patient's knee flexed up off the mattress (Figure 3–3). If no leg movement is noted, the quadriceps muscles of the leg being tested can be palpated to determine if a score of 1 can be given.

Ankle plantar flexion and dorsiflexion are tested. The examiner's hands are placed on the patient's feet and not the toes when testing against resistance.

If the patient is allowed out of bed, lower extremity weakness may be more easily noted by observing the patient's gait and ability to bear weight.

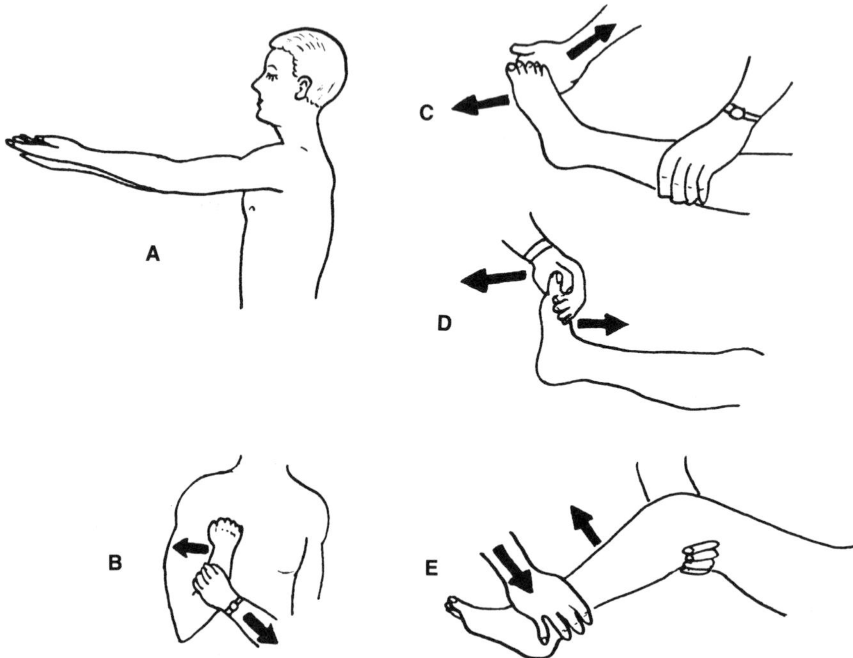

Fig. 3–3—Assessing muscle strength. (A) Testing for arm drift. (B) Flexion of forearm against resistance. (C) Plantar flexion against resistance. (D) Dorsiflexion against resistance. (E) Lower leg extension against resistance.

The facial muscles can be assessed by utilizing a 3-point grading scale. A score of 3 implies normal strength; a score of 2 indicates mild weakness; a score of 1 denotes severe weakness with muscle twitching only; and a score of zero implies complete paralysis. The patient is asked to close both eyes tightly and grimace, then open the eyes widely. The examiner observes for any facial asymmetry, flattening of the wrinkles on one side of the forehead, or an eyelid that does not close completely.

Remember from Chapter 2 that each facial nerve has three branches supplying the muscles of the face. Upper motor neurons of the corticobulbar tracts from both cerebral hemispheres innervate the nuclei for the upper branches of both facial nerves. Because of this dual crossed and uncrossed nerve supply, upper motor neuron lesions occurring in the cerebral cortex may not cause any weakness in the muscles of the upper face. The nuclei of the facial nerve branches that supply muscles to the lower face do not receive bilateral upper motor neuron supply; therefore, a lesion affecting the motor cortex will usually cause contralateral weakness or paralysis of only the lower half of the face. A lesion on a facial nerve (lower motor neuron) will cause ipsilateral weakness or paralysis of all of the facial muscles.

The muscles of the lower face are tested by asking the patient to smile and show the teeth. Again any weakness or asymmetry of the lower face is noted. Weakness of one side of the face may be manifested by flattening of the nasolabial fold (crease between the nose and the corner of the mouth) on the affected side, and the mouth may be pulled away from the weakened or paralyzed side.

The Unconscious Patient. If the patient is unable to follow verbal commands or is unconscious, other methods of testing motor and sensory responses are used. Motor responses should be assessed while a painful stimulus is applied.

The examiner begins by observing the patient's general posture; noting the presence or absence of spontaneous and symmetrical movements before applying stimuli. If the patient does not move to verbal or tactile stimuli, it will be necessary to apply painful stimuli. One should always use the least amount of stimulus required to elicit a response. The strength with which the patient attempts to remove or move away from the stimulus is noted. To rule out any sensory impairment, similar stimuli should be applied to each extremity; comparing the strength and symmetry of responses.

If movement does not occur in response to painful stimuli, the extremities are moved through their range of motion and felt for symmetry of muscle tone. Both arms are lifted and released simultaneously. If the descent of one arm is more rapid and flaccid, paralysis or paresis of that limb is likely. Both legs are flexed so that the soles of the feet rest on the mattress. The legs are released and observed how they respond. The normal leg may hold the position momentarily while the paralyzed or paretic leg may slump into a position of extension with outward rotation of the hip.[7(pp106–147)] Facial muscle symmetry can be tested by applying painful supraorbital pressure and then observing facial grimacing.

Abnormal Motor Responses. Common abnormal motor responses include flexor and extensor posturing. They may occur in response to painful stimuli or may occur spontaneously. Hemispheric lesions affecting the pyramidal (facilitory) and extrapyramidal (inhibitory) tracts may result in an imbalance between these two effects leading to an abnormal motor response known as flexor or decorticate posturing (see Figure 3–4). This is characterized by flexion of the arms, wrists, and fingers, with the hands folded inward and curled together across the chest. The legs and feet are often rigidly extended and plantar flexed.[3]

Extensor or decerebrate rigidity is seen with lesions at the level of the diencephalon or brainstem. It implies a more serious brain dysfunction.[8] Again there is loss of extrapyramidal inhibition, but this is combined with stimulation of extensor muscles. Decerebrate rigidity is characterized by rigid extension, adduction, and internal rotation of the extremities. It is often accompanied by other signs of brainstem dysfunction such as deep coma, rapid breathing, and pupillary dilation.

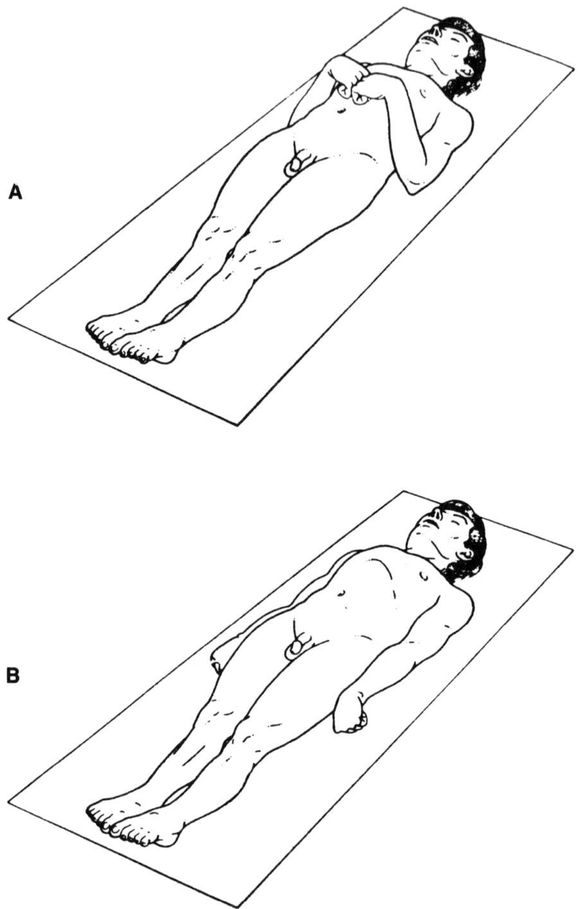

Fig. 3–4—Position assumed by patient with (A) decorticate rigidity, (B) decerebrate rigidity. *Source:* Reprinted from *Emergency Nursing: Principles and Practice* (p 276) by Susan Budassi and Janet Barber with permission of the CV Mosby Company, © 1981.

Decerebrate rigidity may be so severe that the patient assumes a backward bowed position called opisthotonos. Opisthotonos may also be seen in meningitis.[9(p392)]

Occasionally abnormal flexor responses are observed in the extremities of one side of the body while extensor rigidity is seen on the other side. This is caused by different degrees of pathology on each side of the brain. If this phenomenon is observed, a Glasgow Coma Scale best motor response of 3 is given. While the right and left sides of the body may be scored separately if they react differently, the best motor response should always be used in determining the total score.

Flaccidity of all extremities in response to painful stimuli implies very severe brain injury and often carries a poor prognosis.[8]

If meningeal irritation or inflammation is suspected, the patient can be tested for nuchal rigidity. With the patient lying supine and relaxed, the examiner's hand is placed under the patient's occiput and a gentle attempt to flex the neck is made. The neck should normally bend freely. If nuchal rigidity is present, the patient will complain of pain and the neck will not flex. Unfortunately, a deeply comatose patient will not show nuchal rigidity. Blood in the subarachnoid space or meningitis are the most common causes of nuchal rigidity.[9(p391)]

If, when testing for nuchal rigidity, the patient's legs adduct and flex (Brudzinski's sign), further evidence of meningeal irritation exists. The flexion of the legs relaxes the tension on the spinal cord and nerve roots. The patient with meningeal irritation will also resist straight leg raising or extension of the lower leg when the thigh is flexed on the abdomen (Kernig's sign).[9(p392)]

Sensory Function

Depending on the urgency of the neurological emergency, a brief sensory examination may or may not be performed. It should always be performed in patients suspected of having injury to the spinal cord. Testing the sensations of touch, pain, and position sense (proprioception) constitutes a basic sensory examination. These tests evaluate the integrity of the anterior spinothalamic and lateral spinothalamic tracts and the posterior columns, respectively. Sensory tests are performed with the patient's eyes closed, again comparing one side of the body to the other.

Touch. The distal and proximal portions of each extremity and the trunk are touched with a wisp of cotton. The patient is asked to identify when and where he or she is being touched, to report if all areas feel the same, and to indicate any areas where touch could not be felt.[10]

Pain. A clean safety pin is used to test the sensation of superficial pain. The distal (including the hands and feet) and proximal portions of each extremity and the trunk are touched with the sharp and, periodically, the dull part of the pin. The patient is asked to identify the place being touched and if the sharp or dull part of the pin is being used. If the patient is unable to identify superficial pain, deep pain is tested by squeezing the calf, biceps, and trapezius muscles.

When a spinal cord lesion is suspected and sensory losses are evident, using a dermatome chart (Figure 3–5) assists in identifying the level of the lesion. Starting distally and working up the body including the perineal and perianal areas; the patient is asked to identify when the pinprick can be felt. Using the dermatome chart, the examiner notes which spinal nerve root innervates the region in which sensation is first felt. Combined with the results of the motor exam, a more accurate estimate of the level of the spinal cord lesion can be made.

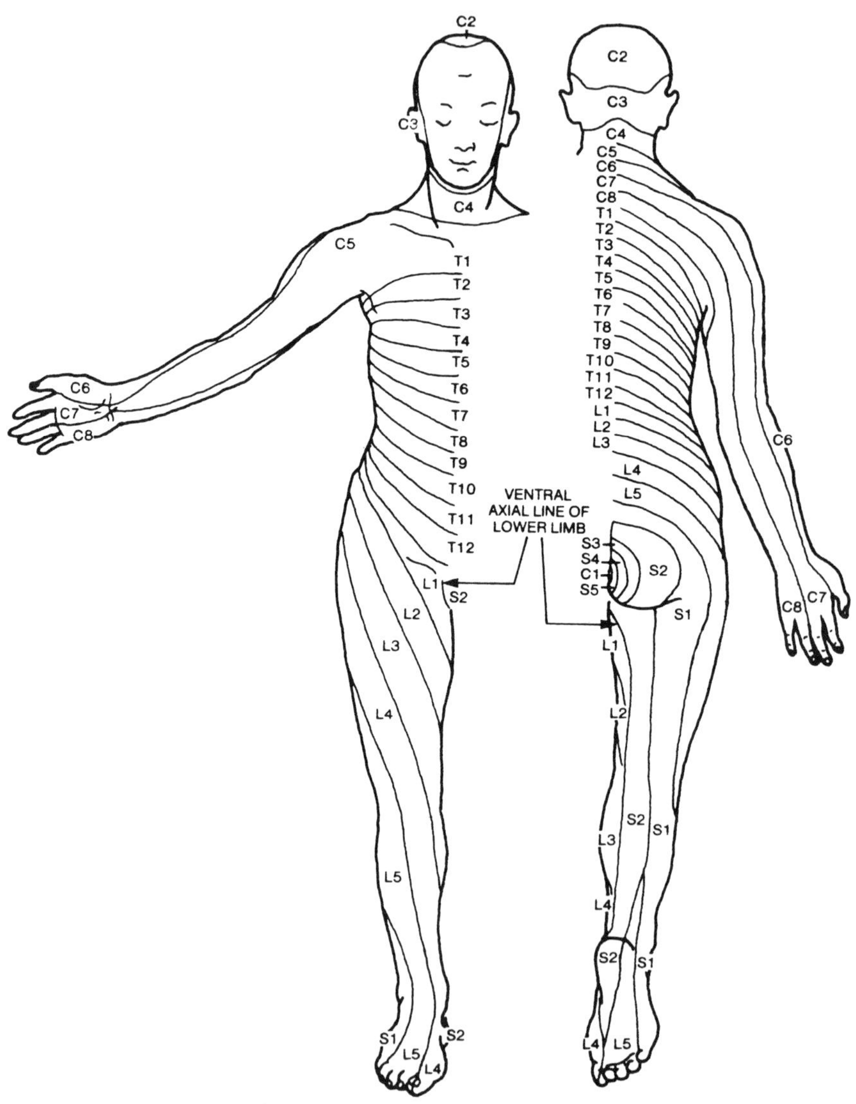

Fig. 3–5—Sensory dermatomes of upper and lower limbs.

Source: Reprinted from *Topics in Emergency Medicine* (1979; 1:1:69), Copyright © 1979, Aspen Systems Corporation.

The sensation in the face can be tested in the same manner, using touch and pinprick. The areas of distribution of all three branches of the trigeminal nerve: the brow, the maxillary, and the mandibular areas are tested.

Position Sense. Position sense or proprioception is tested by gently grasping (on the sides) the distal portion of a finger or a toe and moving it in different directions. The patient is asked to identify if the digit is being lifted up or down. This test is repeated in all four extremities. The patient's eyes should be closed.

Cerebellar Function

Tests of the patient's balance and coordination evaluate cerebellar function. Cerebellar testing begins by asking the patient to outstretch the arms, then touch the nose alternately with each index finger. The test should be performed first with the eyes open then closed. The patient is asked to again put the finger to the nose, and touch the examiner's finger while it is moved to various positions. The patient alternatively touches his or her nose, then the examiner's finger. Have the patient repeat this with the opposite hand.

If the patient can sit up, rapid alternating movements of the upper extremities are tested. The patient is asked to pat the knee while rapidly pronating and supinating the hand and forearm.

If the patient can stand, the Romberg test is performed. The patient is asked to stand with his or her feet together, first with the eyes open, then with them closed. The patient's ability to maintain an upright posture and balance is observed.

If the patient is confined to bed, coordination is tested by asking the patient to move one foot down the shin of the opposite leg. The action is repeated with the other leg. Any tremors or uncoordinated movements are noted.[7(pp84–85)]

Reflexes

Reflexes can be evaluated in both the conscious and the unconscious patient. Hyperactive reflexes in the extremities of one side of the body may indicate upper motor neuron pathology affecting the corticospinal tract arising from the opposite cerebral hemisphere. Decreased or absent reflexes may indicate lower motor neuron pathology, possibly due to spinal cord injury.

Deep Tendon Reflexes. Deep tendon reflexes (DTRs) are also known as muscle stretch reflexes. The biceps, triceps, brachioradialis, quadriceps (knee jerk) and Achilles (ankle jerk) are the most common DTRs tested (see Figure 3–6). The patient's muscles should be relaxed with the joints in midposition.[7(p851)] Using a reflex hammer, the appropriate tendon is tapped directly and the muscle is observed for contraction. The muscle responses are graded as follows: grade 0 = absent reflexes; grade 1 (+) = diminished reflexes; grade 2 (+ +) = normal reflexes; grade 3 (+ + +) = brisker than normal reflexes; and grade 4 (+ + + +) = hyperactive reflexes.[3]

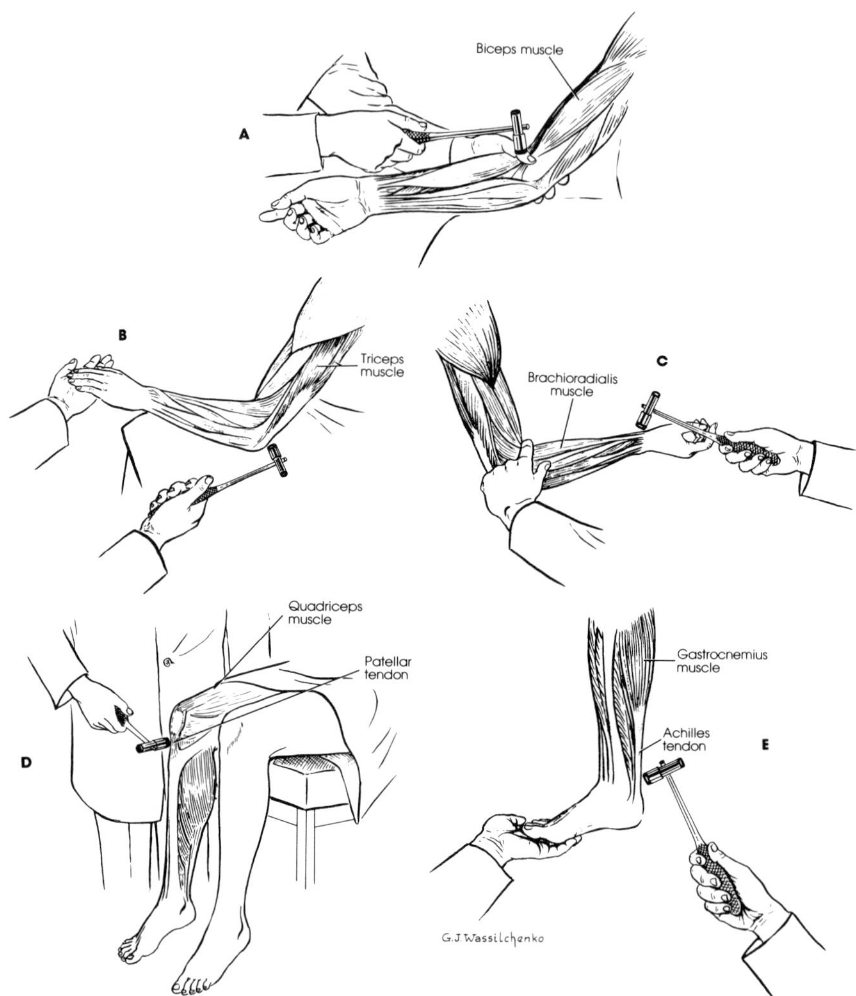

Fig. 3–6—Deep tendon reflexes: (A) biceps, (B) triceps, (C) brachioradialis, (D) patellar, and (E) Achilles.

Source: Reprinted from *Advanced Neurological and Neurosurgical Nursing* (p 77) by Ellen Rudy with permission of the CV Mosby Company, © 1984.

Clonus represents a hyperactive reflex. It can be tested by sharply dorsiflexing the patient's ankle and observing for spasmodic contraction and relaxation of the ankle.

Superficial Reflexes. Superficial reflexes are tested by stroking the skin with a moderately sharp object. When either side of the upper abdomen is stroked, the umbilicus should move toward the quadrant tested. This tests nerve roots T-7 through T-9. The same response should be seen when the lower abdominal quadrants are stroked. This tests nerve roots T-10 and T-11.

In the male patient the cremasteric reflex tests nerve roots T-12 through L-2. It consists of stroking the inner thigh and observing elevation of the ipsilateral testicle.

Stroking the lateral aspect of the sole of the foot normally causes plantar flexion of the great toe. An abnormal response, extension (dorsiflexion) of the great toe with the fanning of the toes (Babinski's sign), indicates contralateral upper motor neuron (pyramidal tract) pathology (Figure 3–7).[10]

Abnormal dorsiflexion of the great toe may also be tested for by stroking the lateral aspect of the foot below the lateral malleolus. This is called the Chaddock's reflex. Oppenheim's reflex also demonstrates dorsiflexion of the great toe in response to stroking the anteromedial tibial surface. These reflexes also indicate pyramidal tract disease.[7(p86)]

Vital Signs

Although the assessment of vital signs is important in the neurological patient, changes in vital signs can be unreliable and even late indicators of deteriorating neurological status. A change in vital signs without a change in level of consciousness suggests the presence of other medical problems.[3]

Increased intracranial pressure can cause specific systemic responses. The classic triad of rising systolic blood pressure, bradycardia, and respiratory changes (the Cushing response), may be seen with ischemia and hypoxia of the brain stem.

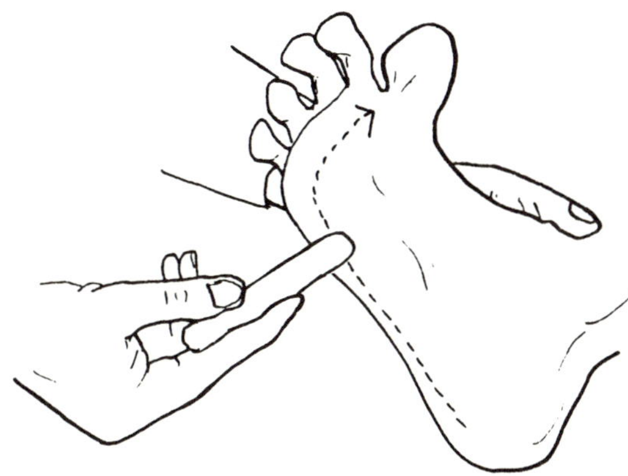

Fig. 3–7—Babinski reflex. Extension (dorsiflexion) of the great toe in response to plantar stimulus.

Direct compression or injury to the brainstem without elevated intracranial pressure can also produce the Cushing response. These changes reflect compensatory brainstem actions. As the patient's condition deteriorates and decompensation occurs, the blood pressure falls, the pulse rises, and the respirations become irregular.

Alterations in Blood Pressure. Ischemia of the brainstem causes a generalized sympathetic response leading to peripheral vasoconstriction and an elevation of the blood pressure. This reflects an attempt by the brain to maintain blood flow to ischemic areas that are in need of both glucose and oxygen. The systolic pressure rises more than the diastolic pressure, leading to a widening of the pulse pressure. Hypotension usually indicates other system injury with blood loss but could represent a terminal neurological event.

The examiner should indicate which arm was used to measure blood pressure and compare current readings with previous readings to identify changes or trends.

Alterations in Pulse. The pulse rate may slow to less than 60 per minute but is usually full and bounding. Blood is being pumped to an edematous brain against great pressure. Baroreceptors in the aorta and carotid bodies sense the increased blood pressure and stimulate the vagus nerve to slow the pulse rate.

A tachycardia may also indicate poor cerebral oxygenation, decompensation of the brain, or the presence of other injuries associated with blood loss.

Cardiac dysrhythmias are common in patients with brain pathology, especially if intracranial hypertension exists. Disturbances of both rate and conduction are seen with atrial and ventricular ectopy, atrial fibrillation, sinus tachycardia, sinus bradycardia, atrioventricular block, and bundle branch block all being reported. Patients with subarachnoid hemorrhage are particularly prone to develop cardiac dysrhythmias, some of which are lethal. S-T and T wave abnormalities have also been reported in patients with brain pathology. Autonomic dysfunction in patients with intracranial lesions can lead to myocardial damage.[11(pp64–67)]

Documentation of the patient's ECG should be a part of the assessment of vital signs. The nurse should also be prepared to treat serious cardiac dysrhythmias when they occur.

Alterations in Respirations. Although mentioned in the last section of the neurological examination, assessment of respiratory status remains the first priority in any patient assessment. Respiratory patterns are best assessed quietly with the patient at rest, before applying any stimuli. There are a number of abnormal respiratory patterns seen in patients with intracranial lesions, and they reflect dysfunction at various levels of the brain (see Figure 3–8). The nurse must be careful in interpreting abnormal respiratory patterns because other factors such as acid-base disturbances can also influence respiratory patterns. The analysis of arterial blood gases helps rule out other causes of respiratory abnormalities while providing information on the adequacy of oxygenation and carbon dioxide

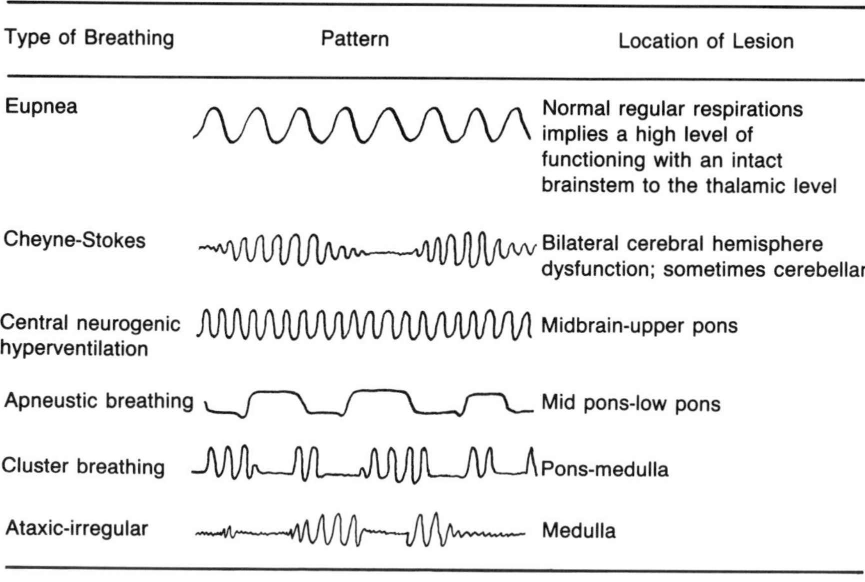

Fig. 3–8—Abnormal respiratory patterns in neurological disorders.[1(p125), 3, 7(p122)]

removal. The detrimental effects on the brain of hypoxemia and carbon dioxide retention are discussed in Chapter 4.

Excessive sympathetic discharge associated with intracranial hypertension can lead to shunting of blood to the pulmonary vascular bed overloading its capacity and resulting in neurogenic pulmonary edema. Pulmonary capillary damage can lead to respiratory distress syndrome. Severe impairment of oxygenation can result from these disorders.[11(pp82–85)]

When assessing respirations, the rate, rhythm, and depth of respirations are recorded as well as the quality of breath sounds.

Alterations in Temperature. It is important that the patient's temperature be monitored in the emergency department. Extremes of hyperthermia or hypothermia can indicate destructive lesions of the brainstem or hypothalamus. Hyperthermia can greatly increase the metabolic demands of a compromised and ischemic brain and should be treated aggressively with antipyretics, tepid sponge baths, and hypothermia blankets if necessary. Infectious processes must of course be ruled out as causes of febrile reactions.

The temperature should be closely monitored because subnormal temperatures can result from hypothermia therapy, especially in patients with hypothalamic damage.[3] Hypothermia may also be seen in spinal shock and metabolic or toxic coma.[7]

Table 3–3 Twenty-four Hour Neurological Flow Sheet

DATE:

Time			0700	0800	0900	1000	1100	1200	1300	140
Level of Consciousness 0 - 3										
PUPIL SIZE N-Normal REACTION S-Sluggish F-Fixed C-Closed	Size/Reaction									
	Size/Reaction									
Eyes Open to 1 - 4 C = 2° Swelling										
Best Verbal Response 1 - 5 T = Trache Tube										
Best Motor Response 1 - 6										
Total GCS Score										
Intracranial Pressure (ICP)/CPP										
Respiratory Pattern R Regular H Hypervent I Irreg. V Vent										
Movement N = None C = Command P = Posturing S = Spontaneous W = Withdrawal	RA	LA								
	RL	LL								
EQUALITY OF STRENGTH = Equal <Less than >Greater than	RA VS LA		RA LA	RA LA	RA LA	RA LA	RA LA	RA LA	RA LA	RA
	RL VS LL		RL LL	RL LL	RL LL	RL LL	RL LL	RL LL	RL LL	RL
Other										
FACE 0-3	Close Eyes Tightly Grimace	R L								
	Smile	R L								
ARMS 0-5	Hand Grips	R L								
	Arm Lift	R L								
	Elbow Flexion	R L								
LEGS 0-5	Ankle Dorsiflexion	R L								
	Ankle Plantarflexion	R L								
	Lower Leg Extension	R L								

Glasgow Coma Scale

Eyes Open To

SPONT. eyes open, does not imply awareness	= 4
SPEECH - responds to any speech or shout, not nec. to command	= 3
PAIN - should apply stimulus to limbs, not face	= 2
NEVER - self explanatory	= 1

Best Verbal

ORIENTED - aware of self & environment; should be oriented x 3	= 5
CONFUSED - attention can be held; responds to questions in conversational manner, but with varying degrees of dis-orientation & confusion	= 4
INAPPROPRIATE WORDS - intelligible articulation, but no sustained conversation possible; usually shouting or swearing	= 3
INCOMPREHENSIBLE SOUNDS - moaning and groaning without recognizable words	= 2
NONE - self explanatory	= 1

Best Motor

OBEYS COMMANDS - self explanatory; do not interpret grasp reflex as response to command	= 6
LOCALIZES PAIN - pain stimulus causes limb to move as to attempt to remove it	= 5
FLEXOR WITHDRAW - withdraws from pain. Flexes arms and legs	= 4
ABNORMAL FLEXION - decorticate; flexion of arms, extension of legs & feet (unless S.C.I. also present)	= 3
EXTENSION - decerebrate; extension of arms, legs, feet with internal rotation of hands and feet	= 2
NONE — flaccid, important to R/O S.C.I.	= 1

Level of Consciousness

ALERT: Responds immediately to command; maintains wakefullness.	= 3
LETHARGIC: Sleepy; response to command may be slow or incomplete; needs stimuli but does obey; returns to sleep when not stimulated.	= 2
STUPOROUS: Does not obey commands; needs vigorous stimulation; spontaneous or purposeful movement may be present.	= 1
COMATOSE. Does not respond to command or in meaningful way to stimuli; may decorticate or decrebrate	= 0

Motor Strength

Face

Normal Strength	= 3
Mild Weakness	= 2
Severe Weakness (Muscle Twitch Only)	= 1
Complete Paralysis	= 0

Arms - Legs

Normal strength against full resistance	= 5
Full range of motion against mild resistance	= 4
Full range of motion against gravity only may drift after several seconds	= 3
Some movement, but limited, may not be able to lift against gravity	= 2
Visible or palpable muscle contraction: No movement	= 1
No muscle contraction, complete paralysis	= 0

PUPIL SIZE: 2 3 4 5 6 7 8

Source: Reprinted with permission of Beverly Means, Lynn Taplett, and Jeanne Raimond. Courtesy of Grossmont District Hospital, La Mesa, Ca.

ONGOING NEUROLOGICAL ASSESSMENT

Ongoing neurological assessments provide information that may indicate improvement or deterioration in neurological status when compared to the baseline and subsequent assessments. Ongoing assessments include evaluations of level of consciousness, orientation, pupillary signs, motor function, and vital signs. Sensory examinations should be included on patients with known or suspected spinal cord lesions.

Ongoing assessments should take no more than two minutes to perform, yet should be sufficiently detailed to allow for accurate assessment of the patient's current neurological status. Use of a neurological flow sheet standardizes the way in which neurological assessments are performed, facilitates the recording of these assessments, and allows for early detection of trends in patient improvement or deterioration (Table 3–3).

Performing a neurological assessment may at first seem difficult, but the ability to perform these examinations improves quickly with practice. Using the assessment data obtained, the nurse can then plan and implement specific nursing interventions.

REFERENCES

1. Conway BL: *Carini and Owens' Neurological and Neurosurgical Nursing,* ed 7. St Louis, Mosby, 1978.

2. Walleck CA: A neurologic assessment procedure that won't make you nervous. *Nursing 82* December 1982;50–56.

3. Rudy EB: *Advanced Neurological and Neurosurgical Nursing.* St Louis, Mosby, 1984, chap 2.

4. DeGown EL, DeGown RL: *Bedside Diagnostic Examination,* ed 3, New York, Macmillan, 1976.

5. Plum F, Posner JB: *The Diagnosis of Stupor and Coma,* ed 3. Philadelphia, FA Davis Co, 1980, pp 101–113.

6. Jones C: Glasgow coma scale. *Am J Nurs* September 1979;1551–1553.

7. Hickey JV: *The Clinical Practice of Neurological and Neurosurgical Nursing.* Philadelphia, Lippincott, 1981.

8. Nikas DL: Neurological assessment of altered states of consciousness: Part III. *Focus Crit Care* 1984;11:54–58.

9. DeMeyer W: *Techniques of the Neurological Examination,* ed 3. New York, McGraw-Hill, 1980.

10. Nikas DL: The nervous system, in Borg N, Nikas DL, Stark J, et al: *Core Curriculum for Critical Care Nursing,* ed 2. Philadelphia, WB Saunders, 1981, pp 201–203.

11. Nikas DL (ed): *The Critically Ill Neurosurgical Patient.* New York, Churchill Livingstone, 1982.

Part II

Special Problems Related to Neurological Disease

Chapter 4

Intracranial Hypertension

DYNAMICS OF INTRACRANIAL PRESSURE

Intracranial pressure (ICP) refers to the pressure within the cranium. It is determined by the amount of brain substance, intracranial blood volume, and cerebrospinal fluid (CSF) present within the cranium at any one time and by the relationship of these components to the capacity of the cranium. The amounts of the three components vary from time to time but generally remain as follows: brain tissue 88 percent; intravascular blood 2–11 percent; CSF 9–10 percent.[1(p38)]

Recall from Chapter 2 that the brain and spinal cord are surrounded by meninges and are contained within bony structures (the skull and vertebral column). Both the skull and the meninges form rigid barriers that prevent expansion of the intracranial contents.

Compensating Mechanisms

If any one of the three intracranial components increases in volume, there must be a reciprocal decrease in the volume of another component or else the ICP will rise. This concept is part of the modified Monro-Kellie hypothesis.[2] This hypothesis does not apply to infants since their skulls are not rigid and are capable of expansion.[3]

Normal ICP is 0–15 mm Hg (80–180 mm H_2O). Intracranial hypertension is said to exist when the ICP exceeds 15 mm Hg or 200 mm H_2O. In an effort to maintain ICP equilibrium and prevent intracranial hypertension, the three intracranial components adjust to changes in volume in one of three ways: by displacement of cerebrospinal fluid, reduction of cerebral blood volume, or by displacement of brain tissue.

Displacement of Cerebrospinal Fluid

Of the three mechanisms, displacement of CSF occurs the most rapidly. This compensatory mechanism allows the shunting of some of the CSF from the cerebral subarachnoid spaces into the more distensible spinal subarachnoid space.[4] There is also an increase in the absorption of CSF into the venous sinuses.[5]

Reduction of Cerebral Blood Volume

Intracranial blood volume can decrease via enhanced drainage into the venous sinuses, which then empty into the extracranial vascular system.

Intracranial blood volume can also be reduced through the constriction of cerebral blood vessels. Some pathological conditions, especially CSF acidosis and midbrain lesions, induce central neurogenic hyperventilation, a breathing pattern characterized by sustained, rapid, deep respirations. This breathing pattern leads to a respiratory alkalosis, which induces cerebral vasoconstriction.

Displacement of Brain Tissue

In the presence of a slow increase in ICP, brain tissue becomes compressed, ischemic, and eventually atrophies.[3] If the pressure continues to rise, or in the presence of acute increasing ICP, the brain ultimately moves through the openings in the ''rigid box,'' the tentorium incisura or the foramen magnum (Figure 4–1). This is termed brain herniation; it is usually fatal for the patient.

Decompensation

A state of decompensation occurs when CSF and blood displacement can no longer maintain ICP equilibrium. Intracranial pressure rises when the increase in volume within the cranium exceeds the compensatory decrease in volume. This concept is best explained by the intracranial volume-pressure curve (Figure 4–2). Because of the capacity for compensation for increasing intracranial volume, the volume-pressure relationship is not a linear one. Slower-growing mass lesions such as certain tumors may produce little change in ICP because of compression and atrophy of adjacent brain. In Figure 4–2, point A represents compensation for increasing intracranial volume. The ICP remains normal. Point B represents a point at which the capacity for compensation has been strained and volume increases begin to cause elevation of the ICP. Point C represents the critical point at which the compensation capacities are exhausted and small increases in volume cause drastic increases in ICP.

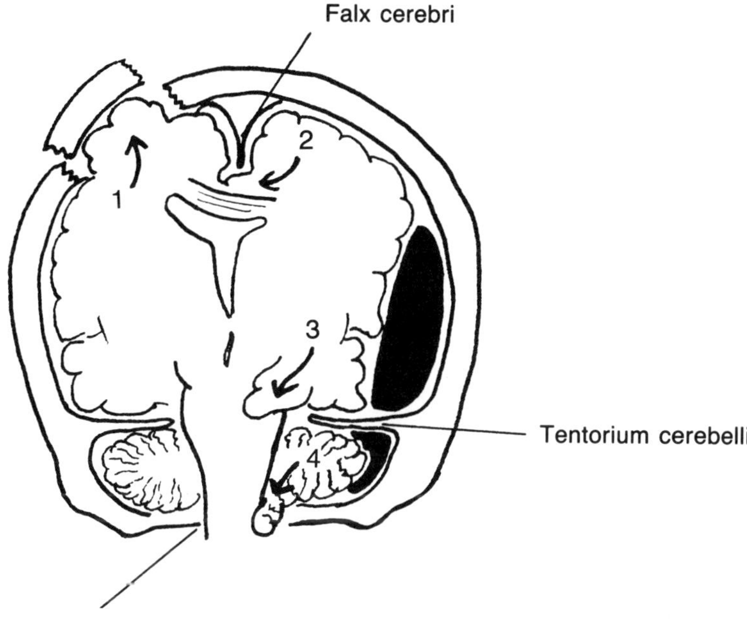

Fig. 4–1—Brain herniation syndromes. (1) Herniation of brain tissue out through a bony defect in the skull, (2) herniation of the cingulate gyrus under the falx, (3) herniation of the uncus through the tentorial notch, and (4) herniation of a cerebellar tonsil through the foramen magnum.

Increased Volume of Cerebrospinal Fluid

Displacement of CSF can be impeded by the blockage of normal CSF circulation within the subarachnoid pathways. Increasing pressure or mass lesions can cause obstructions in the foramina, aqueducts, or at the basal cisterns.

Impedance of CSF reabsorption into the venous system can occur because of compression of the arachnoid villi or by their obstruction with debris within the CSF.

Obstruction of venous drainage from the head can cause a retrograde impedance of the reabsorption of CSF into the venous sinuses. Enhanced CSF production can occur in the presence of choroid plexus papillomas, leading to intracranial hypertension. This is a rare occurrence.

Increased Intracranial Blood Volume

Several factors can influence the volume of blood within the brain such as disorders of cerebral autoregulation, carbon dioxide, and oxygen levels, and

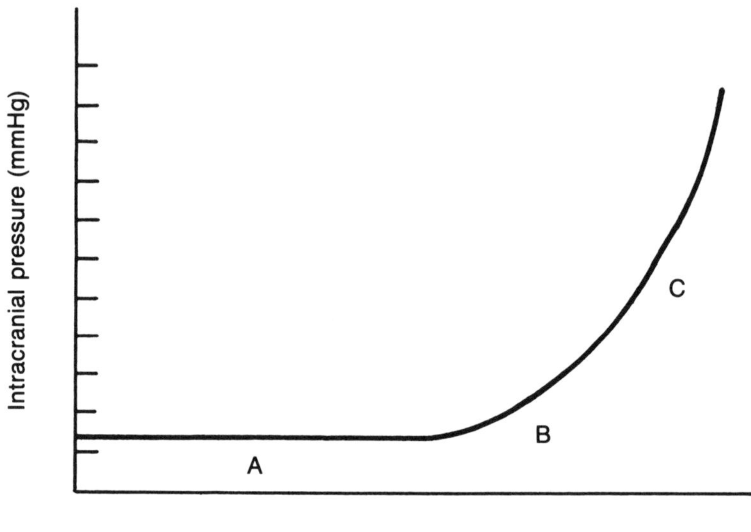

Fig. 4–2—Volume-pressure relationship. At point A, compensation is occurring for increasing intracranial volume. Point B represents the point at which the capacity for compensation is strained and ICP begins to rise. Point C represents decompensation, when even small increases in volume can cause drastic increases in ICP.

---

obstruction of venous drainage. Complicated hemodynamic and blood chemistry factors are involved in the maintenance of normal cerebral blood flow.

Disorders of Cerebral Autoregulation. Cerebral autoregulation is the process by which cerebral blood flow remains relatively constant in the presence of fluctuations in mean systemic arterial blood pressure. In normal persons, fluctuations of mean systemic arterial pressure (MSAP) between 50–150 mm Hg do not alter cerebral blood flow.[5(p35)]

In the presence of systemic hypertension, cerebral arterioles normally constrict in an effort to spare the brain from excessive perfusion and pressure. Low MSAP may cause dilation of these same vessels as a means of ensuring an adequate blood supply to the brain.

Brain injury can cause a loss of autoregulation of cerebral blood flow. Following some head traumas, such as acute subdural hematoma, a hyperemia or increase in cerebral blood flow occurs leading to vascular congestion. This probably accounts for the early "brain swelling" seen on computerized tomography (CT) scans of head injury patients and precedes the development of cerebral edema.

With the loss of cerebral autoregulation, blood flow to the brain will become dependent on the systemic arterial blood pressure. This can have a devastating effect on the brain. It becomes readily apparent that the brain could receive excessive amounts of blood during hypertensive states and inadequate blood supply with ischemia during hypotensive states. Either instance can contribute to the formation of intracranial hypertension.

In localized brain trauma, or ischemia, dead tissue is surrounded by an ischemic trouble zone. Autoregulation within these areas is lost because the blood vessels are paralyzed. Hyperventilation therapy may improve circulation into the ischemic area by constricting blood vessels in the surrounding healthy tissue. This constriction causes a shunting of blood to the ischemic zone. This is known as the "Robin Hood" phenomenon although its evidence remains controversial. In contrast, CO_2 retention with arterial acidosis may actually steal blood from the already ischemic tissue because it results in the dilation of blood vessels in the surrounding healthy tissue. This has been described as the "intracerebral steal" phenomenon.[6]

Effects of Carbon Dioxide and Oxygen. Cerebral arterioles are responsive to arterial Pa_{CO_2} and, to a lesser extent, arterial Pa_{O_2}. Retention of carbon dioxide leads to respiratory acidosis. The excess hydrogen ion (H^+) that accumulates as a result has a profound effect on the diameter of cerebral arterioles. Excessive levels of hydrogen ions cause a relaxing effect on the smooth muscles of the cerebral blood vessels, leading to dilation. This can greatly increase cerebral blood flow and cerebral blood volume. A low Pa_{CO_2} results in respiratory alkalosis, which has the opposite effect, cerebral vasoconstriction.

Arterial hypoxemia, to a lesser extent, can also increase the diameter of cerebral blood vessels. This is usually not evident until the Pa_{O_2} falls to 50 mm Hg or lower.[5] The nursing implications of CO_2 retention and hypoxemia in the neurological patient are great. Maintenance of the patient's airway and breathing remain the nurse's first priority.

Obstruction of Venous Drainage. Any obstruction to venous drainage from the brain can contribute to the development of intracranial hypertension. Compression of intracranial veins by edematous brain will lead to pooling of blood in the capillaries. This increases the total blood volume within the brain.

Any factor that obstructs internal jugular or vertebral venous return can raise the intracranial pressure. Lateral head rotation and flexion or extension of the neck have been shown to retard venous return from the head.[7]

Elevated intrathoracic or intraabdominal pressure can be transmitted in retrograde fashion via the jugular veins to the intracranial venous system. Straining, coughing, breath holding, vomiting, extreme hip flexion, or positive end expiratory pressure (PEEP) on a ventilator are all examples of mechanisms that can increase either intrathoracic or intraabdominal pressure.[5] Nursing care should be directed toward preventing these activities when possible.

Increased Brain Volume

Brain volume may be increased because of tumor, abscess, hematoma, or edema. Cerebral edema is a frequent complication of neurological disease processes. While the initial brain swelling seen immediately following head injury is due to cerebral vascular congestion, cerebral edema follows, with a peak of swelling usually evident in 48–96 hours.[2] Cerebral edema can be either localized or generalized, but both contribute to intracranial hypertension if there is not a compensatory drop in CSF and/or intracranial blood volume. Two pathophysiologically distinct types of cerebral edema have been described by Klatzo.[8] These are vasogenic edema and cytotoxic or metabolic edema. A third type, interstitial edema, has also been described.[9]

Vasogenic Cerebral Edema. Vasogenic cerebral edema starts locally, around the area of brain injury, but may spread to become generalized. Vascular damage interrupts the permeability pattern of the blood vessels in the injured area of the brain. There is disruption of the normal blood-brain barrier, with leakage of plasma proteins out of the blood vessels into the extracellular space. This is followed by an osmotic influx of water into the area. Most vasogenic edema fluid accumulates in the white matter of the brain, because of the white matter's less closely interwoven cellular structures. Vasogenic edema can cause focal neurological deficits as well as disturbances of consciousness.[9] Like a leaking water pipe, the higher the patient's blood pressure, the greater the potential for vasogenic edema. Nursing actions may need to be directed toward preventing and treating hypertensive episodes.

Cytotoxic Cerebral Edema. Cytotoxic edema refers to the actual swelling of brain cells. It is more generalized and is thought to be due to some toxic factor that causes destructive alteration of brain cellular elements. While neuronal, glial, and endothelial cells are all affected, it occurs most often in the gray matter. It may be due to failure of the sodium pump, a situation that results in abnormal distribution of electrolytes and water across the cell membranes.

Most cytotoxic edema occurs as a result of hypoxia and hypercapnia, as seen following cardiac arrest. It also occurs in conditions associated with low serum levels of sodium. These include the syndrome of inappropriate antidiuretic hormone secretion (SIADH), severe sodium depletion, and water intoxication.[9]

Brain ischemia can result in both vasogenic and cytotoxic edema. Progressive ischemia causes cytotoxic edema, which leads to brain cell death. This contributes to the disruption of the blood-brain barrier and the formation of vasogenic edema.

Interstitial Cerebral Edema. Interstitial or extracellular cerebral edema forms as a result of hydrocephalus with leakage of CSF from the ventricles into the surrounding tissues. This edema may develop as a result of impaired CSF reabsorption in the arachnoid villi.[9]

The ultimate outcome of untreated intracranial hypertension from any of the aforementioned causes is brain herniation (see Figure 4–1). Priorities in the management of the brain-injured patient are directed toward preventing this occurrence.

Brain Herniation Syndromes

Locked within the cranium, the semiliquid gelatinous brain is partitioned into various subcompartments by the infoldings of the dura: the falx cerebri and the tentorium cerebelli (see Figure 2–7). When there is a regional increase in the mass of the brain and compensatory mechanisms are exhausted, that portion of the brain attempts to move from its compartment of high pressure to a compartment of lower pressure. This movement of a portion of the brain under or through one of the dural partitions is referred to as brain herniation. Common areas of herniation are movement of the medial portions of the frontal lobe under the falx, movement of the medial temporal lobe through the tentorial incisura, movement of the cerebellum through the foramen magnum, and movement of brain out through a bony defect in the cranium (see Figure 4–1).

Supratentorial Herniation Syndromes

Pathological processes involving those portions of the brain lying above the tentorium may cause tissue reactions that result in displacement of brain tissue.

Cingulate Herniation. The cingulate gyrus is located over the corpus collosum. An expanding mass lesion in one cerebral hemisphere causes movement of the cingulate gyrus under the falx. Compression of brain tissue and cerebral blood vessels, especially the ipsilateral anterior cerebral artery, occurs, causing cerebral ischemia, congestion, and edema.[10]

Central or Transtentorial Herniation. Central herniation occurs as downward displacement of the cerebral hemispheres compresses and eventually displaces the diencephalic structures. Compression of the midbrain occurs as the brain attempts to move downward through the tentorial incisura. Figure 4–3 depicts the changes frequently associated with rostral caudal deterioration seen in central herniation.[10]

Uncal Herniation. Uncal herniation refers to movement of the uncus and the hippocampal gyrus toward the midline and eventually through the tentorial

Area of Involvement	Level of Consciousness	Respiratory Pattern
Upper Thalamic (Early Diencephalon)	**Lethargic** Sleeps when left alone. Disinterested. Easily aroused. **Obtunded** Asleep and hard to arouse. Answers questions monosyllabically, appropriate but inaccurate.	Eupnea 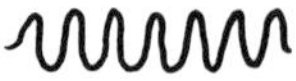 Cheyne-Stokes 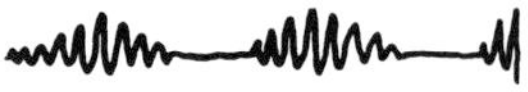
Lower Thalamic (Late Diencephalon)	**Stuporous** Cannot be aroused to communicate. Moves purposefully to pain.	Cheyne-Stokes
Midbrain (Mesencephalon)	**Coma** Unable to awaken. No speech. Abnormal or no response to pain.	Cheyne-Stokes Central Neurogenic Hyperventilation
Pons Medulla	**Coma**	Apneustic 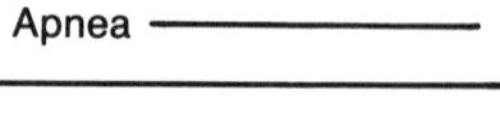 Ataxic 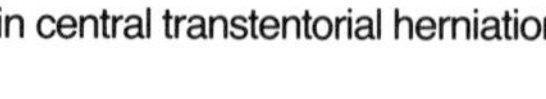 Apnea

Fig. 4–3—Rostral caudal progression in transtentorial herniation. This chart represents the possible sequence of clinical signs that may appear as supratentorial pathological changes radiate progressively downward, terminating in central transtentorial herniation.

Pupils	Oculocephalic Reflex	Response to Pain
Small (2-3mm) Reactive 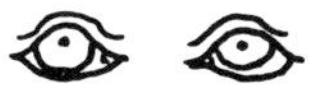	Present 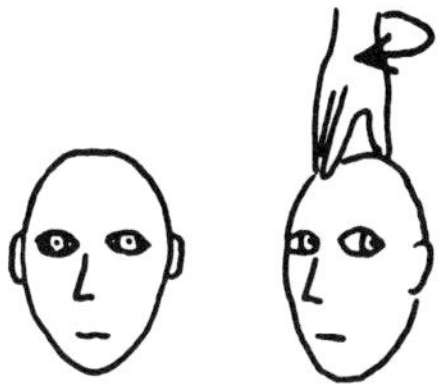	Appropriate 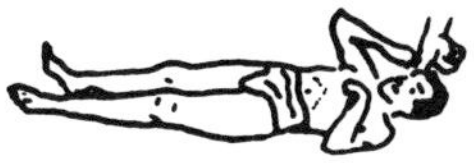
Small (2-3mm) Reactive	Present	Approp. or decorticate 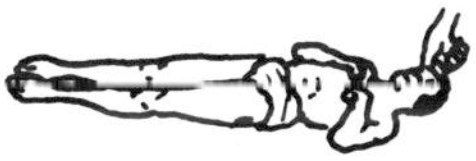
Mid-position Fixed 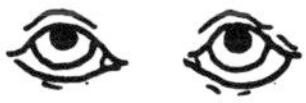	? Present + Caloric 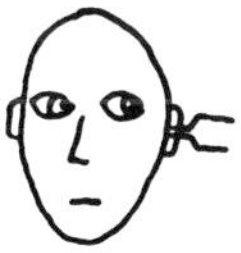	Decerebrate 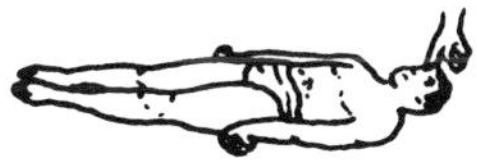
Dilated-fixed 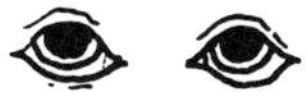	Absent, − Caloric 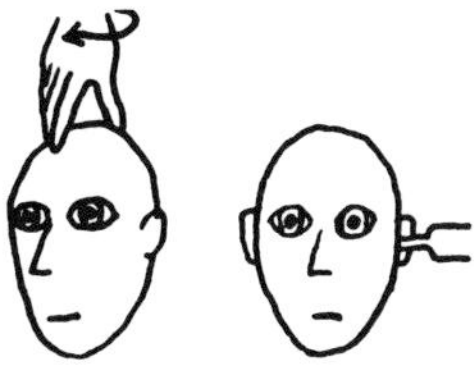	No Response or Flexion at Knee 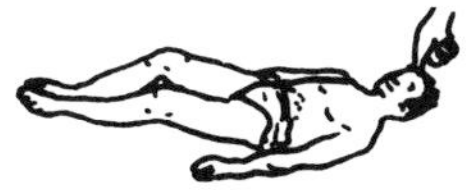

Source: Adapted from *The Diagnosis of Stupor and Coma,* ed 3 (pp 103–108) by Fred Plum and Jerome Posner with permission of the FA Davis Company, © 1980.

incisura. It is caused by expanding lesions in the temporal lobe or lateral portion of the middle fossa. Lateralizing neurological signs are seen with this type of brain herniation.[10]

Subtentorial Herniation Syndromes

Expanding lesions in the posterior fossa compress the brainstem and may cause an upward transtentorial herniation. Asymmetrical signs of focal brainstem dysfunction appear. Signs and symptoms are not consistent, but may include vomiting, coma, hyperventilation, miotic fixed pupils (pontine compression), and unequal pupils, loss of upward gaze, and extensor posturing (midbrain compression).[10] Death usually follows respiratory arrest.

Herniation of the cerebellum through the foramen magnum does not consistently induce clear-cut warning signs and symptoms. Patients may exhibit nuchal rigidity, paresthesias in the shoulders, coma, respiratory abnormalities, and widely variable pulse rates.[2]

Clinical Features

Although signs and symptoms do not always occur in any particular order, the nurse should be aware that symptoms of brain herniation can occur rapidly. Prompt action is necessary at the first sign of neurological deterioration if brain herniation is to be prevented. Nausea and vomiting and/or increased restlessness and confusion may be the earliest signs.

Decreased Level of Consciousness. Decreasing level of consciousness is usually the first sign of neurological deterioration. This occurs because of compression of the reticular activating system (RAS) located in the diencephalon and brainstem.

Alteration in Respiratory Pattern. Abnormal respiratory patterns develop depending on the area of the brain or brainstem being compressed (see Figure 4–3).

Pupillary Changes. Pupillary changes also depend on the area of brain compression. Midbrain compression affects the third cranial nerve, which may initially cause the appearance of oval pupil. This can progress to a dilating, nonreactive pupil, usually on the same side as the expanding lesion. Pontine compression causes small, fixed pupils. There may be paralysis of eye movements and loss of upward gaze. Bilateral dilated and fixed pupils imply bilateral brainstem compression and usually indicate a fatal outcome for the patient.

Motor Deficits. Hemiparesis or hemiplegia occurs as the descending motor fibers passing through the brainstem are compressed. Paralysis often begins in a lower extremity, progressing upward to include the arm and face. Most often the motor deficit is noted on the side opposite the brain pathology as the corticospinal motor fibers have not yet crossed to the opposite side in the medullary region. Ipsilateral motor deficits may occur from displacement of the brain medially, compressing the contralateral motor fibers. Abnormal posturing may be seen (see Figure 4–3). Flexor or decorticate posturing is due to hemispheric compression of corticospinal tracts. Extensor or decerebrate posturing is due to diencephalic or upper brainstem compression. Medullary compression causes flaccidity in all extremities.

Alterations in Blood Pressure and Pulse. Changes in blood pressure and pulse rate and rhythm are often seen in progressive compression of the brainstem. As intracranial pressure rises, the brain and brainstem become increasingly more ischemic. Sympathetic stimulation induces a systemic vasoconstriction and an increase in cardiac output, which increases the blood pressure in an effort to perfuse the tight brain. Bradycardia ensues because of pressoreceptor responses and stimulation of the vagal nuclei in the brainstem. Respiratory variations are often seen in combination with the elevating blood pressure and slowing pulse rate. This triad of clinical signs is known as the Cushing response. It is felt to be due to ischemia of the medulla.

NURSING MANAGEMENT

Nursing responsibilities include identifying those patients at risk for developing intracranial hypertension, early detection of intracranial hypertension, undertaking nursing measures to reduce and control intracranial pressure, and delivering nursing care with the goal of minimizing or eliminating increases in intracranial pressure.

Identification of Patients at Risk

Any patient with a space-occupying lesion in the cranium, such as a tumor, abscess, cyst, hematoma, or hemorrhage is at risk for developing intracranial hypertension. Patients at risk for developing cerebral edema include those with hypoxia, fluid and electrolyte imbalances, cerebral ischemia or infarction, central nervous system (CNS) infection, or trauma to the brain.[11]

Early Recognition of Intracranial Hypertension

Neurological signs and symptoms can be unreliable indicators of early developing intracranial hypertension. Classic signs such as decreasing level of consciousness, pupillary changes, elevated systolic blood pressure with a widened pulse pressure, bradycardia, and changes in respiratory pattern are actually late signs and represent brainstem compression. By the time many of these signs appear the opportunity to prevent permanent brain damage may be lost. When these same signs are found in a patient with normal ICP, they represent primary brainstem damage.[5(p37)]

Patient assessment has been greatly augmented with the advent of direct ICP monitoring. Although clinical signs and level of ICP do not always correlate, direct measurement of ICP provides the medical team with one more tool for early detection and treatment of intracranial hypertension. Direct monitoring of ICP is covered in detail at the end of this chapter.

Control of Intracranial Hypertension

Foremost in the nurse's mind should be the prevention of intracranial hypertension. While this is not always possible, there are numerous nursing measures that help to minimize its development. Intensive medical management of intracranial hypertension is covered in more detail in Chapter 5, which deals with brain resuscitation.

Many necessary nursing procedures have a tendency to cause transient increases in ICP. For this reason, whenever possible, nursing activities should be spaced to allow the patient time to rest and time for the ICP to return to its previous level. Of course this is not always possible, especially in emergency situations, but the nurse should remember that the simultaneous performance of several activities may have a compounding effect on increased ICP.

The following nursing measures are undertaken to control intracranial hypertension.

Maintain Respiratory Function

Maintain patency of airway and ensure adequate ventilation. Assess rate, depth, and pattern of respirations, and administer oxygen as ordered. Assess skin and mucous membrane color and auscultate lung sounds. Obtain arterial blood gases (ABGs) and maintain the patient's Pao_2 over 85 mm Hg and $Paco_2$ under 35 mm Hg. The physician may prescribe hyperventilation therapy to maintain the $Paco_2$ at 25–30 mm Hg and the Pao_2 at or above 100 mm Hg. If suctioning is needed, hyperoxygenate and hyperventilate with 100 percent o_2 before and after suctioning. Suction no more than 15 seconds per catheter insertion. Be alert for the development of cardiac dysrhythmias during suctioning (see Chapter 11). Recognize the effects that PEEP has on elevating ICP and try to avoid its use when possible.

Perform Frequent Neurological Assessments

Perform a rapid, yet thorough assessment of level of consciousness, including Glasgow Coma Scale, pupils, motor function and vital signs to establish a baseline. This must be done before the administration of any sedatives, narcotics, paralyzing agents, etc. Compare subsequent, timely assessments to this initial assessment and report any noted deterioration to the physician.

Facilitate Venous Return

Maintain the patient in a semi-Fowler's position with the head of bed elevated to 30–45 degrees unless contraindicated. Avoid neck flexion or extension, or rotation of the head to either side. If the patient has a tracheostomy, make sure that the ties are not too tight.[11] Avoid hip flexion of 90 degrees or greater as this can increase intraabdominal pressure. Assist the patient in moving in bed. Instruct the patient to avoid any isometric exercise. Ask the patient to exhale on turning or moving to prevent the initiation of Valsalva's maneuver.[2(p163)]

Control Seizures

Anticonvulsants such as phenytoin (Dilantin) can be administered prophylactically to prevent seizures. Diazepam (Valium) may need to be administered if seizures occur. See Chapter 5 for further details on anticonvulsant therapy.

Control Pain and Hyperactivity

The manner in which the patient is assessed and the nursing procedures performed can influence the patient's response to stimulation. All procedures and treatments should be explained, even if the patient is unconscious. Perform procedures in a gentle and unhurried manner. Avoid using wrist or arm restraints if at all possible as they may increase agitation. Assist the family in communicating with the patient in a calm manner. Excessive patient activity can lead to increases in ICP. Try to determine the cause of hyperactivity and eliminate it if possible. It may be due to confusion, fear, or even a full bladder.

Increasing headache may indicate increasing ICP, but sometimes mild analgesics such as codeine are indicated. Mild tranquilizers or short-acting barbiturates may be necessary to treat hyperactivity.[12] Try to decrease sensory input if possible. In extreme cases it may be necessary to paralyze the agitated patient with pancuronium bromide or succinylcholine. This necessitates intubation, mechanical ventilation, and direct ICP monitoring.

Administer Intravenous Fluids

An infusion pump should be used to ensure accurate intravenous (IV) fluid intake and prevent accidental overinfusion. Generally these patients will receive limited fluid intake using 5 percent to 10 percent dextrose solutions in 0.45 percent or 0.2 percent NaCl. Hypotonic IV solutions tend to worsen cerebral edema. In patients with multiple trauma, the restoration of adequate circulatory volume takes priority over the prevention of brain edema. These patients require the amount of fluids necessary to overcome hypovolemia. Hypovolemia contributes to decreased cerebral perfusion and will only worsen brain ischemia and intracranial hypertension.

The patient should be assessed carefully for the development of neurogenic pulmonary edema (see Chapter 11), which may necessitate further fluid restriction.

Maintain Adequate Cerebral Perfusion Pressure

Cerebral perfusion pressure (CPP) is the product of the mean systemic arterial blood pressure (MSAP) minus the ICP (CPP = MSAP − ICP). It represents the amount of pressure needed to maintain adequate blood flow to the brain. The brain needs a CPP of at least 60 mm Hg. Normal CPP is 80–90 mm Hg. Cerebral perfusion pressure can be reduced because of increased ICP or decreased blood pressure. Nursing and medical measures are directed toward reducing ICP as well as maintaining an adequate systemic blood pressure. If the patient's ICP is elevated or, in the absence of direct ICP monitoring, is suspected to be elevated, some elevation of the systemic blood pressure may be necessary to ensure adequate CPP. Hypotension may need to be treated with pressors such as dopamine. A CPP below 30 mm Hg may lead to irreversible brain hypoxia.[13] In brain injury, altered metabolism within the brain may require that a minimal CPP of at least 50 mm Hg be maintained.[5(p33)]

The development of hypertension can increase the formation of vasogenic cerebral edema. Antihypertensive medications such as trimethaphan camsylate (Arfonad) or hydralazine may need to be administered.

Administer Medications to Reduce Intracranial Volume

Corticosteroids such as dexamethasone (Decadron) or methylprednisolone (Solu-Medrol) may be prescribed. Osmotic agents such as mannitol and diuretic agents such as furosemide (Lasix) may also be used. Nursing responsibilities include administering these medications and monitoring for their effects and/or side effects.

Reduce Intracranial Volume by Withdrawing Cerebrospinal Fluid

On a physician's order the nurse may be directed to slowly and carefully withdraw CSF from a direct ICP monitoring line as a means of reducing intracranial pressure. The nurse should strictly follow the medical institution's policy regarding this procedure. The physician must specify either to withdraw a prescribed amount of CSF or to withdraw fluid until a specified ICP reading is obtained. Refer to the procedure for monitoring intracranial pressure later in this chapter.

Control Temperature

Extremes of hypothermia or hyperthermia may be seen early in the patient's illness. Fever increases oxygen consumption by the brain and is to be prevented. If treatment with hypothermia is instituted, shivering is to be avoided. Wrapping the patient's hands and feet in soft blankets or towels before the start of hypothermia therapy may prevent shivering. Medications such as chlorpromazine may be required to abolish shivering.

Prevent Urinary Retention

The patient may require an indwelling catheter, especially if osmotic or diuretic agents have been administered. Maintain accurate records of intake and output. If osmotic agents or diuretics have not been administered, report urinary output in excess of 200 ml per hour and of low specific gravity as this may indicate the presence of diabetes insipidus.

Prevent Gastric Retention

The patient with a decreased level of consciousness is at risk for the aspiration of gastric contents. Vomiting also increases the ICP. Assess for the presence of bowel sounds and for abdominal distention. A nasogastric tube may be required. In head trauma patients, rule out the possibility of anterior basal skull fracture before inserting the nasogastric tube. An anterior basal skull fracture that extends into the nasal sinuses can provide an errant pathway for the nasogastric tube. The nasogastric tube can actually be diverted up into the brain with disastrous consequences. Oral gastric intubation may be required in these patients.

Emergency Interventions in Impending Brain Herniation

Prompt nursing intervention can reverse a potentially fatal brain herniation syndrome. When neurological signs indicate that brain herniation is imminent or is occurring the nurse should take the following actions:

- Notify the physician STAT.
- Elevate the patient's head to 30–45 degrees (if there is no spinal injury).
- Maintain the patient's head in neutral plane (no flexion or rotation).
- Slow the IV infusion to keep open rate.
- Hyperventilate and hyperoxygenate patient.

- Prepare to administer mannitol and furosemide.
- Prepare patient for emergency CT head scan and/or emergency surgery.

MONITORING INTRACRANIAL PRESSURE

CSF pressure was measured through lumbar puncture as early as the 19th century. This procedure remains an unreliable indicator of actual intracranial pressure because any blockage between the spinal and cranial subarachnoid spaces can result in an erroneous reading of CSF pressure. Even in the absence of such blockage, lumbar puncture provides only a single measurement of CSF pressure. Lumbar puncture can be dangerous in patients with increased intracranial volumes that have been compensated for by CSF displacement into the spinal subarachnoid spaces. As CSF is drawn off in the lumbar area, there can be downward herniation of the brain because of the sudden change in CSF pressures between the cranial and the lumbar areas.[5(p37)]

Experimental techniques of monitoring ventricular fluid pressure were begun in 1929. Not until the 1950s did the technique of direct ICP monitoring become a widespread, acceptable practice.[14] Direct ICP monitoring provides not only continuous information on ICP and brain compliance, but also allows for early intervention to prevent and treat intracranial hypertension. CSF can be drawn off as a treatment for elevated ICP. Direct ICP monitoring provides an ongoing assessment of the effectiveness of therapy aimed at preventing or controlling intracranial hypertension. It also permits measurement of CPP, which is made even easier by the insertion of an arterial line for the continuous display of arterial blood pressure. One cannot rely on ICP readings exclusively to evaluate the patient's condition. There is no substitute for the clinical examination in patient evaluation. This is particularly true in patients with brainstem disorders. Significant clinical deterioration can occur with little or no change in ICP readings.

Patient Selection

Monitoring of ICP is used in patients with a wide range of intracranial disorders. It has proved useful in patients with head injury, hydrocephalus, diffuse encephalopathies, encephalitis (especially Reye's syndrome), subarachnoid hemorrhage, and lesions of the posterior fossa in which direct compression of the brainstem can occur rapidly and with little warning.

Contraindications to direct ICP monitoring include abnormalities of blood clotting, collapsed or displaced ventricles (if intraventricular monitoring is considered), and a cerebral aneurysm in or near the pathway the monitoring catheter must follow. Some prefer that the patient have an intact skull before performing a twist drill hole through which the monitoring device must pass.

Techniques

Direct, continuous ICP monitoring involves the use of the following: an implantable intracranial device (the sensor), pressure monitoring tubing, prefilled with sterile preservative-free normal saline (preservative alters pH), a transducer to convert the mechanical pressure into electrical impulses, and a pressure module that converts the electrical impulse into an oscilloscopic display and provides a numerical display in mm Hg.

Implantable transducers are not used as frequently because the transducer cannot be recalibrated once implanted. Three basic techniques are widely used in continuous ICP monitoring (Figure 4–4): a subarachnoid screw (or bolt), an intraventricular catheter, and an epidural sensor.

Subarachnoid Screw

A small twist drill hole is made into the skull, usually behind the hairline in the frontal bone lateral to midline in the nondominant hemisphere. The dura is incised

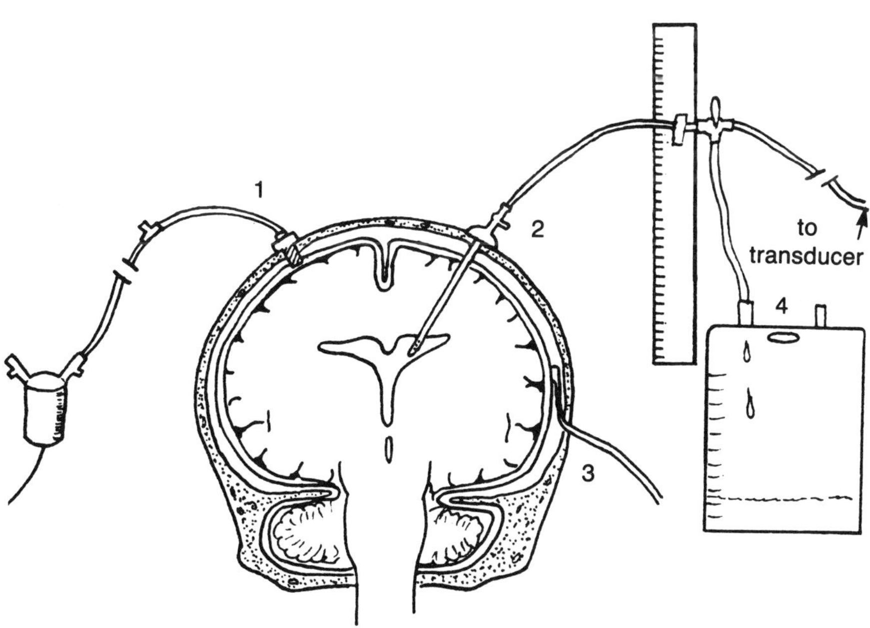

Fig. 4–4—Intracranial pressure monitoring techniques. (1) Subarachnoid screw or bolt, (2) intraventricular catheter, (3) epidural sensor, and (4) optional continuous overflow drainage system attached to the intraventricular line.

and a hollow screw, bolt, stopcock, or other device is firmly placed into the skull with the base of the device resting in the subarachnoid space. It is then connected to the transducer via the saline-filled pressure tubing.

Advantages of the subarachnoid screw include speed and ease of placement without penetration of brain tissue and direct measurement of CSF pressure. Disadvantages include the risk of infection because of its invasive nature, limited ability to drain significant amounts of CSF, limited ability to test the volume-pressure response, the requiremnt of an intact skull (generally used in patients over six years of age), and the possibility of occlusion of the screw by brain tissue or blood.

Intraventricular Catheter

A small silicone rubber or polyethylene catheter, approximately 7 cm long, is introduced via a small twist drill hole in the skull and advanced into the frontal or occipital horn of a lateral ventricle, usually in the nondominant hemisphere. The catheter is connected to saline-filled pressure tubing, which is attached to the transducer. This system provides the most accurate method of measuring ICP and facilitates the easy withdrawal of CSF. The volume-pressure response can be readily tested. Contrast material or air can be injected through the intraventricular catheter for radiological assessment of ventricular size.

Disadvantages of this system include an increased risk for infection, which could result in ventriculitis. It requires a more difficult technique to ensure proper placement of the catheter, especially if the ventricles are small, displaced, or collapsed because of cerebral edema. There is also an increased risk of leakage of CSF,[15] ventricular collapse, and a small risk of hemorrhage and functional damage from traversing brain tissue during insertion.[5(p38)]

Epidural Sensor

A tiny fiberoptic sensor is inserted through a small burr hole into the epidural space just under the skull. Sensor cables attach directly into the monitor. Advantages include the ease of placement and reduced risk of infection because it is less invasive and is not a fluid-filled system. It also cannot become occluded with brain tissue or blood. Disadvantages include questionable accuracy (because it does not measure ICP directly from a CSF space) and the inability to either drain off CSF or test the volume-pressure response.[15]

Testing the Volume-Pressure Reponse

The volume-pressure response is used to evaluate intracranial compliance, or the degree of compensation existing within the cranium. It involves instilling, over one second, a small, known fluid volume into the system, or withdrawing a small, known amount of CSF and then observing the pressure change. Compliance is reflected by the change in pressure in response to the known change in fluid volume. In Figure 4–2, point A represents normal compliance, point B reflects minimal remaining compliance, and point C represents loss of compliance. A pressure change of 1 mm Hg after the instillation of 1 ml of preservative-free sterile saline equals a volume-pressure response (VPR) of 1 (1 mm Hg per 1 ml saline). If, for example, the ICP rises by 2 mm Hg in response to the instillation of 0.5 ml saline, the VPR equals 4. A VPR greater than 2 is considered abnormal and reflects limited compensation reserve.[5(p39)] In performing the test, it is best not to use a tuberculin syringe because of the high pressure that can be generated by such a small-diameter syringe. This could injure the brain. Since this test could prove dangerous in the maximally compensated patient, it should be performed only in the presence of a physician. One must be prepared to immediately withdraw CSF if there is a precipitous rise in ICP during the test.

Equipment and Procedure

Equipment and procedures vary from hospital to hospital, so a step-by-step procedure for setting up and maintaining the ICP monitoring system are beyond the scope of this book. In general, the subarachnoid screw and intraventricular catheter require a fluid-filled system (Figure 4–4). Preservative-free sterile normal saline can be used to minimize possible pH changes to the CSF. The preservatives contained in ''normal saline for injection'' are also toxic to the brain. An antibiotic can be added to the saline that is used to expel air from the system before the system is attached to the patient. Never connect a continuous flush or irrigation system to a ventricular line or subarachnoid screw. Strict asepsis is mandatory. Keep all stopcocks covered and maintain a sealed, sterile dressing around the insertion site. Maintain strict asepsis and the watertight integrity of the system upon transfer of the patient to another area of the hospital.

A word of caution is warranted concerning the withdrawal of CSF from an ICP monitoring system. Withdrawal is best accomplished with an intraventricular catheter. Fluid should be withdrawn only through a stopcock in the tubing and not directly from the intraventricular catheter; this method lessens the possibility of causing collapse of the ventricles or the aspiration of brain tissue into the catheter. Too rapid removal of fluid can lead to brain herniation if the intracranial pressure is significantly elevated. If you withdraw fluid with a syringe, allow CSF pressure to fill syringe rather than aspirate. The physician may choose to have a continuous drainage system attached to prevent too rapid decompression of the ventricles. With this method, a drainage bag is placed at a level, measured in centimeters above the foramen of Monro, above which the physician does not want the ICP to rise. If the ICP rises to the level of the drainage bag, CSF spills over into the bag. In this way the CSF in the ventricles is vented and a predetermined level of ICP can be maintained. By turning a stopcock, the drainage bag can be temporarily "turned off" while a pressure reading is recorded.

Measuring ICP

The patient is usually positioned with the head of the bed elevated to 30–45 degrees. Be consistent in taking pressure readings. The patient's head should be at the same level in relation to the transducer for each reading. The stopcock that will be opened to air to balance and calibrate the transducer should be placed at the level of the foramen of Monro, found by approximating the intersection of imaginary lines drawn down from the vertex of the cranium and back from the outer canthus of the eye.

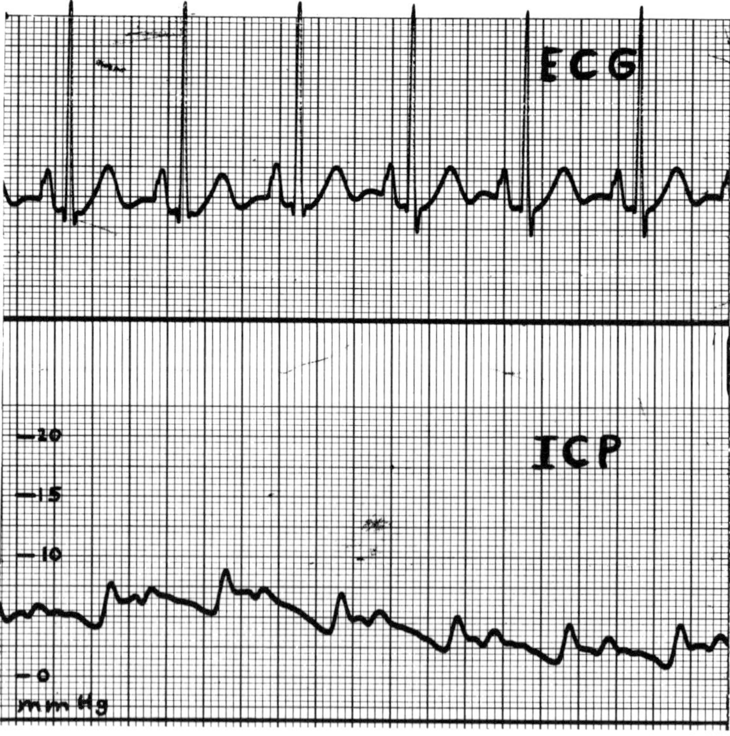

Fig. 4–5—Normal ICP waveform. The simultaneous recordings of electrocardiogram and ICP demonstrate the influences that cardiac pulsations and respiratory variation (note wandering baseline) have on ICP waveforms. If cardiac pulsations are not visible, suspect an occluded ICP monitoring system.

Normal ICP is 0–15 mm Hg. Pressures of 15–40 mm Hg are considered moderately elevated, while pressures greater than 40 mm Hg are markedly elevated and may be accompanied by changes in clinical signs.[16] Any increase in ICP of more than 4–5 mm Hg should be reported to the physician. More important than the actual ICP reading is the measurement of cerebral perfusion pressure (CPP = MSAP − ICP). This measurement provides the best approximation of the adequacy of cerebral blood flow. A poor prognosis is usually seen when the CPP is less than 30 mm Hg and when the ICP continues to rise despite treatment.[14] The nurse needs to recongize and understand the clinical significance of the various waveforms depicted in Figures 4–5 and 4–6.

Patient assessment for intracranial hypertension has been greatly enhanced by direct ICP monitoring. Although clinical signs and symptoms and level of ICP do not always correlate, ICP monitoring has proved useful in facilitating the early diagnosis, treatment, and evaluation of therapy of intracranial hypertension. ICP monitoring can also aid in determining patient prognosis.

While complications do occur infrequently, the most common ones are infection, CSF leakage, and hematoma. Increasing numbers of clinicians believe that the benefits of ICP monitoring often outweigh the risks.

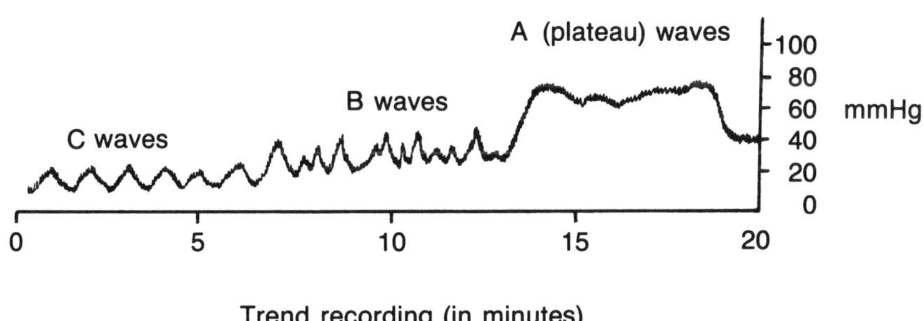

Fig. 4–6—Variations of intracranial pressure waveforms. As intracranial pressure rises, these variations of waveforms may be observed. C waves occur four to eight times per minute and correlate with normal fluctuations in blood pressure. They are not necessarily clinically significant. B waves represent transient, short (one-half to two minute) increases in ICP up to 50 mm Hg probably related to blood pressure changes, or more commonly, respiratory changes, such as Cheyne-Stokes breathing. A waves, or plateau waves, are transient, recurrent elevations of ICP from 50 to 100 mm Hg lasting from 5 to 20 minutes. They may be related to patient activities such as coughing or straining, but if recurrent or sustained, may indicate reduced ability of the brain to compensate and may be associated with concurrent changes in clinical neurological signs.

REFERENCES

1. Snyder M, Jackle M: *Neurological Problems, a Critical Care Nursing Focus*. Bowie, Md, Brady Co, 1981.

2. Hickey JV: *The Clinical Practice of Neurological and Neurosurgical Nursing*. Philadelphia, Lippincott, 1981.

3. Howe JR: *Patient Care in Neurosurgery*. Boston, Little, Brown, 1977.

4. Price SA, Wilson LM: *Pathophysiology: Clinical Concepts of Disease Processes*. New York, McGraw-Hill, 1978.

5. Nikas DL (ed): *The Critically Ill Neurosurgical Patient*. New York, Churchill Livingston, 1982.

6. Meyer JS, Marx P: Cerebral autoregulation and ''dysautoregulation'' and their relation to cerebral vascular symptoms. *Curr Concepts Cerebrovasc Dis: Stroke* 1971;6:1–5.

7. Lipe HP, Mitchell PH: Positioning the patient with intracranial hypertension: How head turning and head rotation affect the internal jugular vein. *Heart Lung* 1980;9:1031–1077.

8. Klatzo I: Presidential address on the neuropathological aspects of cerebral edema. *J Neurosurg* 1967;26:1–4.

9. Speers I: Cerebral edema. *J Neurosurg Nurs* 1981;13:102–114.

10. Plum F, Posner JB: *The Diagnosis of Stupor and Coma*, ed 3. Philadelphia, FA Davis Co, 1980.

11. Nikas DL: The nervous system, in Borg N, Nikas DL, Stark J, et al (eds); *Core Curriculum for Critical Care Nursing*, ed 2. Philadelphia, WB Saunders, 1981.

12. Rudy EB: *Advanced Neurological and Neurosurgical Nursing*. St Louis, Mosby, 1984.

13. Taylor JW, Ballenger S: *Neurological Dysfunctions and Nursing Intervention*. New York, McGraw-Hill, 1980, p 149.

14. Hanlon K: Description and uses of intracranial pressure monitoring. *Heart Lung* 1976;5:277–282.

15. Millar S (ed): *Methods in Critical Care*. Philadelphia, WB Saunders, 1980.

16. Mauss NK, Mitchell P: Increased intracranial pressure: An update. *Heart Lung* 1976;5:919–926.

Chapter 5

Brain Resuscitation

The concept of brain resuscitation has grown out of research conducted since the 1970s on patients who have developed global brain ischemia-anoxia as a result of cardiac arrest. Following cardiac arrest, restoration of spontaneous circulation will not benefit the patient if the brain does not remain viable. Brain resuscitation is the restoration of neuronal and glial cell functioning after a global ischemic-anoxic event. While several treatment modalities remain controversial and are still being researched, clinicians are currently adapting many brain resuscitation guidelines to patients with traumatic brain injuries. Likewise, several standard treatments for head injury are being applied to patients with anoxic brain injuries.[1]

PATHOPHYSIOLOGY OF GLOBAL ISCHEMIA-ANOXIA

Definitions of acute cerebral failure and resuscitation differ among investigators and clinicians. Global ischemia-anoxia refers to the effects of the cessation of cerebral blood flow (CBF) that is seen in cardiac arrest. Focal ischemia-anoxia results from disorders such as stroke or vasospasm in which there is localized brain tissue damage. Brain hypoxia-anemia can result from carbon monoxide poisoning, head injury, hemorrhage/aneurysm, infection, etc.[1] Whereas each type of pathological process may affect the brain in its own particular way, the ultimate outcome of brain ischemia is neuronal damage and death.

Cardiac Arrest Phase

Cardiac arrest results in the total cessation of blood flow. Within 10–15 seconds of cessation of CBF, the brain's oxygen stores are depleted and consciousness is lost. In approximately five minutes, glucose and glycogen stores are used up and even low energy yielding anaerobic glycolysis comes to a halt. Intracellular ATP is exhausted, so all energy-requiring cellular reactions stop. Among these is the cell-membrane sodium pump. Intracellular sodium concentrations increase, leading to intracellular (cytotoxic) cerebral edema.[2] In five to seven minutes, histological and functional changes take place in neuronal cells due to the formation of calcium deposits in the mitochondria. This leads to scattered necrosis, which causes various neurological deficits. If circulatory arrest continues for more than 30 minutes, there is breakdown of the blood-brain barrier followed by the leakage of proteins into the brain.[3] This results in vasogenic cerebral edema.

Closed chest cardiopulmonary resuscitation (CPR), performed under the best circumstances, is inadequate to sustain normal aerobic cerebral metabolism and cerebral activity, even in the presence of adequate hemodynamic and respiratory control.[4]

Postresuscitation Encephalopathy

Once spontaneous circulation is restored, it takes approximately two minutes for carbohydrate metabolism to return to aerobic pathways with the resumption of ATP production. Restoration of suboptimal circulation to the brain can result in more damage than no blood flow. This may be due to continued glucose transport in the presence of inadequate oxygen, resulting in continued anaerobic metabolism and the accumulation of lactic acid.[5] Lactic acidosis will continue until there is a full return to aerobic metabolism, which may take up to one to two hours. Normalization of cerebrospinal fluid (CSF) pH lags behind that of arterial blood, and may take up to 72 hours.[4] Meanwhile, CSF acidosis has a depressant effect on neuronal function.

It appears that reperfusion may induce additional damage. There is a brief 10 to 20 minute period of hyperperfusion with loss of autoregulation with vasodilation and possible breakdown of the blood-brain barrier. This is followed by the appearance of multifocal areas of hypoperfusion and no-reflow because of blood sludging and pressure on capillary walls from tissue edema. A multifocal hypermetabolism occurs in which oxygen and glucose are used faster than they can be supplied. There is also a release of free chemical radicals, which further damage lipoprotein membranes. Some of these reactions may be mediated by certain of the brain's neurotransmitters.[6] The diffuse and multifocal nature of these changes is probably due to variations in the ratio of oxygen consumption to blood flow in certain regions of the brain. Susceptible areas include the cerebral cortex (primarily the occipital area) and the midbrain, both known to have high metabolic rates.[4]

In summary, the changes occurring in the brain during and after cardiac arrest appear to be a combination of the primary insult, the arrest, and the secondary postischemic changes. These include multifocal hypoperfusion and areas of no-reflow, hypoxia, and hypermetabolism. A severe mismatch exists between oxygen supply and metabolic demand.

Clinical Aspects of Global Ischemia-Anoxia

During cardiac arrest, cortical functions cease first with cessation of CBF. The last areas of the brain to cease functioning are the respiratory and vasomotor centers in the lower brainstem. Following restoration of spontaneous circulation, those brain areas that ceased functioning last usually resume functioning first. For example, after restoration of a cardiac rhythm, agonal, gasping respirations may be seen, with eventual return of a normal respiratory pattern. Cranial nerve function then recovers, manifested by the return of corneal reflexes and pupillary constriction to light. Muscle tone also returns. The cerebral cortex recovers more slowly. Coma may resolve, but residual neurological dysfunctions such as memory loss, intellectual impairment, and speech problems may remain. Safar states that up to 20 percent of all successfully resuscitated patients may be left with various degrees of permanent brain damage.[2]

Errors in resuscitative efforts such as uncorrected hypotension, hypertension, hypoxemia, hypercarbia, elevated CVP, or changes in blood osmolality may all negatively influence the chances for normal brain recovery.[3]

Prognostic Indicators

If the cardiac arrest is brief and resuscitation is successful, the patient usually shows no signs of central nervous system (CNS) disturbances. The longer the period of absent or inadequate blood flow to the brain, the greater is the risk of permanent brain damage.

A complete clinical examination of the CNS is indicated following resuscitation. A history of events leading up to the arrest should be obtained. Physical signs seen after resuscitation can be influenced by preexisting conditions and can lead to misinterpretation of prognostic indicators. For example, some drug intoxications can induce coma and result in dilated, fixed pupils. Prolonged coma can also be caused by a preexisting metabolic disorder.

The electroencephalogram (EEG) remains controversial as a prognostic indicator because it appears to be able to predict only brain death and not survival.[7] The length of the comatose state remains one of the best prognostic indicators. Use of the Glasgow Coma Scale is taking on greater significance in predicting the outcome of patients with global ischemia-anoxia. Higher mortality is associated with patients having scores of 3–5 and who remain comatose for over 24 hours.[7]

Evoked potentials are sometimes used as prognostic indicators of brain viability. Evoked potentials test the integrity of neural pathways and brainstem integrity by recording (similar to EEG) the cortical responses to peripheral stimuli.

The stimuli may be visual, auditory, or somatosensory. A grading system is used to analyze responses.[7]

Favorable Indicators. Favorable prognostic indicators include the appearance of signs related to the return of brainstem function. These can be rapidly assessed by observing for the return of pupillary constriction to light, the return of the ciliospinal reflex, the return of additional cranial nerve function, and the return of spontaneous respirations. Abnormal posturing such as extension (decerebration) or flexion (decortication) are commonly seen shortly after arrest. They usually subside within 24 hours.[8(p254)] They imply that messages from the periphery are being processed at least by the brainstem.

Signs of improving cortical function include the appearance of localized responses to stimuli, such as reaching for the site of an applied painful stimulus. Of course the return of consciousness is the best indicator of a recovering cerebral cortex and brainstem.

Unfavorable Indicators. Unfavorable prognostic indicators include prolonged unconsciousness after restoration of spontaneous circulation, the absence of spontaneous respirations, cranial nerve function, or motor response. All of these indicate severe brainstem compromise.

Prearrest Factors Contributing to Cerebral Viability

Many preexisting factors can influence the degree to which the brain is able to recover from a global ischemic-anoxic insult. There seems to be some degree of neuronal protection in younger patients, particularly infants. This may be due to incomplete maturation of CNS neurotransmitters and thus lower cerebral metabolic rates.[6]

The length of time the patient is in cardiac arrest before resuscitation begins certainly influences outcome. The quality of prehospital care becomes a critical factor. It is hoped that improvements in cardiopulmonary and cerebral resuscitation (CPCR) may actually allow an extension of the length of ''down'' time from the traditional four to six minutes.

The presence of hypothermia before or during cardiac arrest has a protective effect on the brain. Hypothermia, as may be experienced by the near drowning victim, reduces cerebral metabolic demand, helps preserve adenosine triphosphate (ATP), and lessens cerebral edema, permitting the brain to survive longer periods of anoxic arrest. Animal research has shown, though, that this brain protection is most effective when hypothermia occurs before the onset of cardiac arrest.[9]

The presence of an elevated blood sugar before the arrest may have a detrimental effect on cerebral viability. With the breakdown of the blood-brain barrier, glucose may leak out into the brain and osmotically pull water to it, increasing the formation of cerebral edema. Cerebral ischemia coupled with hyperglycemia contributes to severe cerebral lactic acidosis.

Barbiturates have been shown to have a therapeutic effect on the brain by decreasing cerebral metabolic rate. Although barbiturates have shown beneficial effects on the brain after focal ischemia or incomplete global ischemia, animal studies indicate that their cerebral protection is also most effective when given before the arrest.[10] They have not been shown to be effective following global ischemia.[11]

A major determinant of survival and cerebral viability lies in the efficacy of CPR. Normal CPR, at its best, usually yields a cerebral blood flow of only 30 percent of normal. This may still be inadequate, so anything less than near perfect CPR is unacceptable.

BRAIN RESUSCITATION

Medical efforts during and after cardiac arrest must be directed toward brain as well as cardiopulmonary resuscitation. Since the major problems following global ischemia-anoxia are scattered hypermetabolism, hypoperfusion, and no-reflow phenomena, restoration of optimal cerebral blood flow is paramount. In addition to correcting acidosis and reducing cerebral edema, treatment guidelines for brain resuscitation include measures aimed at protecting neurons by restoring the balance between cerebral metabolic rate and oxygen delivery.[2] Table 5–1 summarizes the following goals and therapeutic modalities that constitute brain resuscitation.

Maintain Adequate Cerebral Perfusion Pressure

Cerebral perfusion pressure (CPP), as recalled from Chapter 4, is the product of the mean systemic arterial pressure minus the intracranial pressure (CPP = MSAP − ICP). Maintenance of adequate CPP then must involve efforts to maintain adequate systemic blood pressure as well as control ICP.

Maintain Normotension

Extremes of hypotension or hypertension can have harmful effects on the postanoxic brain. A smooth return of blood pressure to normotensive levels with mean arterial blood pressure (MAP) of 90–100 mm Hg and systolic arterial blood pressure (SAP) of more than 100 mm Hg are desired. In previously hypertensive individuals, higher MAPs should be maintained. Severe hypertension may require the administration of hypotensive agents. Hypotension may need to be treated with plasma volume expanders, or vasopressors.[3] Some of the options that may help ameliorate post arrest brain damage include induced mild hypertension (MAP

Table 5–1 Suggested Guidelines for Brain Resuscitation Following Global Ischemia-Anoxia[2,4,11,12,13,14]

Goal	*Therapy*
Maintain adequate CPP maintain MSAP 90–100; SAP>100	Maintain normotension with volume expanders, vasopressors, antihypertensives prn Maintain normovolemia or plasma volume expansion
reduce ICP	Elevate head of bed to 30–45 degrees Osmotic and diuretic agents as needed: • mannitol 0.25–0.5 gm/kg IV prn • furosemide 0.5–1.0 mg/kg IV, then 0.3 mg/kg every 4 hr prn Corticosteroid of choice • dexamethasone 1.0 mg/kg IV, then 0.2 mg/kg every 6 hr (for 2–5 days) • methylprednisolone 5 mg/kg IV, then 1 mg/kg every 6 hr

Control respiratory variables
   maintain Pa_{CO_2} 25–35 mm Hg
   maintain Pa_{O_2} > 100 mm Hg
   maintain pH 7.3–7.6
	Intubation following preoxygenation
	 • mechanically controlled moderate hyperventilation
	 • adjust FIO_2, cautious PEEP, titrate to avoid increase in ICP
	 • monitor ABGs, adjust tidal volume or rate prn

Maintain normothermia	Control temperature with external cooling measures • hypothermia if necessary • prevent shivering, wrap hands and feet, chlorpromazine prn • may use short-term hypothermia (30–32°C)
Control seizures	Prophylactic phenytoin, up to 1.0 gm loading dose IV • treat seizures with diazepam, barbiturates prn

Control blood variables
   maintain hematocrit 30–35%
   normalize electrolytes
   maintain blood sugar 100–300 mg%
   maintain serum osmolality 280–330mosm/L
   maintain normal oncotic pressure (>15)
      albumin > 3g/dL
	Monitor lab studies daily and prn
	 • give RBCs sparingly, MD may prefer hemodilution
	 • supplement IV with electrolytes prn
	 • 50% dextrose to replenish depleted brain stores
	 • adjust electrolytes, blood sugar prn
	 • assure normal serum albumin level > 3 gm%

Table 5-1 continued

Goal	Therapy
	IV fluids and alimentation • dextrose 5–10% in 0.25–0.5% NaCl @ 30–50 ml/kg/24 hr, 100 ml/kg/24 hr in infants • 2000–4000 cal/24 hr/70 kg + amino acids and vitamins
Reduce cerebral metabolic rate	Barbiturate therapy • thiopental or pentobarbital up to 5 mg/kg IV, then 1–2 mg/kg/hr, maintain serum barb level of 2–4 mg/dL • Immobilize with sedatives, barbiturates, or pancuronium 0.04–0.1 mg/kg IV, then 0.01 mg/kg every 30–60 min
Perform CNS evaluation	Frequent neuro assessment including Glasgow Coma Scale, EEG, CT scanning, evoked potentials prn Neuropsychiatric evaluation after awakening

120–140 mm Hg) for 1 to 5 minutes immediately after restoration of circulation. Intracarotid hypertensive hemodilution has also been used to promote reflow.[11]

Cardiac dysrhythmias that disturb cardiac output need to be controlled.

Reduce ICP

After control of the MAP and the SAP, efforts are directed towards preventing or reducing intracranial hypertension.

Facilitate Venous Return. Facilitating venous return from the head is best accomplished by elevating the patient's head to 30–45 degrees, maintaining the head and neck in a neutral plane, and avoiding flexion of the hips beyond 90 degrees.

Osmotic and diuretic agents are frequently used to reduce increased intracranial pressure. The most commonly used agents are mannitol and furosemide.

Osmotic agents. Mannitol is classified as an osmotic agent. It raises serum osmolality and draws water from the intracellular and interstitial compartments into the vascular space. The secondary plasma expansion and hemodilution may improve microcirculation in the brain.[12] The reduction in cerebral edema and ICP may be only transient and is often followed by a rebound brain edema. The brain cells produce "ideogenic" osmoles in response to the increased extracellular osmolality induced by the mannitol.[4] These osmoles then draw water to them, causing the rebound swelling. In addition, some of the mannitol may leak out through the disrupted blood-brain barrier, eventually leading to a greater concentration of the drug in the tissues than in the blood. This also results in a rebound brain edema.

Dosage regimens vary. Marshall et al[13] reported sustained ICP reduction for up to six hours after a high dose regimen of 1 gm/kg body weight. ICP reduction for two to four hours was sustained by a low-dose regimen of 0.25–0.50 gm/kg. Fewer complications of rebound edema were noted with the low-dose regimen.

Because mannitol temporarily increases circulating blood volume, the patient must be carefully assessed for signs of volume overload and congestive heart failure.

Diuretic agents. Furosemide (Lasix) is a loop diuretic. It and the lesser used loop diuretic, ethacrinic acid, are also used to reduce cerebral edema. They act primarily on the ascending loop of Henle in the kidney. The resulting diuresis creates a pressure gradient for edema fluid to diffuse from the brain tissue into the blood. Intracranial venous dilation occurs following the administration of furosemide, further enhancing edema reabsorption. Furosemide inhibits the enzyme carbonic anhydrase, which has been linked to CSF production in the choroid plexus. The result is inhibition of CSF production, which helps decrease ICP.[12]

Dosage regimens of furosemide also vary. A recommended dosage is 1 mg/kg IV, followed by 0.3 mg/kg every four hours as needed.[14] The combination of an osmotic agent and a diuretic agent appears to produce a greater decrease in ICP.

Corticosteroid Therapy. Although scientifically unproven, corticosteroid therapy is popular for the treatment of cerebral edema. Following the administration of corticosteroids, intracellular sodium concentrations and water volume are decreased, while intracellular potassium is increased, through reactivation of the sodium pump.[4] It is also believed that steroids help stabilize vascular membranes, reducing and sometimes reversing leakage through the blood-brain barrier. Corticosteroids may also decrease CSF production. Although these agents have shown their greatest effectiveness in controlling the cerebral edema accompanying brain tumor, they appear to have minimal effect in reducing cytotoxic edema.[15] Nevertheless, they are often used following global ischemia-anoxia.

Suggested dosages of cortiocosteroids are dexamethasone (Decadron) 1.0 mg/ kg IV, then 0.2 mg/kg every six hours or methylprednisolone (Solu-Medrol) 5 mg/kg IV, then 1.0 mg/kg every six hours.[11] Corticosteroids are given for 2–5 days.

Control Respiratory Variables

Moderate hyperventilation therapy is instituted as a means of reducing ICP. Patients will often hyperventilate spontaneously because of CSF acidosis or increased intracranial pressure, but when this does not occur, it should be induced mechanically. Hypocapnia enhances cerebral vasoconstriction which reduces cerebral blood volume. The Pa_{CO_2} is kept between 25 and 35 mm Hg. Hypoxemia is to be avoided. It is desirable to maintain the Pa_{O_2} above 100 mm Hg. It is best if this can be achieved without the use of positive end expiratory pressure (PEEP) as it can cause elevation of ICP. Pulmonary edema or aspiration may necessitate the cautious use of PEEP.[3] Safar[3] also recommends maintaining the pH between 7.3 and 7.6.

Maintain Normothermia

The maintenance of normothermia is desired because hyperthermia increases cerebral metabolism approximately 10 percent per degree centigrade of temperature elevation.[4] Fever should be treated vigorously with external cooling measures. Pharmacological agents such as chlorpromazine may assist in fever control by inducing vasodilation and controlling shivering. Hypothalamic depression with barbiturate administration may also help control fever.[3]

Hypothermia therapy reduces cerebral metabolic rate, offering protection against ischemic damage. The temperature may be maintained at 30°–32° C for up to 12 hours, although hypothermia can be maintained for 48–72 hours.[9] Shivering is to be avoided because it causes vasoconstriction, increases cerebral metabolic rate, and leads to increases in ICP.

Hypothermia therapy has not gained widespread acceptance because of its many complications. These include an increased risk of cardiac dysrhythmias, hypotension, pH changes, and increased blood viscosity. Hypothermia therapy in conjunction with barbiturate coma therapy remains controversial.[9]

Control Seizures

Convulsive seizures can increase cerebral metabolic rates by 300–400 percent. This cerebral hyperactivity needs to be suppressed, or better still, prevented. Diazepam (Valium) and thiopental afford short-term management while phenobarbital and phenytoin (Dilantin) are used for long-term management.[4]

Phenytoin

Phenytoin may be administered prophylactically to prevent seizures and to reduce neurological deficits in the early postresuscitation period. It stabilizes neurons against hyperactivity by preventing the rise in intracellular sodium and extracellular potassium that follow ischemia-anoxia. It is also thought to increase cerebral blood flow by vasodilation, to decrease cerebral oxygen consumption, and to increase brain energy reserves of glucose, glycogen, and phosphocreatine.[16]

Phenytoin is recommended for those patients who, following resuscitation, have evidence of complete unconsciousness, dilated and unresponsive pupils, and abnormal posturing.[17] Dosage regimens vary. Up to as much as 1.0 gm has been used as an IV loading dose. Reduced doses are then given every six hours. Administration of phenytoin should always be preceded and followed by normal saline to prevent precipitation of the medication. It must not be given any faster than 50 mg per minute to avoid serious cardiovascular side effects.[17(p136)]

Diazepam

Diazepam is sometimes used in the short-term management of seizures. It may also be used to produce relaxation and sedation. Like barbiturates, it promotes de-afferentation, the reduction of sensory input into the brain. Dosage regimens vary depending on their intended use.

Control Blood Variables

Adequate oxygen carrying capacity of the blood is enhanced by maintaining the hematocrit between 30 and 35 percent. Serum electrolytes should be normalized. Serum osmolality should be maintained between 280 and 330 mosm/L to prevent additional causes of cerebral edema. Maintenance of normal albumin levels normalizes oncotic pressure and may help in tissue recovery.[11]

Fifty percent glucose may be administered during resuscitation to replenish the depleted brain glucose stores. Continuous, markedly elevated blood glucose levels are to be avoided because of potential glucose leakage through the disrupted blood-brain barrier.[12]

Reduce Cerebral Metabolic Rate

Depression of the cerebral metabolic rate for oxygen (CMR_{O_2}) is desirable for minimizing the oxygen supply/demand mismatch.

Barbiturate Therapy

Short-acting barbiturates such as thiopental sodium and pentobarbital sodium are being used increasingly in brain resuscitation. The exact mechanisms by which barbiturates afford protection to the brain and improve neuronal survival are not fully understood. It is believed that a reduction in CMR_{O_2} is not the only effect. Theories of other possible effects include supression of catecholamine-induced hypermetabolism, vasoconstriction in undamaged areas of the brain, which shunts blood to ischemic areas, and the mopping up of dangerous free chemical radicals thereby preventing destruction of cellular membranes. In addition, seizure activity is suppressed and the patient is immobilized. Barbiturates may also reduce vasogenic and cytotoxic cerebral edema.[3] Barbiturates have been demonstrated to be more beneficial in focal cerebral ischemia than in global ischemia-anoxia.[11]

Data show that high-dose barbiturate therapy (barbiturate coma therapy) may be necessary to achieve beneficial effects and should be started early. Intubation and ventilatory support are of course mandatory.

Significant side effects are associated with barbiturate coma therapy and mainly involve the cardiovascular system. Hypotension and cardiac dysrhythmias may occur and may require treatment with vasopressors and antiarrhythmics. Intraarterial pressure monitoring should be instituted.

Evaluation of neurological function is made difficult to impossible with high-dose barbiturate therapy. Barbiturates can decrease electrical activity in the brain, resulting in abnormal EEG recordings. Pupils may become constricted, but at high doses may dilate. Loss of muscle tone may occur. Glasgow Coma Scale scores of 3 are the norm.

Since intracranial hypertension is not consistently seen in global ischemia-anoxia, ICP monitoring has not been widely used in these types of patients. In the presence of intracranial hypertension, ICP monitoring would be an effective means of evaluating those therapeutic interventions aimed at reducing ICP. Of course it is not of value in evaluating neuronal function.

Dosages of thiopental or pentobarbital of up to 5 mg/kg IV followed by hourly reduced dosages to achieve and maintain a serum barbiturate level of 2–4 mg/dL have been used.[11] High loading doses of up to 30 mg/kg have been used in controlled studies.[4]

Immobilization

Barbiturates and diazepam may be additionally useful by promoting immobilization. Muscle relaxation reduces oxygen consumption, the work of breathing, intrathoracic pressure, and CVP. All of these effects contribute to ICP reduction.

Pancuronium bromide (Pavulon) is a neuromuscular blocking agent that paralyzes voluntary skeletal muscle. It interferes with the binding of acetylcholine at the motor end plate of the myoneural junction. It is often used to effect immobilization and may be preferred over other agents because it does not produce histamine release, which can increase ICP.[4] It is contraindicated in patients with myasthenia gravis. Pancuronium can induce tachycardia, so it should be administered with caution in the postcardiac arrest patient.

Since pancuronium renders the patient paralyzed and areflexive, intubation and mechanical ventilation are required. In addition, the nurse must take precautions to protect the patient's skin and corneas because of the loss of protective reflexes.

Pancuronium does not depress mental function, so if it is used in the conscious hyperactive patient, concurrent administration of sedation is indicated.

Dosages for pancuronium range from 0.04 to 0.1 mg/kg IV, followed by 0.01 mg/kg every 30–60 minutes. The onset of action is one to three minutes.[18(p351)]

Investigational Pharmacological Agents

Research continues in efforts to find effective therapeutic agents to treat brain ischemia-anoxia and the deleterious changes associated with reperfusion. Desirable agents would increase neuronal survival, yet cause minimal CNS or cardiovascular depression.[2]

Calcium Channel Blockers

Calcium channel blockers, such as nifedipine (Procardia) are receiving increased interest because of their ability to reduce vasospasm and actually dilate some cerebral arteries. These actions may help ameliorate postischemic hypoperfusion. By increasing cerebral blood flow, there is a reduction in platelet aggregation with occlusion of small vessels, a common occurrence during the reperfusion phase that follows the ischemia-anoxic insult. This may help lessen the occurrence of cerebral infarction. It is also theorized that calcium channel blockers protect neuroglia from destructive metabolic processes.[16] The possible detrimental effects of the administration of calcium products during CPR are under investigation.

Dimethyl Sulfoxide

Dimethyl sulfoxide (DMSO) has been found to have several therapeutic effects that may be useful in brain resuscitation. Among these are vasodilation, osmotic diuresis, stabilization of mitochondria, prevention of calcium release, decrease of cellular oxygen demand and consumption, decrease in ICP, and an antiplatelet action that helps prevent the occlusion of small vessels. Additional research is needed to gain a better understanding of the mechanisms involved in its apparent ability to reduce ICP as well as increase cerebral perfusion.[17]

There are some difficulties associated with the administration of DMSO in the research setting. Large volumes of fluid and salt are needed to replace the naturesis and diuresis that occurs with DMSO administration. Hyperosmolality can occur if fluids are not replaced. Electrolyte disturbances occur more frequently than with mannitol administration. Hemolysis has been reported when high concentrations are given. DMSO also requires the use of glass bottles and glass syringes that some may find inconvenient.[18]

It becomes apparent from the foregoing information that conflicting theories exist about what constitutes the best postresuscitation therapy for the brain.

Certain therapies would constrict cerebral blood vessels while others would dilate them. This controversy demonstrates that brain resuscitation has generated a high degree of interest in the medical scientific community. In time, researchers and clinicians will surely show us the correct path to follow.

NURSING RESPONSIBILITIES

Exciting challenges face the nurse participating in brain resuscitation. Competent cardiovascular as well as neurological skills are needed in providing care for these patients. The nurse must understand the pathophysiological events that have occurred as a result of cardiac arrest to better understand the implications for and evaluation of therapeutic interventions. Neurological assessments during and following cardiac arrest are vital. Specific nursing responsibilities in providing intensive brain care were covered in detail in Chapter 4.

Well-informed nurses can be influential patient advocates by encouraging CPCR and not just CPR for victims of cardiac arrest.

In responding to the needs of the patient's family or significant others, the nurse should anticipate their feelings of fear, anxiety, grief, disbelief, and, possibly, guilt. Verbalization should be encouraged, with all questions answered honestly. Share with them the difficulty encountered in predicting ultimate outcome and/or survival. Offer hope, but do not encourage denial. Providing privacy and comfort needs will be greatly appreciated by family members. Try to identify the quality of the family's support system, and enlist the assistance of clergy, social service personnel, or counselors if indicated.

REFERENCES

1. Safar P: Introduction: On the evolution of brain resuscitation. *Crit Care Med* 1978;6:199–202.

2. Safar P: Dynamics of brain resuscitation after ischemia anoxia. *Hosp Pract*, February 1981, pp 67–72.

3. Safar P, Bleyaert A, Nemoto E, et al: Resuscitation after global brain ischemia-anoxia. *Crit Care Med* 1978;6:215–225.

4. Abramson N: Brain function in resuscitology. *Curr Top Emerg Med* 1981;1(no5).

5. Siesjo B, Carlsson C, Hagerdal M: Brain metabolism in the critically ill. *Crit Care Med* 1976;4:283–292.

6. Nemoto E: Pathogenesis of cerebral ischemia-anoxia. *Crit Care Med* 1978;6:202–212.

7. DeBard M: Predictors in brain resuscitation. *Crit Care Q* 1983;5:91–97.

8. Rudy EB: *Advanced Neurological and Neurosurgical Nursing*. St Louis, Mosby, 1984.

9. Jagger J, Bobovsky J: Nonpharmacologic therapeutic modalities. *Crit Care Q* 1983;5:31–39.

10. Barson W: Pharmacologic therapeutic modalities: Barbiturates. *Crit Care Q* 1983;5:63–69.

11. Safar P: Recent advances in cardiopulmonary-cerebral resuscitation: A review. *Ann Emerg Med* 1984;9:856–860.

12. Eilers M: Pharmacologic therapeutic modalities: Osmotic and diuretic agents. *Crit Care Q* 1983;5:44–50.

13. Marshall LF, Shapiro HM, Rauscher AL: Mannitol dose requirements in brain injured patients. *J Neurosurg* 1978;48:169–172.

14. Walleck C: Central nervous system effects postresuscitation. Presented before the American Association Of Critical Care Nurses National Teaching Institute, Dallas, 1984.

15. Hoffman JR, Orban DJ, Podolsky S: Pharmacologic therapeutic modalities: Corticosteroids. *Crit Care Q* 1983;5:52–59.

16. Aldrete JA, Romo-Salas F: Phenytoin for brain resuscitation post cardiac arrest: An uncontrolled clinical trial. *Crit Care Med* 1980;6:474–477.

17. Martin M: Pharmacologic therapeutic modalities: Phenytoin, dimethyl sulfoxide, and calcium channel blockers. *Crit Care Q* 1983;5:72–79.

18. Wagner M (ed director): *Nursing 82 Drug Handbook*. Springhouse, Pa, Intermed Communications, 1982.

19. Marshall LF, Bowers SA: Medical management of intracranial pressure, in Cooper PR (ed): *Head Injury*. Baltimore, Williams & Wilkins, 1982, pp 129–144.

Chapter 6

Brain Death and Organ Donation

BRAIN DEATH

The determination of death has persistently presented considerable controversy for the medical, legal, and theological communities. For centuries the cessation of breathing was considered the indicator of death. With the advent of auscultation, death was determined by the absence of heart sounds and palpable pulse.[1]

Effective cardiopulmonary resuscitation (CPR) came into widespread use in the middle of the 20th century. Common law then defined death as the cessation of the vital functions of respiration, heart beat, and circulation.[2] With successful restoration of cardiac function and mechanical maintenance of respiratory function now possible, it became obvious that many ''successfully'' resuscitated patients were left with nonfunctioning or ''dead'' brains.

Increased attention then became focused on redefining criteria for determining death based on cessation of brain function as well as cessation of respiratory and cardiac function. These efforts were spurred on by the increasing demand for donor organs for expanding organ transplantation programs. Legal and ethical issues relating to organ donation necessitated more than a common-law approach to the determination of death.

In 1968 the Uniform Anatomical Gift Act was adopted, which made brain death the standard of death when dealing with donor/donee situations.[3] In responding to a continued need for a brain death standard to be used in other situations, the medical community enlisted the assistance of a Harvard University Ad Hoc Committee to Examine the Definition of Brain Death. The Harvard Criteria for Determining Brain Death was published in 1968 and eventually became a widely accepted standard for determining brain death. It states, in brief, that irreversible coma or brain death exists if there is (1) absence of reflexes, (2) absence of spontaneous respirations or muscular movements, and (3) unresponsiveness to externally applied stimuli and inner need. Further diagnostic studies such as eletroencephalogram (EEG), computed tomography (CT) scan, and radioisotope tests were frequently done to confirm the diagnosis of brain death. These tests were often repeated 24 hours later to confirm that no change had occurred. These additional tests supported decisions to terminate life support systems.[3] While this additional testing continues to be used, controversy exists about the need to repeat the tests and the minimum time interval between tests.

Uniform Determination of Death Act

In 1980 the National Conference of Commissioners on Uniform State Laws passed the Uniform Determination of Death Act, which includes many aspects of the Harvard Medical School's criteria. This expanded definition of brain death states:

> An individual who has sustained either 1) irreversible cessation of circulatory and respiratory function, or 2) irreversible cessation of all functions of the entire brain, is dead. A determination of death must be made in accordance with accepted medical standards.[4(p257)]

Note that this act states irreversible cessation of *all* functions of the *entire* brain. Patients with functional loss of the cerebral cortex but with intact life sustaining reflexes of the brainstem are not considered brain dead and are known to be capable of existing in persistent vegetative states.[3]

According to the Uniform Determination of Death Act, two groups of criteria exist and physicians can apply either or both depending on the clinical situation. In cases where respiration and circulation have irreversibly ceased, in-depth assessment of brain function is unnecessary. When circulation and/or respiratory function are artificially maintained, it becomes paramount that brain functions be carefully assessed. Only when brain functions have been determined to have irreversibly ceased can death be determined.

Determination of Brain Death

Brain death exists when there is irreversible cessation of all functions of the entire brain, including the brainstem. To confirm cessation of all functions of the brain, certain evaluations can be performed that will demonstrate cessation of function of the cortex, while other methods will demonstrate cessation of brainstem function.

Absence of Cerebral Cortical Function

Confirmation of cortical death can be made by three methods: the clinical neurological examination, electroencephalography, and cerebral blood flow studies.

The Neurological Exam. The neurological exam will reveal the patient to be in deep coma, with no verbal response and no response to stimuli such as light, noise, motion, or deep pain.[4(p258)] Some spinal reflexes may remain, but should not be interpreted as evidence of brain functioning.

Electroencephalogram. Circumstances and individual institutional protocols may require additional confirmation of brain death through the recording of one or two (24 hours apart) EEGs demonstrating electrocerebral silence (isoelectric). The EEG is always silent in brain death, but electrocerebral silence does not always mean brain death.[2]

Cerebral Blood Flow Studies. The absence of cerebral function can also be demonstrated by four vessel angiography which demonstrates an absence of cerebral blood flow. This test however is not without risk to the critically ill patient. Radioisotope studies can also demonstrate the absence of cerebral blood flow and testing can be performed at the bedside at less risk to the patient.[4] An isotope is injected intravenously and the brain is scanned. Absence of the appearance of the isotope in the brain confirms the absence of cerebral blood flow.

Absence of Brainstem Function

The absence of brainstem function can be evaluated by the neurological examination and by apnea testing. Additional confirmation can be obtained through testing for evoked responses.

The Neurological Exam. The neurological exam of the brain-dead patient will reveal deep coma and absence of pupillary responses to light, ciliospinal reflex, and oculocephalic and oculovestibular reflexes. Of course all other brainstem reflexes will also be absent (corneal, gag, cough, etc.).[2]

Apnea Testing. Apnea, or cessation of respiration, must be confirmed. This is done by removing ventilatory support for three or more minutes until the $Paco_2$ rises to 55–60 mm Hg. In previously hypocapneic patients this may take up to 10–15 minutes. To help allay the fear of inducing further brain hypoxia, passive administration of 100 percent oxygen may be done simultaneously. A $Paco_2$ level of 55 mm Hg should stimulate the respiratory centers in the brainstem to resume spontaneous respirations if they remain viable. Absence of the return of spontaneous respirations helps confirm brainstem death.[2]

Evoked Response Testing. Some physicians include a test of the brainstem auditory evoked response (BAER) to help determine brain death. An auditory stimulus is delivered to the ear and surface electrodes on the scalp record any electrical evoked responses. When combined with the other criteria for brain death, the absence of BAERs is consistent with brain death.[3]

Special Consideration in Determining Brain Death

The nature of any comatose state must first be determined to rule out any reversible causes such as CNS-depressant drugs or metabolic state, neuromuscular blockade, hypothermia, or shock. Certain CNS-depressant drugs and profound hypothermia can cause prolonged unconsciousness, loss of reflexes, and at times have produced isoelectric EEG recordings.[5]

It is also important to remember that the brains of infants and young children, especially those under the age of 5 years, have an increased resistance to damage and have a greater ability to recover function after exhibiting unresponsiveness than do the brains of adults. Extra care must be taken in determining brain death in infants and young children.[5]

Nursing Responsibilities

The nursing staff plays an important role in brain death. It is often the nurse who initiates discussion among medical team members about the need for a brain death determination. Nurses may also assist in performing brain death tests. Advanced technical skills are required to provide intensive nursing care, and psychosocial skills are needed to provide the patient's family with empathy and understanding. In addition, nurses must deal with their own feelings about the moral, ethical, and legal issues involved in brain death.

Medical-Legal Implications

Nurses participating in procedures to determine brain death need to be aware of their potential liability.

Most states have adopted the Uniform Determination of Death Act or have similar statutes, but variations exist and medical personnel need to be familiar with the laws or statutes of the state in which they practice. For instance, it may be necessary to have brain death confirmed by a second physician, especially if the patient is to serve as an organ donor. Generally, the criteria for determining brain death are left up to medical experts and must meet the standards of medical practice in the community. Also, individual medical institutions may set additional criteria of their own for the determination of brain death.

Nurses must be familiar with their own institution's policies and procedures and strictly abide by these in their clinical practice. The nurse must accurately document physical assessment data and the patient's responses or lack of responses to tests performed to determine brain death.

Often the decision to determine brain death is made after the patient is in the intensive care unit. It is here that the patient's family and physician may reach an agreement to not resuscitate the patient or declare the patient a ''no code.'' Nurses should accept only written ''no code'' orders from a physician. This may require active participation on the part of nurses to sit on appropriate committees within the hospital that create policies and procedures dealing with patient care.

If a decision is made by the physician and the patient's family to terminate life support systems, it is imperative that all members of the medical team understand the medical-legal implications of such action. The termination of life support systems in patients who are declared brain dead differs medical-legally from the termination of life support systems in patients who have altered states of consciousness but who are not brain dead.[2]

The emergence of the concept of the living will has added controversy to the issue of discontinuing or withholding resuscitation from patients who have declared their right to decide how they would like to die. Not all states recognize living wills. Furthermore, if the patient is unresponsive, family members can disagree about whether or not to continue resuscitation efforts. The attending physician, in conference with the patient's next of kin, should make the decision of whether to allow the patient to die. Emergency medical personnel should make all possible resuscitation efforts in the absence of these decisions.

Physical Care

Until a determination of brain death is made, the nurse continues to provide intensive brain care and supportive nursing care with the goal of preserving remaining functional body systems. Prevention of respiratory failure and infection are primary concerns. The nurse also anticipates the loss of autonomic regulation and resulting alterations in blood pressure, cardiac rhythm, and temperature control.

An isoelectric EEG in the presence of drug intoxication or hypothermia is not a valid measure of brain death. It is not uncommon for a patient to become hypothermic preceding death. The nurse must then use external warming devices to restore normothermia or near normothermia before obtaining the EEG.[5] The potential for organ donation should be considered, and once brain death has been confirmed, should be pursued.

Nursing Interventions for the Grieving Family

When devastating neurological injury and brain death occurs suddenly, family members have not had the opportunity to prepare themselves or work through the stages of grief. They may display emotional reactions ranging from sobbing, to fainting, to stunned silence.[6] Emergency department medical personnel have not had the opportunity to establish a caring, trusting relationship with the family and are probably not the best qualified, at that time, to deal with the many needs of family members. Staff social workers, counselors, or clergymen may be better qualified to provide this necessary emotional and spiritual comfort. Information about the patient's condition and what is being done should be communicated frequently to the family. This reassures the family that the medical personnel are interested and concerned and are doing everything possible to save the life of the family's loved one.

It is important for nurses and physicians to realize that they also experience some degree of loss and grief when caring for this type of patient. Staff members with good working relationships can be effective in providing mutual support. It is comforting for nurses and physicians to reassure one another that each did everything possible to save the patient. Periodic meetings with counselors or psychiatric nurses may also be beneficial for the emergency department staff.

ORGAN DONATION

Each year, tens of thousands of people in the United States need organ transplants. While there are at least 17 transplantable organs or tissues, we are most aware of the needs for blood products, kidneys, livers, hearts, lungs, corneas, pancreas, bone, and skin. Most organ transplant needs go unmet.

Attitudes Affecting Organ Donation

The lack of sufficient organ donors can be attributed to many factors. Historically, the removal of one's organs before or after death has been a controversial issue, culturally, morally, and ideologically. The resistance to the medical ''spare parts'' program comes mainly from deep-seated feelings about the body. People of many religions who believe in an afterlife still may harbor beliefs that to lose a limb, organ, or cornea is to enter the next life maimed.

The population in general may still not fully accept and understand the concept of brain death and there may be refusal on the part of the family to allow organ donation from a loved one. There is also hesitation and a lack of awareness in the medical community caused by dislike in discussing such matters with a family at a time of intense grief, lack of knowledge of procedures to follow, difficulty perceiving the patient as merely an organ donor, lack of time, and concern regarding legal matters.[7] The legal position may be so unclear and the emotions so involved that hospital personnel and physicians often find it easier to fail to obtain donor organs, at the expense of a potential recipient's life.

Uniform Anatomical Gift Act

The Uniform Anatomical Gift Act, enacted in 1968, has since been adopted in some form by all 50 states. This act legally provides for persons aged 18 years or older to donate their bodies or certain organs or tissues for the purposes of transplantation or other scientific uses. This act also authorizes the next of kin (in order of priority starting with the spouse, then an adult son or daughter, either parent, an adult brother or sister, a guardian of the decedent, or any other person authorized to dispose of the body) to grant authority. This intent is made known in the form of a signed document, witnessed by two people. The Uniform Donor Card can be carried with the driver's license and provides legal authorization to remove organs. While this ''pocket will'' is a legal document, transplant centers feel a moral obligation to also obtain permission from the legal next of kin.

Recognizing the Potential Organ Donor

Critical care nurses in emergency departments and intensive care units can play a primary role in facilitating organ donation by recognizing potential organ donors. General criteria for various organ donors are summarized in Table 6–1.

A study by Stark et al[7] noted that a nurse was the first person to recognize the patient as an organ donor in 44 percent of the cases. A physician first recognized the patient as an organ donor in thirty-three percent of the cases. They also pointed out that families of donor patients are relatively unable to recognize the potential for organ donation, being either unaware of the criteria for organ donation, or so grief stricken that thoughts of organ donation do not occur.

Often by the time a potential donor is identified and a decision to donate is made, it becomes too late, for medical reasons, to harvest the organs. Intensive medical intervention can often maintain the viability of transplantable organs while the diagnosis of brain death is being made and the decision to allow organ donation is being reached.

Medical personnel need to be able to identify potential organ donors and to recognize that the same donor can donate many organs. Even though a patient may not meet the criteria for kidney donation, the same patient may well be suitable as a heart, bone, skin, and/or eye donor.

Facilitating Organ Donation

As soon as it is recognized that the patient may be appropriate for organ donation, the regional transplant center or transplant coordinator should be notified. The transplant coordinator can provide information about legalities, will often speak to the family of the potential donor, assist in obtaining necessary permissions, and facilitate the process of screening of donors.

Although the transplant team cannot be involved in the direct care of the donor patient, the ICU team will often respond to suggestions for interventions to maintain organ function.

Table 6–1 Criteria for Organ Donors[7,9]

Organ	Age of Donor	Disqualifying Conditions
Kidney	1½–55 years	Active hepatitis within the past 6 months History of hypertension Untreated systemic infection Neoplasm (other than intracranial) Significant diabetes Poor renal function* Diseased or damaged kidneys
Heart	Male: 15–35 years Female: 15–40 years (Height and weight of donor is most important)	Active hepatitis within the past 6 months History of myocardial infarction, heart trauma, or other heart disease or anomaly Untreated infection Neoplastic disease Long-term pulmonary artery catheter placement
Liver	6 months to 45 years	Active hepatitis within the past 6 months Diseased or damaged liver Neoplastic disease Untreated infection Long-term alcohol abuse
Eyes†	Any age	Active hepatitis within the past 6 months Damaged corneas or frontal eye neoplasms Any infectious disease needs to be evaluated
Skin‡	16–70 years (Depends on skin condition)	Active hepatitis within the past 6 months Jaundice Untreated systemic infection Untreated venereal disease Malignancy (other than intracranial) Skin disease Skin conditions unsuitable for cutting split thickness grafts
Bone§	18–45 years	Active hepatitis within the past 6 months Jaundice Untreated infection or venereal disease Cancer (other than intracranial)

*A period of hypotension or oliguria is acceptable provided that resuscitation is followed by normal renal function.

†Eyes can be taken for donation up to 4 hours after death, but the sooner the better.

‡Skin can be taken up to 12 hours after death, but the sooner the better.

§Bone can also be taken after death.

Supportive Measures for Major Organ Donors

Supportive medical measures are taken to maintain homeostasis and perfusion of organs so that they remain in optimum physiological condition. Urinary output should be maintained at a minimum of 50 ml per hour. This is usually ensured if the patient is adequately hydrated and the kidneys are being well perfused. If perfusion cannot be maintained in spite of adequate hydration, vasopressors should be considered. Intropin (dopamine) is the preferred drug because it does not decrease renal blood flow except at high doses. Vasopressors that decrease renal blood flow, such as metaraminol bitartrate (Aramine) and levarterenol bitartrate (Levophed), are to be avoided if possible.[8]

Administration of mannitol and/or furosemide may be needed to ensure adequate urinary output and protection against acute tubular necrosis. Pitressin may be needed if the patient develops diabetes insipidus. The patient is closely observed and treated for any electrolyte imbalance. Rising levels of blood urea nitrogen (BUN) and creatinine may make the patient an unacceptable kidney donor.[8]

In addition to the aforementioned, arterial blood gases and cardiac enzymes are monitored in the potential heart donor.[9] In potential liver donors, the serum glutamic-oxaloacetic transaminase (SGOT), serum glutamic-pyruvic transaminase (SGPT), lactic dehydrogenase (LDH), and bilirubin levels are monitored.[9]

Strict measures are taken to protect all organs against potential infectious processes. Culture and sensitivity tests should be done on any suspicious drainage. Prophylactic antibiotics are sometimes used. The nurse maintains strict aseptic technique when handling vascular invasive lines, catheters, endotracheal tubes, wounds, etc. All unnecessary invasive lines should be removed.[9]

Eye Care

Eyes as well as skin and bone are body tissues that can be obtained from a deceased person, although harvesting of eyes must be carried out within four hours of death. If the patient is to be an eye donor for corneal transplant or other purposes, special consideration is given to protecting the eyes from injury and infection. The eyes must be kept moist with artificial tears or sterile saline. At the time of death the eyes should be moistened with a few drops of sterile saline or artificial tears, taped shut, and covered with light ice packs.[9]

Each organ donor referred to the transplant coordinator is evaluated on an individual basis. Lymphocyte typing is started as soon as next-of-kin permission has been granted or has been determined likely to be granted.

Requesting an Organ Donation

The patient's family is approached about organ donation only after the physician makes them aware of the patient's prognosis. Sometimes family members offer clues to their potential willingness to consent to organ donation by making statements such as, "he was always so willing to help others" or "what a wasted life." Ask family members if they had ever considered organ donation. They may find comfort in being told that their loved one's life is, in a way, being continued by giving the gift of life to another through organ donation. If the family expresses the desire for spiritual support, a clergyman should be summoned. Most major religious groups are not opposed to organ donation. The majority of families will consent to organ donation from their loved one if approached in a sensitive, sincere manner. They realize that the giving of life to another through organ donation may be the only positive thing to come out of a tragic situation.

Families may have questions about disfigurement, especially if skin is donated. They should be reassured that the removal of donated organs does not cause disfigurement of the body and does not interfere with funeral arrangements. Skin is removed at a thickness similar to that of a sunburn peel, is not taken from any exposed areas, and does not interfere with open viewing of the deceased.

The family should also be assured that the patient incurs no added costs because of organ donation. Generally, the transplant recipient or the transplant hospital incurs the cost of organ procurement, not the donor hospital or donor patient. These costs may include tests, drugs and fluids specifically requested by the transplant team, operating room costs, and surgeon and anesthesiologist fees for harvesting the organs.[9]

Conclusion

Attitudes and beliefs about brain death and organ donation are changing, but many medical personnel and clergy remain ignorant of or indifferent to the need for donor organs. These same people should be leading and educating the public about these critical issues. The national government has become actively involved in issues related to organ transplant technology. Among several items called for by the National Organ Transplant Act (PL 98-507) of 1984 is the establishment of the Organ Procurement and Transplantation Network which will maintain a national registry of persons awaiting transplantation, and a system to match available organs with these persons.[10]

Critical care nurses in EDs and ICUs can exert leadership roles by making people more aware of the need for donor organs. Critical care nurses caring for patients with neurological trauma must understand brain death and the importance of organ transplant needs. The nurse often needs to remind the physician of this need. Adept nursing care has kept many patients stable and free from sepsis until brain death is declared, making a potential donor an actual one. The nurse can establish a trusting relationship with the family members. In this way the family can be supported in reaching their decision, realizing that their decision to allow their loved one's organs to be donated can bring comfort to them and may lessen their grief.

REFERENCES

1. Walker EA: Current concepts of brain death. *J Neurosurg Nurs* 1983;15:261–264.

2. Daly K: The diagnosis of brain death: Overview of neurosurgical nursing responsibilities. *J Neurosurg Nurs* 1982;14:85–89.

3. Brent NJ: Uniform Determination of Death Act: Implications for nursing practice. *J Neurosurg Nurs* 1983;15:265–267.

4. Rudy EB: *Advanced Neurological and Neurosurgical Nursing.* St Louis, Mosby, 1984, pp 257–259.

5. Guidelines for the Determination of Death: Report of the Medical Consultants on the Diagnosis of Death to the President's Commission for the Study of Ethical Problems in Medicine and Biomedical and Behavioral Research. *Crit Care Med* 1982;10:62–64.

6. Taylor JW, Ballenger S: *Neurological Dysfunctions and Nursing Intervention.* New York, McGraw-Hill, 1980, p 324.

7. Stark JL, Reiley P, Osiecki A, et al: Attitudes affecting organ donation in the intensive care unit. *Heart Lung* 1984;13:400–404.

8. Reiley PJ: Organ donation, in Millar S, Sampson LK, Soukup M, et al (eds): *Methods in Critical Care: The AACN Manual.* Philadelphia, WB Saunders, 1980, pp 463–467.

9. *Cadaver Donor Protocol.* San Diego, San Diego and Imperial Counties Regional Transplant Center, University Hospital, UCSD Medical Center, 1981.

10. *AACN News.* American Association of Critical-Care Nurses Vol II, No. 6, July 1985.

Chapter 7

Neurological Infections

There are an almost infinite number of bacterial, viral, and fungal processes that can affect the nervous system. Only those most commonly seen in the emergency department are discussed in this chapter.

BACTERIAL MENINGITIS

Bacterial meningitis is essentially an infection of the pia and arachnoid meningeal coverings (leptomeninges) that surround the brain, spinal cord, and optic nerves,[1] and thus may be referred to as a cerebrospinal infection. The infection spreads rapidly throughout the subarachnoid spaces and into the cerebral ventricles.

The most common infectious agents are (1) *Hemophilus influenzae,* (2) meningococcus (*Neisseria meningitidis*), and (3) pneumococcus (*Streptococcus pneumoniae*). Staphylococci, streptococci, *Klebsiella,* and other organisms may also be seen, usually when meningitis is a complication of head injury, brain surgery, or other invasive procedures.[1,2] Children are the most common victims of meningitis, although pneumococcal meningitis is seen frequently in older adults. Epidemics of meningitis tend to be seasonal, occurring most often during the cold months.

Pathophysiology

Bacteria invade the nervous system by extension from contiguous areas such as the ears, sinuses, mastoids, or skull, or by infected emboli or thrombi in the circulating blood.[1,3] Sources for emboli may be the lungs, heart, or major blood vessels. Even though the common pathogens are found in the nose and throat of many healthy individuals, most do not contract meningitis. It is assumed that bacteria spread into the meninges only when there is some breakdown of tissue or disruption of the blood-brain barrier by an initial viral infection.

The mortality rate for meningitis remains 5–15 percent and is even higher in infants and neonates.[1] With fulminating disease, death occurs from vasomotor collapse, septic shock, adrenal hemorrhage (Waterhouse-Friderichsen syndrome), or respiratory failure.

Pathological changes early in the disease include hyperemia of the meningeal vessels and an inflammatory reaction with exudate of white blood cells into the subarachnoid spaces. This purulent exudate collects around the base of the brain and may extend into the sheaths of the cranial and spinal nerves, and even into the perivascular spaces of the cortex, resulting in an associated encephalitis.[2] The exudates draining into the ventricles may cause blockage of the tiny connecting pathways, resulting in hydrocephalus. Inflammation and irritation cause brain swelling and increased intracranial pressure, thus compounding the danger of permanent brain damage.[2]

With early and adequate treatment, the inflammatory cells begin to decrease, intracranial pressure returns to normal, and exudates are absorbed. There may be complete resolution with little or no residual damage. However, if the disease continues for several weeks, formation of fibrous tissue (scarring) occurs in the arachnoid layers, leading to permanent hydrocephalus with severe mental retardation. If fibrosis forms around the cranial or spinal nerves, there may be permanent blindness, deafness, ocular palsies, or paralyses.[3,4]

Clinical Features

The initial signs and symptoms of bacterial meningitis may include fever, severe headache, photophobia, confusion, obtundation, or seizures. There will usually be signs of meningeal irritation such as nuchal rigidity and inability to completely extend the legs (Kernig's sign). In addition, many patients will have a petechial or purpuric rash with ecchymosis and lividity of the skin in the lower extremities.[1] Less often there will be focal neurological signs such as ocular palsies, facial weakness, blindness, or deafness.

In infants and young children the classic signs and symptoms may be absent or difficult to elicit. The child may have a high fever or an abnormally low temperature; may be irritable or listless and display a shrill cry; may be vomiting; may have bulging fontanels; or may have seizures.

As the disease progresses, the patient will show increasing evidence of high intracranial pressure with deepening coma, papilledema, respiratory irregularities, and even decorticate or decerebrate posturing. Inappropriate secretion of antidiuretic hormone with hyponatremia or diabetes insipidus with hypernatremia are not uncommon complications. Death occurs from respiratory failure, septic shock, or circulatory collapse.[1]

The differential diagnosis of meningitis depends on the results of a lumbar puncture and examination of cerebrospinal fluid (CSF). When intracranial pressure is elevated (and especially when a mass lesion is present) a lumbar puncture can precipitate cerebral herniation. Therefore, in cases where increased intracranial pressure is suspected, computed tomography (CT) scanning may be done before a lumbar puncture is performed.

CSF findings consistent with meningitis include the following:[1,3,4]

- Elevated CSF pressure (180–400 mm H_2O)
- Elevated white blood cell (WBC) count (1000–100,000/mm)
- Elevated protein (above 50 mg/mL)
- Decreased glucose (below 40 mg/dL)
- Decreased chloride (usually below 700 mg/dL)
- Positive gram stain for causative organism
- Positive culture for causative organism
- Cloudy or turbid CSF

In addition, blood cultures; nose and throat cultures; and chest, skull, and sinus films may be helpful in identifying an underlying infectious process, which may also require therapy. Elevated serum enzymes may indicate progressing brain damage and may also have prognostic value.[1,4]

Medical and Nursing Management

Management of the patient with bacterial meningitis is directed toward adequate antibiotic therapy, control of intracranial pressure, and respiratory and circulatory support. Since the prognosis for morbidity and mortality depends on rapid resolution (before permanent brain damage has occurred), diagnostic procedures must be expedited so that appropriate therapy can be initiated. Usually a ten-day course of parenteral or intrathecal antibiotics is required. If fever or other symptoms persist, a longer course may be indicated.

Intracranial pressure is treated with hyperosmolar diuretic agents such as mannitol. Fever should be aggressively managed with cooling blankets and antipyretic agents. Headache is controlled with analgesics. Seizures should be controlled (see Chapter 16). Intubation and ventilatory support may be needed as well as drugs to maintain blood pressure.

Nursing care includes careful ongoing assessment so that late complications such as hydrocephalus or brain abscess will be recognized early. Nursing care may need to be given in a darkened room because of the patient's severe photophobia. Reduction in stimuli helps to prevent seizures and control intracranial pressure.

The most infectious period for meningitis is during the prodromal stage and before antibiotic therapy has been initiated. The need for isolation of the patient to protect health-care personnel, visitors, and other patients depends on the type of invading organism and the stage of the illness. Therefore, any patient coming into the emergency department who has a high fever and other evidence of meningitis should be isolated from other patients. Special care is taken against infecting others with secretions from the nasopharynx and droplets from the respiratory tract. Good handwashing technique must be maintained along with other techniques to minimize cross contamination.[2]

Because many of the victims are children, and serious sequelae are common, family members will need supportive care and counseling throughout the illness.

ASEPTIC VIRAL MENINGITIS

A relatively benign condition, sometimes referred to as benign lymphocytic meningitis, may resemble bacterial meningitis in the early stage, and may appear in epidemic form. Children are the most common victims, but the condition may appear at any age and often breaks out in families.[4]

A variety of viral agents may be responsible, and often the precise organism is never established. Enteroviral infections, infectious mononucleosis, nonparalytic polio, mumps, herpes simplex infections (Epstein-Barr virus), and hepatitis may all be involved. The pathological changes usually involve only the meninges, although there may be a mild associated encephalitis. The course is usually benign, with gradual recovery over a week or two and without residual effects. The patient often will feel tired and depressed for several weeks after the acute phase of the disease appears to have ended.[4]

Clinical Features

The history may include an upper respiratory infection, mumps, or other infection prior to the onset of neurological signs. Signs and symptoms include fever, photophobia, headache, backache, nuchal rigidity, and sometimes confusion and somnolence. Especially in children there may be a papulomacular rash on the head and neck or grayish-white spots on the mucous membranes of the mouth.[1,4]

Findings on lumbar puncture will usually show normal pressure, elevated WBC count, normal or slightly elevated protein levels, normal glucose levels, and the CSF may appear clear. It is rare to find the organism in the spinal fluid.

Medical and Nursing Management

There is no specific treatment, so the management is largely supportive, once the diagnosis is established. As with bacterial meningitis, the patient may need protection from bright lights and other environmental stimuli. Food and fluids should be given as tolerated, with particular attention to avoiding dehydration caused by fever and vomiting. Mild analgesics will usually be adequate to control headache and backache. It may be best to avoid aspirin, particularly in children, since there is evidence that connects aspirin with the onset of Reye's syndrome.

Meticulous nursing care is designed to maintain comfort and to prevent complications and intercurrent infections. Family members and staff may need to be protected from exposure to secretions and body excreta, but other isolation precautions are not required.

REYE'S SYNDROME

Reye's syndrome is an acute toxic encephalopathy most often seen in children.[5] The disease has a very high mortality rate, and a high rate of permanent brain damage in survivors. The prognosis improves markedly with early diagnosis and aggressive treatment. The cause is unknown, but the onset is usually associated with an antecedent viral infection such as an upper respiratory infection, gastroenteritis, or chicken pox (varicella).[5] The possibility exists that an interaction between the virus and an unidentified toxin is the cause of the disease. Aspirin and perhaps other medications used during the prodromal illness have also been linked to onset of the illness [5] (For this reason, aspirin should not be prescribed for the minor illnesses of childhood.)

Pathophysiology

While the exact cause remains problematical, it is believed that the pathology involves an injury to the mitochondria of the cell with compromise of the metabolic pathways within affected tissues.[1,5,6] Pathological changes are seen in almost every body system, and include:[1,5]

- The brain is edematous, with vascular congestion and vascular degeneration.
- The liver is swollen and increases in weight, with evidence of fatty deposits.
- The kidneys are infiltrated with fatty droplets.
- There are fatty deposits in the bundle of His and bundle branches of the heart, and petechiae may be seen throughout the epicardium.

Clinical Features

Several days after the onset of a nonspecific viral illness, the child begins to vomit. This is followed shortly by mild to severe changes in mental status, which may vary from somnolence to restlessness, hyperactivity to delirium. There may also be sympathetic nervous system signs such as diaphoresis, tachycardia, pupil dilation, and tachypnea. Papilledema may be present or may develop as the cerebral edema persists. The liver is usually enlarged, and gastrointestinal bleeding is common. The child may have seizures, and may alternate between hypertonicity and hypotonicity, with decortication and decerebrate posturing.[1,5]

Laboratory findings include a high serum ammonia, elevated liver enzymes and creatine phosphokinase (CPK), elevated blood urea nitrogen (BUN) and creatinine, prolonged clotting time, hypoglycemia, increased free fatty acids, respiratory alkalosis, and metabolic acidosis. Cerebrospinal fluid (CSF) studies are usually normal except for elevated pressure.[5]

Medical and Nursing Management

Recovery from Reye's syndrome depends both on the severity of the disease and on early and aggressive treatment. Management is based on the need to protect the brain from permanent damage and to support other organ functions during the acute phase of the disease.[5] Control of intracranial pressure (see Chapter 4), restoration of fluid and electrolyte balance, and correction of hypoglycemia and hyperammoniemia take high priority. Meticulous nursing care to prevent complications is essential. The critical nature of the illness and the fact that most of the victims are young children accentuates the need for family support and teaching. Children who survive the acute phase of the illness may need a protracted period of rehabilitation.

TETANUS (LOCKJAW)

Tetanus is one of several diseases believed to result from a bacterial toxin. The organism associated with tetanus is an anaerobic, spore-forming rod, *Clostridium tetani*. This organism is a common contaminant of soil and animal excreta. The spores may remain dormant for extended periods until introduced into a wound, where they produce a toxin that invades the nervous system. The incubation period may be from a few days to several weeks.

With modern methods of immunization, tetanus has become relatively rare in developed countries. When it is seen in the United States it is most often the result of the use of contaminated needles by users of illicit drugs.[1]

It is believed that the offending toxin enters the nervous system either by direct invasion along the neuronal sheaths or through the blood and lymph. The exact mode of action is poorly understood, but the toxin appears to act in a manner similar to strychnine, interfering with the inhibitory neurons within the reflex arc at both spinal cord and brainstem levels.[1] There may also be a direct effect on the skeletal muscles, the sympathetic nervous system, and the hypothalamus.[1]

The disease does not result in permanent damage to either the nerves or muscles, and patients who survive recover completely unless anoxia becomes severe enough to cause brain damage. Death is usually due to asphyxia or circulatory collapse.

Clinical Features

Tetanus can occur in either a localized or generalized form. The localized disease may become generalized as the disease progresses. There may be a history of injury or drug use, or an injury may have been so slight as to be forgotten.

The localized form affects the muscles in the area of the wound, beginning with involuntary muscle twitching followed by brief spasms. The spasms may then become continuous, resulting in rigidity, which may be referred to as hypertonic contraction or tetanic spasm. In addition to the continuous state of rigidity, any stimulation of the area may cause brief but intense and painful spasms. The symptoms may persist for weeks and then gradually recede; complete recovery is the norm.

When the localized form affects the facial and ocular muscles, it is referred to as cephalic tetanus. Cephalic tetanus usually follows a wound of the head or face and has a very short incubation period.[1] The facial and ocular muscles may be weak, preventing voluntary movement, but contraction occurs during periods of spasm. The spasms involve the tongue and throat, causing persistent difficulty with eating and speaking.

Generalized tetanus causes trismus (inability to open the mouth because of spasms of the muscles of mastication). The patient will also have a fever and rapidly developing stiffness, spasm of bulbar muscles, neck, trunk, and limbs. The entire body becomes rigid with legs hyperextended, a boardlike abdomen, lips pursed and retracted (risus sardonicus), eyes partially closed, and eyebrows elevated.[1] Every slight stimulus percipitates paroxysms of severe, extremely painful tonic contractures, which are sometimes referred to as tetanic seizures or convulsions. These differ from epileptic seizures in that consciousness is not lost. During these episodes the patient's back will arch (opisthotonus), arms flex and adduct, legs extend, and fists clench. Spasms of the glottis, larynx, and muscles of respiration may lead to asphyxiation or respiratory arrest. The effects of the toxin on the sympathetic nervous system may lead to circulatory collapse and death.

Diagnosis is made from the history and clinical picture. There are no definitive laboratory or other diagnostic tests. The symptoms are similar to those seen in strychnine poisoning and have some elements in common with rabies, black widow spider bites, and extrapyramidal disease.

Medical and Nursing Management

Emergency department personnel are, of course, particularly aware of the need to prevent the development of tetanus. Everyone should be immunized for tetanus and should have a regular booster injection of tetanus toxoid. Any patient with a deep wound (particularly with the possibility of contamination) should receive tetanus immune globulin, or tetanus antitoxin if the former is not available. Those with clean minor wounds should receive tetanus toxoid if it has been more than ten years since their last immunization.[7] Tetanus immune globulin may also need to be administered in addition to tetanus toxoid to patients who are uncertain of their immunization history, and who may have never initially received the usual series of tetanus immunization injections as a child. This provides immediate protection by the immune globulin and the ability to produce active immunity to tetanus by the tetanus toxoid.

Treatment for the disease consists of administration of the above and appropriate antibiotics. Wounds should be carefully cleaned and debrided. In symptomatic patients, intubation may be required before breathing is compromised.

Nursing care should be provided in a quiet, darkened room, with every precaution taken to minimize stimulation. The frequency and extent of all movement should be reduced as much as possible. Sedation is given to reduce convulsions, spasms, and rigidity. It should be kept in mind that the patient is not unconscious, and the suffering can be intense. If necessary to control paroxysms of spasticity and prevent asphyxiation, pancuronium bromide (Pavulon) may be given along with ventilatory support and sedation.[1] Such patients will, of course, be completely paralyzed by this drug, although awake, and thus require conscientious nursing care with attention to both preventing complications and maintaining comfort and reassurance.

If there is a history of drug abuse, withdrawal symptoms may complicate the treatment but should be managed in the usual manner.

RABIES (HYDROPHOBIA)

Rabies is an acute, usually fatal viral disease, rarely seen in humans in the United States. It is distinguished by its relatively long incubation period, which may vary from weeks to months. While the disease itself is rarely seen, preventative treatment should be undertaken for any individual who has been bitten by a potentially rabid animal. Because of the long incubation period, the animal should be observed for a period of ten days. Should the animal develop symptoms, its brain must be examined for the presence of rabies, and if present, the patient must receive a course of postexposure prophylaxis. If the offending animal is unknown or cannot be captured, the patient must undergo prophylaxis immediately. Newer immunizing agents have reduced the number of doses required as well as the incidence of allergic reactions, so that the preventative treatment is less arduous than it was in the past.

The prevalence of rabid animals varies widely from location to location and from time to time. Rabid animals are more likely than healthy animals to attack, so every animal bite (particularly one that was apparently unprovoked) should be suspect. The virus enters the body through the bite (or scratch) and spreads along the peripheral nerves to reach the central nervous system. Deep bites around the head, face, or neck are likely to result in rapid spread of the virus.

Clinical Features

The disease usually presents with the onset of fever, headache, and malaise, followed by severe dysphagia and spasms of the throat and mouth resulting in the "frothing at the mouth" and "hydrophobia" commonly associated with the disease. The patient has difficulty speaking due to the facial spasms and numbness. Generalized seizures and an acute confusional psychoses are typical. A less typical form affects the spinal cord and results in paralysis. In either case death usually ensues within a few days, although in recent years a few patients have been known to survive when aggressive respiratory and cardiac support were initiated early.

Medical and Nursing Management

Animal bites should be thoroughly cleaned and, if necessary, debrided. Tetanus prophylaxis should always be given as for any dirty wound. The authorities should be notified, so that the animal can be kept under surveillance for the required time. If this is not possible (a wild animal that has not been captured, for example), anti-rabies anaphylaxis should begin at once. This is particularly essential if there have been reported cases of animal rabies in the area.

Should symptoms of rabies develop, there is no specific treatment, but intensive supportive care should be instituted immediately.

VIRAL ENCEPHALITIS

Unlike meningitis where only the coverings of the brain (the meninges) are involved, encephalitis is characterized by widespread degeneration of nerve cells and necrosis of both gray and white matter of the brain.[1,4] Many viral agents can cause encephalitis, and there are wide variations in the severity of the illness, the prognosis, and treatment modalities. It is not possible to describe all of the viral conditions in the scope of this book. References at the end of this chapter can be used for further study. In this chapter only the general characteristics of acute encephalitis are presented, along with general guidelines for early diagnosis and treatment.

Clinical Features

Adams and Victor[1] described acute encephalitis as a febrile illness with evidence of meningeal involvement and various combinations of cortical symptoms (e.g., seizures, delirium, stupor, coma), focal neurological deficits such as aphasia or hemiplegia, involuntary movements such as ataxia or myoclonus, ocular palsies, nystagmus, and facial weakness. The specific signs and symptoms depend on the specific cortical area most affected, and each of the viral agents appears to have a predilection for a particular location.

Mortality and morbidity rates vary from 5 to 20 percent (30 to 70 percent for untreated herpes simplex encephalitis).[4] Residual effects such as memory defects, personality change, or focal deficits are not uncommon with many forms of the disease.

Medical and Nursing Management

Immediate care is focused on establishing the diagnosis. Only a few forms of encephalitis (herpes being one of them) can be definitely treated, and effective therapy depends on initiating treatment early in the disease. Most helpful in establishing the diagnosis are the history, initial presenting signs and symptoms, the presence of fever, and results of the lumbar puncture and electroencephalogram (EEG). With most forms of encephalitis the CSF shows increased WBC, elevated protein levels, and normal pressure. In some instances, an increase in the level of neutralizing antibodies may help identify the virus.

Except in the few viral infections for which specific drug therapy is available, management is largely supportive and symptomatic. Behavioral abnormalities, including severe personality change, delirium, limbic phenomena, and memory defects, complicate the nursing care and rehabilitation of these patients (see Chapter 13).

BRAIN ABSCESS

Brain abscess is usually secondary to a focus of infection somewhere else in the body. A common source is infection in the ears, nose, or mastoid, which reaches the brain through direct extension or along the venous walls. Abscesses may also be metastatic, that is, infection reaches the brain from a focus in a distant organ such as the lungs, heart, pelvic organs, or large veins.

The most common organisms found in brain abscesses are streptococci, staphylococci, pneumococci, *Klebsiella,* and *Proteus.* Sometimes there will be multiple abscesses ''seeded'' throughout the brain. There may also be an associated meningitis or encephalitis.[4]

Pathophysiology

Early reaction to the bacterial invasion of the brain is localized inflammation with purulent exudate and septic thrombosis of blood vessels. The area around the infected tissue becomes edematous and necrotic. The term cerebritis is often used to describe this stage. After a few days, the infected area begins to be walled off, with the center filled with purulent matter and the periphery formed by a layer of granulation tissue. The infection may then become idle, or it may spread into multiple abscesses or rupture into the ventricles.[1]

The course is variable, with rapid evolution and death, or a more indolent course may develop. Symptoms may appear to abate, only to break out again. Mortality is high and residual disability is common among those who survive.

Clinical Features

Signs and symptoms may vary depending upon the size and location of the brain abscess. In the early stages, signs and symptoms may be similar to those seen in meningitis. Headache, fever, and stiff neck with drowsiness, confusion, seizures, or focal motor and sensory abnormalities may be present. As the abscess becomes more formed, symptoms of a mass lesion will appear, including increased intracranial pressure with papilledema. There is usually a history of an infection somewhere in the body. If no such history is found, a search will need to be undertaken to find the focus.

Lumbar puncture (which should be taken with care when evidence of a mass lesion exists) reveals high pressure, elevated WBC count, elevated protein levels, and normal glucose levels. Organisms may be found on stain or by culture, but may have to be deducted from organisms found in the original infection. CT scans will often show evidence of swelling and a mass lesion.

Medical and Nursing Management

The early stages of treatment should emphasize the use of antibiotics and the aggressive management of intracranial pressure (see Chapter 4). When the abscess has been adequately walled off, surgical drainage or excision may be undertaken. It is important that antibiotic therapy be continued for an adequate period. The signs and symptoms tend to recede with the administration of antibiotics, only to resurge when treatment is discontinued.

Nursing care is similar to that described for patients with meningitis. The patient will be ill for a considerable period of time, so attention to nutrition is especially critical. Meticulous attention to hand washing and wound care is essential, both to protect other patients and to prevent secondary infections in a debilitated patient.

REFERENCES

1. Adams R, Victor M: *Principles of Neurology*, ed 3. New York, McGraw-Hill, 1985.

2. Hickey J: *The Clinical Practice of Neurological and Neurosurgical Nursing*. Philadelphia, Lippincott, 1981.

3. Feigan RD, Dodge PR: Bacterial and fungal infections of the central nervous system, in Tower DB (ed): *The Nervous System: The Clinical Neurosciences,* vol 2. New York, Raven, 1975.

4. Taylor JW, Ballenger S: *Neurological Dysfunctions and Nursing Intervention*. New York, McGraw-Hill, 1980.

5. Miller J, Arsenault L: Reye's syndrome. *J Neurosurg Nurs* 1983;15:154–168.

6. Plum F, Posner J: *The Diagnosis of Stupor and Coma,* ed 3. Philadelphia, FA Davis Co, 1980.

7. Nursing 79 Books: *Nurse's Guide to Drugs*. Springhouse, Pa, Intermed Communications, 1979.

Chapter 8

Neurological Trauma

Trauma ranks fourth in frequency as a cause of death in the United States and represents the leading cause of death in persons between the ages of 1 and 35 years.[1] One-fourth of all trauma deaths occur as a result of head injury. In addition, head injury has been demonstrated in 75 percent of all victims of fatal road accidents.[2(p4)]

Approximately 10,000 spinal cord injuries per year result in paraplegia or quadriplegia in the United States.[3] Of these injuries, approximately 62 percent occur in persons between the ages of 15 to 29 years.[4] Approximately 13 percent of these spinal cord injury victims also sustain head injury.[2(p4)] In the prehospital setting, direct cerebral and high spinal cord injuries cause approximately 50–55 percent of traumatic deaths.[5(p4)]

The extent of neurological deficits that afflict the survivors of neurological trauma varies according to their primary lesion and medical management. Aggressive initial management of patients with neurological trauma is essential and can significantly reduce both morbidity and mortality. Since neurogical trauma often occurs in the young, the emotional, social, and financial implications for the survivors, their families, and society are great.

MECHANISMS OF INJURY

An understanding of the more common mechanisms of neurological trauma allows one to anticipate real and potential injuries to the central nervous system (CNS). Neurological trauma can occur from penetrating injuries such as knife or gunshot wounds, or more commonly from blunt trauma.

Any information available from the patient, witnesses, or prehospital medical personnel regarding circumstances of the accident should be considered. Desired information includes height of falls and points of impact, speed of automobiles or other vehicles, associated findings such as bent or collapsed steering wheels, broken windshields, ejection from a vehicle, and whether or not the victim was a passenger or a pedestrian. In cases of penetrating injuries, the caliber of a gun or size of a knife blade is important information to obtain. All of these aspects take into consideration the amount of energy that was dissipated at the time of the accident which directly can influence the severity of trauma sustained.

Penetrating Injuries

Open or penetrating injuries to the CNS are most often the result of stab or gunshot wounds. As a bullet enters the body, bone and other tissues cause resistance and slowing of the missile, dispelling some of its energy. In gunshot wounds to the CNS, bone fragments are also drawn into the neural structures. In the brain, the tissue itself projects outward radially, creating a cavity much larger than the bullet itself (see Figure 8–1).

Contusions can occur in brain tissue distant to the bullet tract because of the pressure wave that precedes the bullet as it moves through the tissue. Fractures can even occur from this pressure or shock wave. Bullets fired at close range are more likely to cause these fractures than bullets fired at long range. The cribiform plate, oribital roofs, sphenoid ridges, and the tegmental plates of the petrous bones are vulnerable areas.[6]

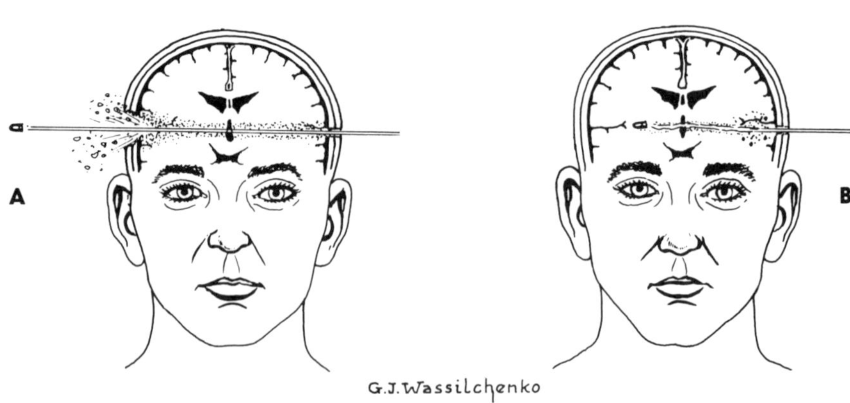

Fig. 8–1—Bullet wound of the head. Bullet wound or other penetrating missile causes an open (compound) skull fracture and damage to brain tissue. Shock wave effects are transmitted throughout the brain. (A) High velocity bullets cause more cerebral damage than (B) low velocity ones.

Source: Reprinted from *Advanced Neurological and Neurosurgical Nursing* (p 119) by Ellen B Rudy with permission of the CV Mosby Company, © 1984.

A high velocity bullet passing near but not through the spine can also inflict serious injury to the spinal cord because of this pressure wave.[7] In through and through bullet wounds, exit wounds tend to be larger than entrance wounds because of this greater release of energy at the point of highest resistance.[8]

Low velocity bullets may not exit the skull if sufficient energy was expelled, but instead may ricochet back through the brain, or may course along the inner table of the skull. Bullets that lodge in the ventricles of the brain or enter the vascular system are capable of migrating.[8]

Tissues disintegrate in the missile tract and acute ischemic nerve cell damage occurs because of the resulting hemorrhage and edema. Within hours, the tissues adjacent to the missile tract also disintegrate. Demyelinization of white matter effected by hemorrhage and edema begins to occur by the second day.[8]

It is important to determine the type of weapon used because the mass, size, and velocity of the bullet influences the extent of injury inflicted. The higher the velocity, the greater the kinetic energy, and therefore the greater the damage. Generally, handguns eject bullets at a low velocity while rifles eject at a high velocity.[8]

The size and shape of the bullet also influences the damage it can do. Bullets with greater mass can be expected to cause greater damage. Hollow bullets that flatten on impact also cause more damage than solid bullets.

Blunt Trauma

Because of the relative inability of the brain or spinal cord to expand within their protective meninges and bony supporting structures, closed trauma can cause concussion, contusion, laceration, bleeding, and swelling within the CNS with devastating consequences.

Acceleration-Deceleration

Acceleration injuries occur when a moving object such as a baseball bat or club strikes a stationary object or slower-moving object, the head or spinal column. These acceleration forces are then transmitted to the neural structures.[9]

Deceleration injuries occur when the moving object, the patient, strikes a stationary or slow-moving object. Falls, automobile, and diving accidents account for most deceleration injuries.

Automobile accidents account for 50,000 deaths annually in the United States with neurological trauma responsible for the greatest percentage of these deaths. Characteristically, automobile accident related deaths are highest on Fridays, Saturdays, and Sundays, with the highest levels recorded in July and August. More than one-third of the fatalities occur between 10 P.M. and 4 A.M. Alcohol impaired driving contributes significantly to these statistics.[10]

The significance of the trauma sustained in an automobile accident can be best understood by considering the following hypothetical situation. A car moving at 30 miles per hour that collides with a solid barrier takes about one-tenth of a second to come to a complete stop. While the front end of the car may be demolished and the passenger compartment remain intact, severe injury and death to the passengers can result from the "second collision" that takes place. This occurs one-fiftieth of a second after the car has stopped and consists of the passengers, still moving at 30 miles per hour, slamming against the dashboard and windshield. A subject weighing 150 pounds continues forward with a force about 30 times his or her weight, or about 4500 pounds.[10]

The advantages of seat belts, airbags, and child restraining seats cannot be overemphasized. A child held in its parent's arms rather than restrained in a child seat moves ahead at 30 times its weight on impact of the car against another object. If the child weighed 20 pounds, it would move at a force of 600 pounds—a weight few adults could hold. This is why injuries to children can be especially severe in automobile accidents.[10]

Hyperextension, Hyperflexion, Lateral Flexion, Rotation, and Vertical Compression

The head and spinal cord also suffer injuries from hyperextension, hyperflexion, lateral flexion, rotation, and vertical compression of the head and neck. The degree of damage experienced by the neural structures often seems out of proportion to the apparent external trauma. The brain can be concussed, contused, lacerated, or can sustain diffuse injury as it moves violently within the skull. The spinal cord can be concussed, contused, and lacerated as well as stretched or disrupted as it becomes entrapped by fractures or dislocations occurring in the vertebral column.[11]

Hyperextension injuries can result from vehicular accidents in which the vehicle is struck from the rear and the head snaps back, or in head-on collisions when the chin is forced against the steering column. Falls in which a person lands on the jaw, diving accidents in which the head strikes the pool bottom, and a severe blow under the chin from an assault can also cause severe hyperextension of the head and neck. Hyperextension injuries are most common in elderly persons with degenerative changes in the cervical vertebrae.[12(p395)]

Hyperflexion can result from diving accidents in which the back of the head hits the diving board. Falling and striking the back of the head on stairs can also cause hyperflexion injuries.[13(p340)] Lateral flexion injuries can occur when a vehicle is hit broadside.

A rotational injury might occur when the impact is at an angle to the head's center of gravity.[9] The cerebral hemispheres may rotate around the relatively fixed brainstem resulting in widespread shearing injuries to axons and loss of consciousness.[14]

Falls in which the victim lands on the buttocks or feet can cause compressive forces exerted on the vertebral column leading to spinal cord injury, often in the lumbar area.[12(p398)] In addition, the spine may impact up against the skull indirectly causing a head injury. In addition to causing head injury, falls onto the top or vertex of the head can cause compression injuries affecting the cervical spine, usually at the C5 to C6 level.[12(p395)]

HEAD INJURY

The term "head injury" encompasses a wide variety of injuries and their consequences. Considerable damage can occur to the scalp, facial structures, and skull, but the amount of damage sustained by the brain is of primary concern.

Scalp Lacerations

Scalp lacerations can be serious because of the extreme vascularity of the scalp with the potential for significant blood loss. Homorrhage can usually be controlled by digital compression along the scalp edges. If the galea, the fibrous sheet of connective tissue that attaches the scalp tissues to the skull, is split, bleeding may be excessive. It may require the placement of hemostatic instruments on galeal edges, and turning the instruments back to tamponade the vessels. Surgical closure of the galea prior to scalp closure is important to ensure hemostasis.[15]

Extensive scalp lacerations may require closure in the operating room. In preparation, an intravenous line should be established, hypovolemia treated, and vital signs and neurological status monitored frequently.

In the presence of an open head wound, a scalp laceration overlying an open skull fracture can contribute to meningitis or brain abscess. Such wounds may need to be closed temporarily if the patient is to be transported to another facility for definitive care.[16]

Skull Fractures

Approximately seven percent of all head injuries result in skull fracture, yet these statistics may not be reliable because many basal skull fractures are not visible radiologically.[17(p231)] This low figure is possible because of the frequency with which skull x-rays are performed, for legal reasons, in even the most trivial head injuries. Serious head injuries are much more often associated with skull fractures, with the incidence approaching 65 percent.[18(p99)]

Classification

The type and extent of skull fractures not only depend on the velocity, direction, and momentum of the impact object, but also vary with the age of the patient. In young children, separation of the sutures may occur. In neonates, the more flexible skull may only be indented, with no actual interruption of the continuity of the bone.[16]

Linear. The simplest form of skull fractures are linear (Figure 8–2). They account for 70 percent of all skull fractures.[17(p231)] These fractures resemble thin lines or single cracks in the skull, without displacement of bone parts.

Comminuted. In comminuted fractures, multiple cracks radiate from the center of impact, with fragmentation of bone into many pieces. The pattern resembles a cracked eggshell.

Depressed. In depressed fractures, the contour of the skull is indented because of the displacement of bone fragments inward toward the brain. Extensive damage to underlying brain tissue can result.

Open. In an open fracture, depressed skull fractures and scalp lacerations exist so that there is a communication pathway to the intracranial cavity. Such fractures are common in penetrating injuries.

Basal. A basal skull fracture frequently results from a linear fracture extending into the base of the skull. Basal skull fractures can also be of the comminuted or depressed type. Most often the anterior or middle fossae are affected. The posterior fossa can be fractured from severe impact upward of the cervical vertebrae against the base of the skull.

Clinical Features

Skull fractures are not always clinically significant and frequently require no emergency treatment. Yet forces strong enough to cause skull fracture can also cause injuries to important structures within the skull such as the brain tissue, meninges, blood vessels, and cranial nerves.

Meningeal Tears. Meningeal tears can occur with basal skull fractures. When the fracture extends into the paranasal air sinuses, there may be leakage of cerebrospinal fluid (CSF) mixed with blood from the nose, referred to as rhinorrhea. Since 75 percent of all basal skull fractures occur in the petrous portion of the temporal bone, there can be injury to the middle ear. When this is combined with a tear in the tympanic membrane, there can be CSF and bloody drainage from the ear, referred to as otorrhea. The irritation and potential for infection from a CSF leak are great and can result in meningitis.[16] A CSF leak may temporarily mask the usual signs of an expanding intracranial lesion by preventing brain compression.

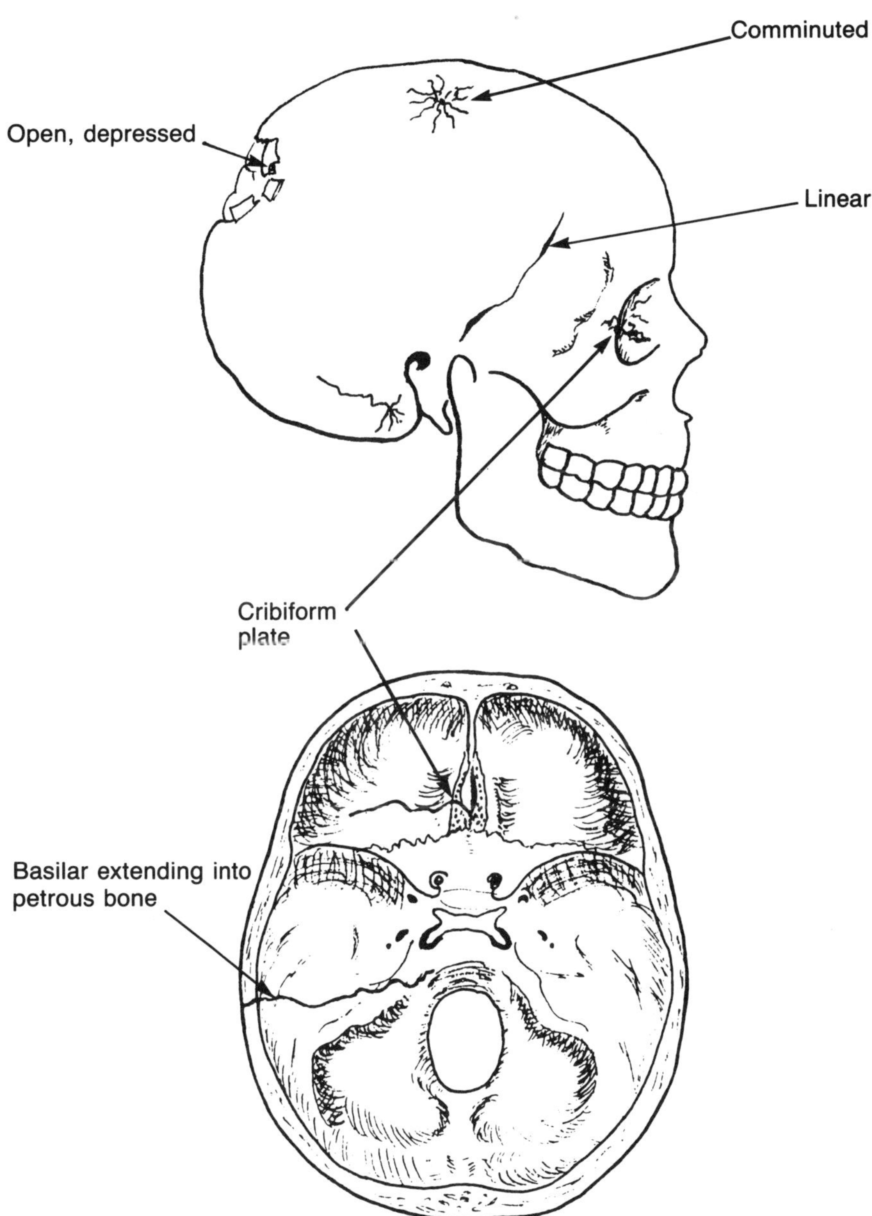

Fig. 8–2—Skull fractures.

Because basal skull fractures are often not visible on x-ray, diagnosis is often made on the basis of signs and symptoms such as rhinorrhea, otorrhea, or visualization of blood behind the eardrum (hemotympanum). Conjunctival hemorrhage, periorbital ecchymosis (raccoon sign) without evidence of direct eye injury, or ecchymosis over the mastoid bone (Battle's sign) are additional clinical signs that may indicate basal skull fractures.

Injury to Cranial Nerves. Skull fractures can also cause injury to certain cranial nerves. Anterior fossa and orbital plate fractures can cause injury to the optic nerve resulting in loss of vision in the affected eye.

Orbital plate fractures can also cause injury to the oculomotor nerve resulting in impaired eye movement, ptosis of the eyelid, and an inability of the affected pupil to constrict to light. Diplopia will also be present because of the impaired eye movements.

The dura overlying the cribiform plate is very fragile and frequently tears, with resulting injury to the olfactory nerves. This causes a loss of the sense of smell.

Temporal bone fractures (middle fossa) with involvement of the petrous portion can cause injury to the facial nerve resulting in paralysis of the facial muscles on the affected side. With injury to the acoustic nerve, both cochlear and vestibular branches are affected. There may be deafness or ringing in the ear and dizziness, with nausea and vomiting. Otorrhea is a common finding.[17(p232)]

Medical and Nursing Management

Because the amount of force necessary to cause a skull fracture is sufficient to also cause injury to the brain and other underlying structures, the patient with a skull fracture is often admitted to the hospital for observation, especially if there was any loss of consciousness.

Diagnosis. The diagnosis of skull fracture is usually based on skull x-rays. In a skull series, the basic projections are posteroanterior (PA), lateral, occipital (Towne), and base views. Sometimes it is advantageous to have the lateral films made with a horizontal beam to detect air-fluid (blood) levels in the sinuses. Depending on the patient's signs and symptoms, projections of the mastoids, sinuses, orbits, facial bones, and optic foramina may also be indicated.[19]

Basal skull fractures are often not visible on skull x-rays. The presence on x-ray of intracranial air, an air-fluid level, or an opaque sphenoid sinus may indirectly indicate basal skull fracture.[20]

Sometimes the diagnosis of skull fracture can be made by visual inspection and/ or careful palpation (with a sterile gloved hand) of a scalp laceration and by certain clinical signs. Inspection should be carried out for the presence of Battle's sign, periorbital ecchymosis, hemotympanum, otorrhea, or rhinorrhea, any of which could indicate basal skull fracture.[20]

If a CSF leak is suspected, the halo test can be performed. Allow bloody drainage from the ear or nose to drip onto a piece of filter paper or the pillow case. Observe for the presence of a double ring as CSF quickly migrates circumferentially around the central blood spot. To further confirm the presence of CSF, the fluid can be collected and tested with a Dextrostix. CSF will show the presence of glucose while mucous drainage will not.[17(p233)]

Emergency Management. Skull fractures usually require no specific treatment unless they are open, communicating with the paranasal or mastoid sinuses, are depressed, or cross major vascular areas such as the middle meningeal artery groove in the temporal bone.

Meningitis is a serious complication of fractures which cause dural tears that communicate with the sinuses. Hospitalization followed by close outpatient observation is required for these patients. Prophylactic antibiotics may be indicated.[16]

If otorrhea or rhinorrhea is present, the ear and nose orifices should not be vigorously cleaned, irrigated, or in any way disturbed until the leak ceases with sealing of the dura. Sterile pads should be placed at the draining orifice and changed frequently. The patient should also be instructed not to put fingers in these orifices, not to blow the nose or sniff.[12(p142)] Leakage of CSF will usually cease in two to four weeks.[16]

Any patient with a suspected anterior basal skull fracture should never be suctioned through the nasal passages and should not have a nasogastric tube passed. There is a chance of inadvertent intracranial intubation with either procedure.[20]

Depressed, open, or comminuted fractures may require surgery to elevate the bone if depressed more than the thickness of the skull; to debride bone fragments which could cause post-traumatic epilepsy; and to repair dural lacerations which may require grafting.[16]

All patients are observed closely for changes in neurological status that could indicate a concomitant epidural or subdural hematoma, or cerebral edema formation. Patients are also assessed for signs and symptoms of meningeal irritation such as headache, nuchal rigidity, photophobia, and fever. Cranial nerve assessment is included because of the high incidence of cranial nerve injuries associated with basilar skull fracture.

Brain Injury

The amount of energy transmitted to the brain is equal to the total force minus the energy dissipated by the disruption of the scalp and skull. A major skull fracture may cause little or no actual brain injury while fatal brain injury can occur without evidence of skull fracture or scalp laceration.

The CSF in the cranial vault helps protect the brain by distributing the force of impact throughout the intracranial space. The brain behaves as a semiliquid, and impact injuries set it in motion. Since different tissues of the brain are of different densities, two areas of the brain may slide across each other, producing injury. In addition, the positive and negative pressure created by impact on the brain within the cranial vault can result in cavitation of brain tissue.[9]

Because the skull cannot expand, closed head injury resulting in intracranial bleeding, brain swelling, and/or edema can be critical. The lack of external signs of serious injury does not preclude the presence of severe brain injury.[14]

Primary brain injuries are those that occur on impact. The resulting lesions can be of a focal nature such as lacerations, cortical contusions, and hematomas. Other injuries can be diffuse or widespread and can range from mild concussion to severe axonal shearing in the white matter of the brain.

Following head injury, several conditions can occur, some almost immediately and others delayed, that contribute to additional insult or secondary brain injury. Intracranial factors leading to secondary brain injury include hematoma formation, brain swelling and edema, infection, subarachnoid hemorrhage, and hydrocephalus. Extracranial factors such as respiratory failure with hypoxemia and hypotension can also induce secondary brain injury. Regardless of the cause, the mechanisms responsible for inflicting secondary injury to the brain are either hypoxia/ischemia or a shift with distortion and compression of brain tissue. These secondary insults account for much of the overall high mortality associated with head injury.[21]

Focal Brain Injury

Focal brain injuries include lacerations and localized space-occupying lesions that cause mass effects such as contusions and hematomas. These lesions may be localized to the site of impact or may be distributed to other areas because of the movement of the brain against the irregular surfaces inside the skull.

Laceration

Brain lacerations can occur in blunt head trauma by tearing and shearing forces within the skull. Direct destruction of brain tissue by laceration also occurs with penetrating injuries and depressed skull fractures.[12(p117)]

Pathophysiology. Brain lacerations, especially from missile injuries, are often accompanied by contusions, hemorrhage, edema, and necrosis.[17(p236)] These add to the degree of destruction and contribute to increased intracranial pressure (ICP), which can ultimately terminate in brain herniation.

The frontal and temporal lobes at the frontal poles are vulnerable areas in blunt trauma. Cerebral lacerations are always considered severe brain injuries, with recovery dependent on the location and extent of the laceration. With missile injuries, infections such as meningitis and brain abscess are ever-present dangers.[17(p236)]

Clinical Features. Signs and symptoms depend on the location and extent of injury or destruction of brain tissue. Symptoms can be severe because there is an actual break in the continuity of the brain tissue. Post-traumatic syndromes are common and may include irritability, memory loss, nervousness, dementia, psychosis, seizures, and focal symptoms such as aphasia, paresis, paralysis, and cerebellar dysfunction.[17(p236)]

Medical and Nursing Management. Surgical intervention is indicated to control bleeding, evacuate blood clots, and debride the wound. Efforts are also directed toward minimizing and treating increased ICP. Recovery is usually very slow with nursing efforts directed toward maintaining body functions and preventing and treating complications.

Contusion

Contusions or bruising can occur anywhere on the cortical surface of the brain where there is tearing of superficial cortical vessels. Contusions are commonly found beneath depressed skull fractures.[17(p235)] Cerebral contusions are the most frequently found lesions following head injury with mortality rates ranging from 25 to 60 percent.[22]

Pathophysiology. Most contusions occur as a result of blunt head trauma. There may be bruising directly under the area of impact called a ''coup'' injury. As the brain moves inside the skull and slaps against the opposite side of the skull, a contusion often occurs on the surface that is opposite the area of initial impact. This is called a ''contrecoup'' injury. For example, occipital fractures are often associated with frontal cortical contusions. Fewer contusions appear in the occipital lobes because of the better protection afforded by the smoother inner surface of the occipital skull and the smooth tentorium cerebelli on which the occipital lobes rest.[9] Contrecoup injuries are seen in acceleration-deceleration and severe rotational injuries.[12(p117)]

Cerebral contusions are often multiple and frequently occur on the undersurface of the frontal lobes and on the anterior poles of the temporal lobes regardless of the site of impact.[18(pp24–25)] Cerebral contusions can manifest themselves as areas of necrosis, pulping, infarction, hemorrhage, and edema. They are most often wedge-shaped with the apex extending into cortical tissues. Secondary events can occur with deterioration in the patient's neurological status. These include hemorrhagic lesions, which can result in bleeding into the subarachnoid space, bleeding into cerebral tissue forming an intracerebral hematoma, and brain swelling and cerebral edema.[22] These secondary events are largely responsible for the high mortality rates associated with cerebral contusions.

Clinical Features. Clinical signs and symptoms are related to the location and extent of the lesion. Localized lesions of the dominant motor cortex can cause motor and speech deficits. While such deficits can be transient, they can also be permanent if brain tissue is irreversibly destroyed by the contusion.[22] Contusions themselves are usually not sufficiently extensive to cause a loss of consciousness, although the patient may be stuporous or confused.

Small frontal lobe contusions can contribute to difficult behavior problems. Larger or multiple contusions, especially those involving the temporal lobe, can act as mass lesions as they initiate the formation of edema, swelling, or hemorrhage. This eventually causes brain shifts with ultimate compression of the brainstem. Patients who may have exhibited little or no neurological deficits may develop increasing deficits with deterioration in level of consciousness as the brain shifts and ICP rises.[22]

Medical and Nursing Management. Accurate diagnosis to rule out an operable lesion is essential. The diagnosis of cerebral contusion is suspected in patients who have sustained head injury that was followed by focal neurological signs. Cerebral contusions are best confirmed by computed tomography (CT) scanning that would show an area of increased density with areas of tissue necrosis and edema.[22]

Clinical management depends on the patient's clinical presentation. Small lesions are usually treated with frequent neurological assessments and measures to control ICP (see Chapter 4). Patients with large contusions with mass effects require immediate surgical intervention.[22] In performing neurological assessment, it is important to always consider the possibility of contrecoup injuries.

Epidural Hematoma

An epidural hematoma refers to bleeding that occurs between the skull and the dura (Figure 8–3). An epidural hematoma can transform a seemingly mild head injury into a life-threatening situation.[18(p153)]

Pathophysiology. An epidural hematoma results from injury to an extracerebral blood vessel, often an artery. Such artery tears are often associated with linear skull fractures of the parietal or temporal bones that cross the groove of the middle meningeal artery.[20] Epidural hematomas can also be venous in origin, although these are less common. A frontal-parietal vertex skull fracture can cause laceration of the superior saggital sinus with venous epidural hematoma formation.

In a multicenter study[23] of severe head injuries (Glasgow Coma Scale scores of 8 or less for at least six hours), the incidence of epidural hematoma was 9 percent, with mortality rates ranging from 9 percent to 36 percent depending on severity.

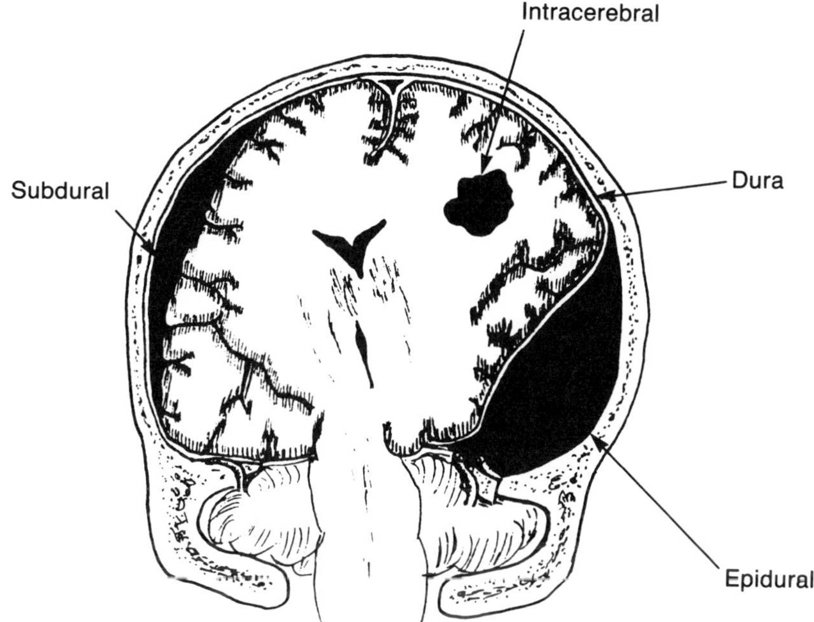

Fig. 8–3—Hematoma sites.

Clinical Features. Often the patient with an epidural hematoma has a history of a head injury that was immediately followed by a brief period of unconsciousness. There is often an associated lucid interval lasting a few minutes to several hours following recovery from the initial unconsciousness. As the hematoma expands, the patient begins to experience headache, vomiting, drowsiness, and stupor. Lateralizing neurological signs appear, such as contralateral hemiplegia and a dilated ipsilateral pupil that becomes fixed. Contralateral Jacksonian seizures might occur. If the mass lesion displaces the brain medially and presses the contralateral cerebral peduncle (ventral part of the midbrain) against the incisural border, hemiparesis ipsilateral to the lesion can occur. This is known as Kernohan's notch phenomenon or "false localizing sign."[18(p65)]

Supratentorial herniation leads to coma. Hemiparesis may progress to bilateral spasticity with Babinski signs. Respiratory changes occur and can terminate in respiratory arrest. The pulse slows while the blood pressure rises as brain herniation progresses. Death results if timely medical and surgical intervention is not taken.[11,12(pp144–145),17(p236)]

Diagnosis of epidural hematoma is made by CT scanning or, if unavailable, by arteriography.

Medical and Nursing Management. Treatment is surgical evacuation of the hematoma and ligation of the bleeding vessel if the lesion is causing a mass effect.[12(p145)] Sometimes emergency twist drill trephination (burr holes) is performed in the emergency department if signs of uncal herniation progress in spite of intensive medical therapy and when there may be a delay in obtaining a CT scan. While this technique may be lifesaving and can be done in less than two minutes, it affords only partial evacuation of the hematoma. The patient must then undergo craniotomy for complete evacuation of the blood collection and ligation of the involved vessel.[24]

Subdural Hematoma

A subdural hematoma collects between the inner surface of the dura mater and arachnoid layers of the meninges (Figure 8–3).

Pathophysiology. Large venous sinuses lie within the dura, therefore subdural hematomas are most often venous in origin. Frequently associated with serious head injury including contusion and laceration, these hematomas are associated with a high mortality rate.[11,23]

Acute subdural hematomas by definition are those that occur within 48 hours of injury. Some acute subdural hematomas occur immediately after the impact. They can occur from skull fractures and high impact injuries in which the violent movement of the brain within the skull leads to shearing and tearing of small vessels that bridge the subdural space. Bleeding edges of a cerebral laceration can also cause a subdural hematoma.

Clinical signs of acute subdural hematoma include gradually worsening headache, drowsiness or agitation, and confusion. Brain shifts lead to dilation of the ipsilateral pupil, contralateral hemiparesis, and decreasing level of consciousness.[17(p239)] Some patients may be deeply comatose on arrival in the emergency department.

Subacute subdural hematomas cause significant neurological deficts more than 48 hours but less than two weeks after injury.[11] The history can vary. Typically the patient with a subacute subdural hematoma shows gradual improvement following head injury, but after a period of time demonstrates signs of deteriorating neurological status, with signs and symptoms similar to acute subdural hematoma.[11]

Chronic subdural hematomas can develop as late as several months after what could have been considered a trivial head injury. The initial trauma ruptures one of the veins traversing the subdural space. Slow bleeding occurs, and within seven to ten days a fibrous membrane forms around the hematoma.[11] The fluid-filled space gradually enlarges for reasons that are not fully understood. Repeated bleeding or osmotic changes may contribute to the gradual enlargement of the lesion. The hematoma then begins to behave like a space-occupying lesion.[18(p185)]

Signs and symptoms of chronic subdural hematoma are often nonspecific and nonlocalized. Typically there is an alteration in level of consciousness including apathy, lethargy, and decreased attention span. Sometimes patients complain of headache. Lateralizing signs such as hemianopsia, hemiparesis, and pupillary changes occur in less than five percent of cases.[11]

The cerebral atrophy that accompanies the aging process places elderly people at risk. They can develop chronic subdural hematomas that remain asymptomatic for a longer period of time because of more available space within the skull. Since the onset of symptoms can be subtle, these patients may be misdiagnosed as exhibiting signs of senility. After surgical evacuation, subdural hematomas tend to recur in the elderly because of this available space within the cranium.[17(p239)]

Chronic alcoholic patients are also at risk because of frequent falls, a decreased production of clotting factors by a cirrhotic liver, and cerebral atrophy. Their symptoms can also mimic the mental deterioration caused by the alcoholism.[12(p147)]

Diagnosis of subdural hematoma is based on the CT scan. A subdural hematoma tends to spread over a considerable portion of a cerebral hemisphere causing a concave or half-moon appearance.[18(p164)] The fresh blood of an acute subdural is of very high density and appears white on the CT scan (see Figure 1–4). A chronic subdural hematoma has decreased density and may actually become isodense with brain tissue, rendering the CT scan less effective. A lesion can be suspected if there is a shift of the ventricles or other mixed density abnormalities evident on the scan. Radioisotope scanning will enhance visualization of isodense subdural hematomas.[18(pp114–121)]

Subdural hematomas can be differentiated from epidural hematomas by the appearance on CT scanning of the shape of the blood collection. An epidural hematoma forms an eliptical or lens shaped opacity against the inner table of the skull with a convex inner margin. Epidural hematomas usually appear in the temporal-parietal area.[18(p164)]

Arteriograms also demonstrate subdural hematomas. While an echoencephalogram can demonstrate a shift of the brain's midline structures, it does not indicate the type of lesion causing the shift.[17(p239)] CSF is rarely helpful in diagnosing subdural hematoma. It may show nonspecific abnormalities such as elevated protein and xanthochromia, and may contain a few red blood cells.[11]

Medical and Nursing Management. Small subdural hematomas that cause no neurological deficits may resolve spontaneously. Patients with progressive neurological signs require surgical evacuation. Jennett reports that about ten percent of patients require a second operation because of evidence of neurological deterioration. Recurrent hematomas and brain necrosis requiring excision constitute the major reasons for reoperation.[18(p178)] Emergency burr hole evacuation may be necessary in acute subdurals. Not all subdural hematomas can be evacuated this way because the blood may have become gelatinous. This necessitates craniotomy. The fibrous membrane encapsulating chronic hematomas also needs to be surgically dissected away.[17(p239)] Some chronic subdural hematomas are successfully treated with burr holes and catheter drainage.[25]

Intracerebral Hematoma

An intracerebral hematoma refers to bleeding into the parenchyma or actual brain substance. It occurs in only one to three percent of head injury patients.[12(p147)]

Pathophysiology. Intracerebral hematomas (Figure 8–3) are frequently found in the frontal and temporal lobes and may result from contusions that are accompanied by significant bleeding. Penetrating missile injuries and laceration of the brain from depressed skull fracture segments can also result in intracerebral hematomas.

Intracerebral hematomas occur singularly or as multiple lesions. These hematomas act as space-occupying lesions appearing immediately after trauma or sometimes not becoming evident until 24 hours or more after injury.[17(p239)]

Clinical Features. Signs and symptoms will vary depending on the location and size of the hematoma. Since intracerebral hematomas are often associated with brain contusions and lacerations, the patient may rapidly deteriorate to a comatose state with contralateral hemiparesis and ipsilateral pupillary dilation. As brain shifts leading to tentorial herniation continue, changes in respirations and other vital signs follow.

Diagnosis of intracerebral hematoma is made by CT scanning or arteriography. On CT scan, an intracerebral hematoma appears as a sharply circumscribed area of increased density. There will be surrounding edema evident on scans taken 24 or more hours later.[18(p166)]

Medical and Nursing Management. Treatment requires surgical evacuation if the lesion is accessible. Because of the need for brain manipulation in order to reach the hematoma and the frequency of multiple hematomas, results are often disappointing.[12(p147)] Patients with stable or improving neurological status may be treated medically.

Diffuse Brain Injury

Diffuse brain injuries encompass injuries from as minor as mild concussion, to as severe as diffuse axonal injury, which is second only to subdural hematoma as a leading cause of death from head injury.[23]

Mild Concussion

Mild concussion is a clinical diagnosis characterized by a temporary alteration in level of consciousness following head trauma from which the subject recovers in minutes.

Pathophysiology. Concussion is caused by acceleration-deceleration forces acting on the brain causing stretching of many axons and the possible shearing of a few axons that make up the white matter of the brain. This results in a temporary failure of conduction in these nerve fibers. Emphasis has shifted away from the belief that temporary brainstem dysfunction causes the brief changes in level of consciousness associated with concussion. The brainstem is actually less vulnerable to axonal injury than is the cerebrum.[23]

Clinical Features. Following a mild concussion, the patient may be briefly dazed or confused. These effects are quickly reversible. There may be an associated post-traumatic amnesia occurring immediately or delayed until 5–15 minutes later at which time the patient is unable to remember events immediately surrounding the accident. This amnesia may persist.[26] There appears to be a cumulative effect of repeated mild concussions indicating that there is structural damage, although slight, with each concussion.[18(p91)]

Medical and Nursing Management. Patients with mild concussion not associated with a loss of consciousness are not usually admitted to the hospital. Following evaluation in the emergency department, the patient is sent home with a responsible adult who can be in attendance. Instructions on patient observation and reportable signs are given to this person (Exhibit 8–1).

Classical Cerebral Concussion

Classical cerebral concussion results from the same pathophysiological events as mild concussion but apparently more axons are affected, leading to more severe clinical manifestations.

Clinical Features. Clinical signs and symptoms include immediate loss of consciousness and reflexes, temporary cessation of respirations (a few seconds), a brief period of bradycardia, and a sudden transient fall in blood pressure. After several minutes to hours, the patient regains full consciousness but memory impairment for the event persists. Vomiting may occur on awakening and the patient may be disoriented for hours or days. It is thought that the duration of unconsciousness and memory loss may indicate the severity of the concussion.[17(p234)]

A postconcussion syndrome has been described. Memory impairment, headache, nervousness, giddiness, inability to concentrate, fatigability, and insomnia have all been reported, with symptoms gradually subsiding with time.[17(p234)]

Exhibit 8–1 Head injury instruction sheet.

HEAD INJURY INSTRUCTION SHEET

Name ____Date _______________________

1. You have been seen at this facility for ____

   At this time, this condition does not require hospitalization. However, you should be aware that this condition could worsen or that another problem could occur. To assure that you receive the best care for these problems, call your referral physician if any of the following occur (even within several months):

   a. Persistent vomiting, stiff neck, fever
   b. Unequal pupils (one pupil large, one small)
   c. Severe, persistent headache
   d. Confusion or any type of unusual behavior
   e. Convulsions, seizure, or unconsciousness
   f. Loss of the use of an arm, hand, or leg
   g. Drainage of clear fluid or blood from ear or nose

2. Referral physician ____

   Address ____Phone _____________________

3. Wake the patient every _____________ hours the first night to check the above signs. Do not take any pain medication stronger than aspirin or Tylenol unless instructed to do so by your doctor. Do not take any sleeping pills, tranquilizers, or sedatives unless instructed to do so by your doctor.

4. Treatment rendered ____
   ____
   ____
   ____
   ____
   ____

   Rx ____

   Pharmacy Called ____

   _______________________________________   _______________________________
   Emergency Nurse Practitioner   Patient

Source: Reprinted from *Protocols for Advanced Emergency Management* (p 135) by Linda L Larson with permission of the Robert J Brady Company, © 1982.

Medical and Nursing Management. Classical cerebral concussion, being associated with a loss of consciousness, warrants hospitalization and observation. The length of time the patient remains hospitalized is often based on the length of time that the patient was unconscious. Generally, a patient unconscious for five or more minutes should be observed in the hospital for at least 24 hours. The length of amnesia (retrograde or antegrade) is also considered.[5(p50)] Because vomiting and/or convulsions may be more common in children, patients under the age of 12 are often admitted for observation.[5(p50)]

Diffuse Injury

Gennarelli[26] described diffuse injury as brain injury that is more severe than classical cerebral concussion, yet less severe than diffuse axonal shearing injury.

Pathophysiology. The causes of diffuse injury are the same as for concussion, but more widespread impairment of physiological function is evident. It may represent a transition between pure physiological dysfunction and anatomical disruption of axons.[26]

Clinical Features. Certain clinical features differentiate this syndrome from classical cerebral concussion. The period of unconsciousness is prolonged beyond 24 hours, often lasting from days to weeks. The patient often arrives in the emergency department with a Glasgow Coma Scale (GCS) score of 4–8 (see Chapter 1 for discussion of GCS). Abnormal posturing and autonomic nervous system signs are usually not evident. The patient will often withdraw from painful stimuli and may exhibit random or purposeful movements. On awakening, the patient will be confused, and this condition may persist for long periods. Post-traumatic amnesia is more pronounced. Although some patients recover sufficiently to resume normal activities of daily living, many are left with permanent intellectual, cognitive, and personality dysfunctions.[26]

Medical and Nursing Management. Treatment consists of measures to promote cerebral oxygenation, reduce intracranial hypertension, and prevent infection and other complications. (See ''Brain Injury: Critical Care Considerations'' later in this chapter.)

Diffuse Axonal Injury

Diffuse axonal injury (DAI) refers to widespread shearing damage that occurs to ascending and descending axons in the white matter of the cerebrum and brainstem following blunt head trauma. It represents the most severe form of diffuse brain injury, resulting in death in 55 percent of the cases.[26]

Pathophysiology. Diffuse axonal injury occurs most often as a result of a motor vehicle accident in which there is severe rotational acceleration of the head. The "swirling" motion of the brain results in mechanical deformation, violent shearing movement between different components of the brain, and severe tensile strain on axons with shearing of some axons within their myelin sheaths. It is believed that this axonal damage occurs at the time of impact rather than as a consequence of secondary events such as hypoxia, brain swelling and edema, or brainstem compression from tentorial herniation.

In comprehensive neuropathological studies of fatally brain-injured patients by Adams et al,[27,28] patients with DAI were found to represent a distinct pathological and clinical group. A lower incidence of skull fracture, intracranial hematoma, cerebral contusion, and elevated ICP was found in patients with DAI than in other fatally brain-injured patients without DAI. Characteristic postmortem pathological findings included microscopic evidence of diffuse axonal tears and petechial hemorrhages in the corpus callosum and dorsal midbrain. The location of these lesions may have resulted from impingement of the relatively mobile brain against the free edges of the falx cerebri and the tentorium cerebelli during maximum acceleration of the head. Axonal lesions in the brainstem alone were not found but were always associated with cerebral hemispheric white matter lesions. Degeneration of nerves distal to the sites of axonal tears, shrunken white matter, and dilation of the ventricles were found in the brains of patients who survived for several weeks.

Clinical Features. Patients with DAI are rendered deeply unconscious at the time of impact and remain so for a long time. Signs and symptoms differ from diffuse injury by the presence of such abnormal brainstem signs as posturing that may occur spontaneously or in response to painful stimuli and may or may not be symmetrical. Autonomic nervous system dysfunction such as hyperthermia, hypertension, and hyperhydrosis (excessive sweating) are common.[26]

Diagnosis of DAI is often made on the basis of the mechanism of injury and the presenting signs and symptoms. Occasionally enhanced CT scanning will show small hemorrhages in the corpus callosum, the supracerebellar peduncles, or in the periventricular areas. Brainstem auditory evoked responses show prolonged transmission of impulses through the pontine-midbrain areas.[26]

Recovery of the brainstem may occur after several weeks, at which time the posturing and abnormal autonomic signs disappear. Of those patients surviving DAI, residual neurological deficiencies are profound. If fewer axons are torn, recovery is better, but severe intellectual or bilateral sensorimotor deficits may persist. The intellectual impairment can be a much greater handicap than the physical neurological deficits. Thirty-six percent of the patients who survive this injury remain in a persistent vegetative state. Most commonly, patients with DAI succumb to this injury.[29]

Recovery of some function following DAI may reflect the use of other undamaged neuronal pathways. Recovery may also indicate that the shearing injury fell short of the total loss of continuity of the axons. Regeneration of neurons is scant in the CNS compared to the peripheral nervous system. It is believed however that if DAI results in axonal damage that leaves the glial sheaths intact, the opportunity for axonal regrowth is possible.[29]

Medical and Nursing Management. Treatment is consistent with that described in diffuse injury. Attention is also given to aggressive treatment of the late rise in ICP associated with DAI.[26]

Complications and Sequelae Following Severe Head Injury

Several complications and other phenomena occur frequently following severe brain injury. Nurses caring for head injury patients can direct their efforts toward preventing complications where possible, and recognizing and reporting the signs and symptoms of complications when they appear. Nursing interventions are then directed toward minimizing the effects of the complications.

Brain Swelling and Cerebral Edema

Brain swelling occurs quickly after head injury and is caused by hyperemia resulting from generalized cerebral vasodilation. This increase in cerebral blood volume can significantly increase the ICP. Brain swelling can be worse in the presence of decreased Pao_2 and/or increased $Paco_2$.

Cerebral edema represents a major cause of increased ICP following head injury. (Chapter 4 covers, in detail, the pathophysiology and treatment of cerebral edema.) Cerebral edema is usually proportional to the severity of the injury and reaches its maximum in 48–96 hours. It can be life threatening because of the pressure that is exerted on brain tissue. Brainstem herniation and death can occur if measures are not taken to minimize its occurrence and maximize its treatment.[17(p146)]

Subarachnoid Hemorrhage and Intraventricular Hemorrhage

In severe head injury, it is not uncommon to have bleeding into the subarachnoid space. Clinical signs consist of headache, nuchal rigidity, and other signs of meningeal irritation. The subarachnoid blood can obstruct the arachnoid villi and/or basal cisterns blocking CSF reabsorption. This will lead to the development of hydrocephalus.[12(p144),17(p240),18(p280)]

Intraventricular hemorrhage can occur from the subarachnoid hemorrhage or as an extension of the bleeding from an intracerebral hematoma. Significant bleeding can cause rostral-caudal deterioration terminating in coma and abnormal brainstem signs, then death.[12(p144),17(p240)]

Clinical diagnosis is made by CT scanning. Lumbar puncture is usually avoided because of the possibility of inducing brainstem herniation from the increased ICP. Subarachnoid precautions are implemented in the care of these patients.

Subdural Hygroma

A subdural hygroma, or effusion, is a collection of CSF and blood in the subdural space. It appears as a clear to yellowish fluid. Subdural hygromas result from small tears in the arachnoid over the sylvian fissure that allow CSF to leak into the subdural space. A ball-valve effect of the tear prevents the fluid from returning to the subarachnoid space. The fluid, which acts as a space-occupying lesion, may be localized or may extend over an entire hemisphere. Symptoms are similar to a slowly developing subdural hematoma. Removal is by aspiration or surgical drainage.[12(p155),17(p239),18(p184)]

Vascular Injury

Extracranial as well as intracranial vessels can be injured in head trauma. Abnormalities include stenosis, occlusion, aneurysm, arteriovenous (AV) fistula, and rupture of a vessel. In addition, vasospasm can occur, resulting in ischemia of portions of the brain.[18(p119)]

A blow to the head, fracture of the sphenoid bone, or a penetrating injury can lacerate the carotid artery within the cavernous sinus. A carotid-cavernous fistula can result. Protruding eyes and ocular palsies may result.[12(p148)]

Trauma to the neck, such as severe whiplash, can accompany head trauma and cause injury to major neck vessels. Spasm or thrombosis of the extracranial portion of a carotid artery can lead to hemiplegia after head injury. The vertebral arteries can be damaged by hyperextension injuries.[18(p119)]

Post-traumatic Hydrocephalus

Post-traumatic hydrocephalus is a common complication of severe head injury. It can occur as a result of shrinking of white matter leading to ventricular dilation, or from adhesions, inflammation, or bleeding causing obstruction of CSF circulation or impairment of its reabsorption. If CSF circulation is obstructed, symptoms of increased ICP appear and the ventricles will appear dilated on CT scan.[18(pp280–281)]

A slower developing hydrocephalus (communicating hydrocephalus) may develop from the impairment of the reabsorption of CSF. Patients who are recovering from head injury began to show signs of deteriorating mental status, confushio, drowsiness, and sometimes complain of headache.[17(p170),18(pp280–281)]

Emergency treatment for hydrocephalus involves a ventriculostomy, which may later require a surgical shunting procedure.[12(p155)]

Post-traumatic Epilepsy

Epilepsy is the most common delayed complication of severe head injury. The incidence seems to be related to the severity of the head injury and resulting disability. Post-traumatic epilepsy occurs in 5 percent of patients with blunt head trauma and in up to 50 percent of patients with penetrating head injuries and open, depressed skull fractures. The formation of a cerebral scar may serve as the epileptogenic focus.[12(p154)]

The interval between the head injury and the first seizure varies. Fifty percent of the patients who develop seizures do so within one to six months after injury. The seizures may be either focal or generalized with loss of consciousness. Seizures may decrease in frequency over time, and some patients are eventually seizure free.[17(p247)]

Most seizures can be controlled by anticonvulsant medication. Focal seizures are sometimes successfully treated by surgical excision if a surgically accessible, discrete focus can be located.[12(p154)] (See Chapters 10 and 16 for the nursing management of the patient with seizures.)

The significance of post-traumatic epilepsy as a physical disability depends on the extent to which it interferes with the patient's lifestyle and whether there are other disabling neurological deficits.[18(p281)]

The nurse should be aware that seizures can also occur within moments of the initial injury. These seizures are often generalized. These early seizures do not necessarily indicate that post-traumatic epilepsy (that occurring several months after injury) will occur. Appropriate seizure precautions should be taken in all head injury patients.

Metabolic Complications

Metabolic complications can also occur in head injury and may contribute to a depressed level of consciousness. Patients with head trauma should have regular determinations of serum electrolytes, osmolality, and values of urinary sodium.

Hyponatremia. Hyponatremia is sometimes seen following head injury and can lead to altered mentation and seizures. A common cause of hyponatremia is an inappropriate secretion of antidiuretic hormone (ADH) with resultant water retention, a reversible condition. Water retention complicates primary brain injury by causing cerebral edema. The diagnosis of the syndrome of inappropriate secretion of antidiuretic hormone (SIADH) is based on a level of serum sodium below 134 mmole/L, a serum osmolality below 280 mosm/kg, a level of urinary sodium above 30 mmole/L, and a urine osmolality higher than the serum osmolality. Treatment consists of fluid restriction, and in some cases, the cautious intravenous administration of hypertonic sodium. Furosemide may be administered to effect diuresis.[30]

Hyperosmolar States. Hyperosmolar states such as hypernatremia and hyperglycemia can also effect changes in the level of consciousness. Hypernatremia can result from diabetes insipidus (DI), an insufficient secretion of ADH with excessive urinary losses of water without adequate water replacement. Functional or structural defects in the osmoreceptor, the ADH-producing area of the hypothalamus, the pituitary stalk, or the posterior pituitary may produce neurogenic DI. Other causes of hyperosmolar or dehydration states include the administration of tube feedings with a high solute content, osmotic diuretics, fever, and hyperglycemia.[31]

Nonketotic hyperglycemic hyperosmolar states may occur in patients with latent diabetes mellitus. Hyperosmolar drugs (mannitol), corticosteroids, and phenytoin can precipitate this syndrome. Massive osmotic diuresis occurs leading to dehydration.[31]

Accurate intake and output records are needed in head injury patients. Any diuresis should be investigated by testing the urine for glucose to rule out the possibility of a hyperglycemic diuresis. Urine specific gravity should also be tested to rule out diabetes insipidus which is characterized by excretion of large volumes of very dilute urine.

The cause of the dehydration state must be treated in addition to supplying necessary intravenous fluid replacement. Treatment of DI consists of exogenous ADH administration if the condition is not self-limiting. Intranasal administration of *d*-amino arginine vasopressin (*d*DAVP), or parenteral administration of aqueous Pitressin or Pitressin Tannate in Oil may be used. Hyperglycemia is treated by both fluid administration and exogenous insulin. In addition, potassium is supplemented as necessary to prevent hypokalemia.[2(pp88–89)]

Brain Injury: Critical Care Considerations

Head injury management should begin as soon as possible if secondary damage to the brain is to be prevented or minimized. Optimally, management begins in the field with paramedics and emergency medical technicians (EMTs). The ABCs of resuscitation, rapid assessment for signs of head injury, and prompt transport to the emergency department for definitive treatment are essential.

The Glasgow Coma Scale (see Chapter 1), combined with pupil and lateralizing signs can serve as valuable triage criteria in ensuring that serious brain injury patients are transported to appropriate medical facilities equipped and staffed to undertake specialized diagnostic studies and render intensive brain care. Jennett and colleagues have shown that mortality exceeds 50 percent in those head injury patients with initial Glasgow Coma Scale scores of 7 or less. These patients often deteriorate in the field, on admission to the emergency department, or during scanning.[2(pp239–240)]

Initial Stabilization

While intensive brain care is required, additional responsibilities include a brief investigation of the mechanism of injury, whether or not a seat belt was worn (automobile accident), and questioning of observers about the patient's condition immediately following the accident. An overall rapid assessment for multisystem trauma must be carried out if the mechanism of injury dictates it (see Chapter 1). This includes examination for entrance and exit wounds if indicated. The patient may need to be rapidly prepared for diagnostic procedures such as skull and C-spine x-rays, CT scan, or for surgery.

Initial emphasis is placed on securing an adequate airway and ensuring proper ventilation. Often this must be done while simultaneously ensuring full C-spine precautions (see Chapter 1). The next priority is assessment for and treatment of hypovolemia that may be the result of blood loss from multisystem trauma. A relative hypovolemia can result from spinal shock caused by cervical or high thoracic spinal cord injuries. Treatment of hypovolemia with fluids and the MAST suit (medical antishock trousers), if indicated, must precede definitive neurological treatment. Uncorrected hypovolemia will only worsen brain injury because of the decreased cerebral perfusion pressure caused by hypotension made even worse by the presence of brain swelling. An isolated head injury in an adult cannot cause sufficient blood loss to induce hypovolemia. Conversely, an epidural hematoma can be large enough to cause significant blood loss in a child.

Preoperative preparation for all head trauma patients should include a type and crossmatch for blood. Transfusions may be required as a result of significant blood loss during surgery.

Ideally, no more than 45 minutes should be required from the time of arrival in the emergency department to the patient's arrival in the operating room (including the performance of the CT scan).[2(p240)] Continuous monitoring of the electrocardiogram (ECG), vital signs, respiratory, and neurological status must be provided during scanning and transport to the operating room or intensive care unit.

Chapters 4 and 5 presented, in detail, the intensive nursing and medical management of intracranial hypertension and brain resuscitation. Most of these treatment modalities are applicable to acute brain injury. The goals and interventions are summarized below.

1. Frequent neurological assessments to identify any progression or regression of neurological deficits. Use of a neurological flow sheet will expedite documentation. The initial neurological examination may need to be brief, as time is critical in patients with rapidly expanding hematomas. A more detailed examination can be postponed until the CT scan is completed.
2. Maintenance of an adequate airway and respiratory function with the prevention of hypoxemia, carbon dioxide retention, and aspiration.

3. Facilitation of venous return by elevation of the head to 30–45 degrees, unless contraindicated by shock or suspected spinal cord injury. Avoidance of neck flexion, entension, and rotation; prevention of hip flexion; and prevention of straining and Valsalva maneuver.
4. Control of hyperactivity by reduction of environmental stimuli when possible. Severely agitated patients may require administration of sedation or paralyzing agents.
5. Maintenance of adequate cerebral perfusion pressure by frequent assessment of vital signs and control of systemic blood pressure at normal levels for patient, and reduction of intracranial pressure.[32]
6. Treatment of impending brain herniation by administration of osmotic agents and diuretics, hyperventilation therapy, and the possible administration of corticosteroids and barbiturates.[32–35]
7. Prevention and control of seizures by administration of anticonvulsant medications.
8. Control of temperature and prevention of fever.
9. Maintenance of an accurate intake and output (I&O) record, with probable fluid restriction if hypovolemia is not present.
10. Prevention of gastric aspiration, in the absence of protective airway reflexes, by nasogastric or oral gastric intubation and suction.
11. Control of bladder dysfunction by insertion of indwelling urinary catheter.
12. Promotion of psychological support to both patient and family by encouraging ventilation of their feelings and concerns. Share with family members the difficulty encountered in predicting ultimate outcome.
13. Follow-up includes protection of integumentary and musculoskeletal integrity through frequent inspection, proper positioning, range of motion exercises, protection of skin, corneas, etc. (see Chapter 15). Institution of a bowel program should take place once gastrointestinal (GI) motility is ensured and a feeding program is commenced. Constipation should be avoided by the administration of stool softeners.

The use of corticosteroids in head injury remains controversial, but they may lessen the cerebral edema accompanying head injury.[36] Cardiovascular and pulmonary complications can accompany serious head injury and are covered in detail in Chapter 11.

Prognosis after Head Injury

Several factors are recognized as having strong influence in outcome following severe head injury.

Age. Age is widely acknowledged to influence both mortality rate and, in survivors, the degree of recovery. Jennett reports a continuous relationship between increasing age and a bad outcome (death or a vegetative state). Younger patients have been found to make a better recovery after deeper and more prolonged coma.[18(pp321–322)]

Severity of Injury. The depth and duration of coma relates to the severity of injury and appears to be directly or indirectly related to outcome. Difficulty comes in defining coma.[18(p322)] Level of consciousness is best assessed using the Glasgow Coma Scale (GCS), noted for its objectivity and reliable reproducibility (see Chapters 1 and 3). A GCS score of 8 or less defines coma. If one looks at severity of injury, there is a consensus that patients who remain in coma for longer than six hours after head trauma have suffered severe brain injury.[23] Mortality rates exceed 50 percent in patients with GCS scores of 7 or less.[2(p240)] The proportion of patients who die or remain in vegetative states approaches 80–100 percent if their best GCS score achieved during the first 72 hours following injury was 5 or less.[18(p124)]

Type of Intracranial Lesion. CT scanning allows for more accurate diagnosis of the types of lesions causing severe brain injury. It is now possible to consider lesion type as well as severity of injury as determined by the GCS score.

The results of a study by Gennarelli et al[23] confirm that the type of lesion is as important in determining outcome as is injury severity. Patients with the same GCS score have markedly different outcomes, depending on the causative lesion. Among patients with GCS scores of less than 9, mortality rates varied from 9 to 74 percent depending on the principal lesion. The worst head injury is the subdural hematoma, accounting for 45 percent of all deaths in this series of patients studied. This lesion also caused the worst quality of survival with only 22 percent of patients having good recovery or moderate disability. Diffuse injury with coma lasting longer than 24 hours represents a major cause of death (32 percent of all deaths).[23]

Evoked Responses. Evoked responses involve scalp recordings of electrical activity following various stimuli presented to the patient. Evoked cortical responses to visual, auditory, and somatosensory stimuli not only indicate the degree of cortical responsiveness, but may help distinguish between dysfunction that is mainly in the brainstem or in the cerebral hemispheres. Sequential evoked responses can be valuable in prognosis since improvement or return of evoked responses would indicate integrity and potential recovery of those portions of the nervous system being tested. Often these changes are manifested before the clinical neurological exam shows improvement.[18(p327)]

The absence of the oculovestibular reflex is also felt to be a significant indicator of poor neurological recovery.[12(p156)]

Quality of Life

The quality of survival is increasingly being addressed as more lives are being saved or prolonged by intensive medical therapy. Often the patient's post-traumatic level of functioning, when compared to the population in general, may seem to be quite high, but to the family and close associates, the patient is changed, possibly quite profoundly for the worse.

The Glasgow Outcome Scale[18(pp304–305)] is based on the overall social capability (or dependence) of the patient, taking into account the combined effect of specific mental and neurological deficits. With assessments being made at both 6 and 12 months after injury, four categories of survivors are described.

Vegetative State. In a persistent vegetative state, the patient shows no evidence of psychologically meaningful activity because of severe dysfunction of the cerebral cortex. Although the eyes may be open, there is no cognition. In head injury, this is often the result of severe shearing white matter damage. The secondary events of widespread hypoxic brain damage, elevated ICP, and brainstem distortion can also result in this form of survival.

Severe Disability. Severely disabled patients are conscious, but cannot function independently. They may have severe physical disabilities, limited communication abilities, and/or severely restricted mental abilities. Some are so severely mentally impaired that institutionalization is required.

Moderate Disability. Patients with moderate disability are independent but disabled. They can take care of themselves and some are capable of work. Often these patients have memory deficits or personality changes, varying degrees of hemiparesis, dysphasia or ataxia, post-traumatic epilepsy, or major cranial nerve deficits.

Good Recovery. Patients making good recovery may be able to participate in a normal social life and may return to work. This does not imply that they are free of neurological deficits. They may have memory impairment or other persistent post-traumatic sequelae.

Conclusion

Many advances have been made in the care of head injury patients. It is apparent that vigorous and aggressive therapy in the emergency department and throughout all phases of care can be extremely important determinants of the patient's survival and ultimate outcome.

SPINAL CORD INJURY

Spinal cord injuries usually result from forces that cause severe hyperflexion, hyperextension, rotation, or vertical compression of the spinal column. Open injuries to the spinal column are less common and usually result from gunshot or stab wounds. The spinal cord injury patient is most often a young male, under age

30, injured during a motor vehicle accident, a fall, or a sporting activity such as diving or skiing.[11]

Because of the circumferential bony protection of the spinal cord by the veretebral column, most spinal cord injuries result from fractures and dislocations occurring at areas of articulation between vertebrae. Most vulnerable are the lower cervical and lumbar regions where relatively mobile segments of the vertebral column meet relatively fixed portions.[11] Injuries to the vertebral column can occur with or without injury to the spinal cord.

Vertebral Injury

Vertebral injury refers only to trauma involving the bony segment of the vertebral column. The cervical and lumbar regions are the most flexible and thus most vulnerable to injury.

Persons with preexisting or degenerative disease processes of the spine such as scoliosis, spondylosis, or arthritis are more vulnerable to the forces that cause vertebral injury.

Simple Fracture

Usually a single fracture occurs across the spinous or transverse process. Alignment of the vertebral column remains intact, and spinal cord injury is usually not present.

Compression Fracture

Hyperflexion and hyperextension coupled with compressive forces can cause wedge-shaped or teardrop fractures (Figure 8–4). A teardrop fracture of the superior aspect of the vertebral body indicates an extension type injury and is usually stable but can cause cord damage. A bone chip off the anterior-inferior aspect often results in spinal cord injury due to displacement of the disk or posterior fragment of the vertebral body into the spinal canal.[20]

Comminuted Fracture

Comminuted fractures, also called bursting or blowout fractures, are often caused by traumatic forces that are directed along the vertical axis of the spinal column. Such an injury might result from hitting the head on the roof of a car. The fifth and sixth cervical vertebrae are the most vulnerable for this severe type of compression fracture. Severe spinal cord injury can occur because of exploding bony fragments.

A Jefferson fracture is a ''burst'' fracture of the first cervical vertebra (Figure 8–5). Because the spinal canal is wider in this region, there may or may not be cord damage seen with a Jefferson fracture.[12(p395)]

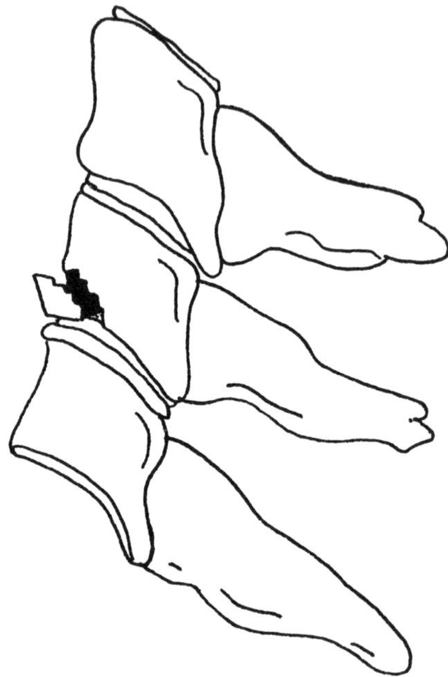

Fig. 8–4—Teardrop fracture of vertebral body.

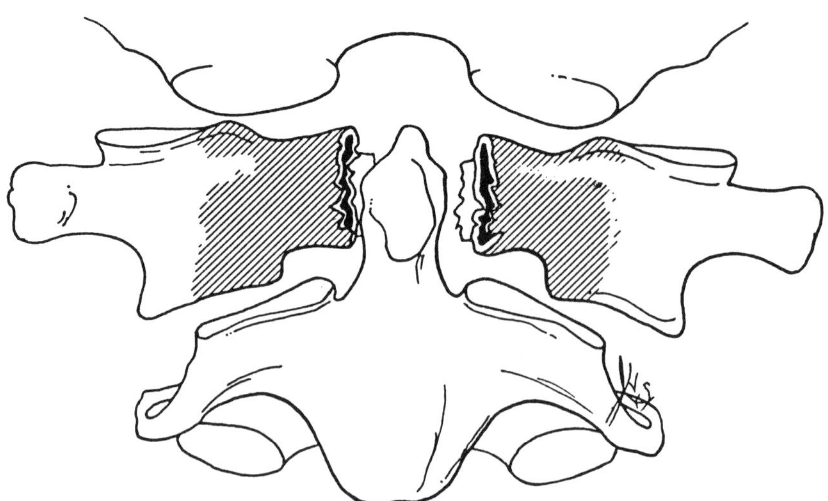

Fig. 8–5—Jefferson fracture with bursting of the ringlike structure of the atlas.
Source: Reprinted from *Emergency Medicine: A Comprehensive Review* (p 619) by TC Kravis and CG Warner (eds), Aspen Systems Corporation, © 1983.

Hangman's Fracture

A unique fracture to include in this discussion is the hangman's fracture (Figure 8–6). Severe hyperextension causes bilateral fractures through the posterior neural arches of the second cervical vertebra. Dislocation of C-2 on C-3 may or may not occur. Death is almost instantaneous if the spinal cord is impinged.[17(p292),37]

Sacral and Coccygeal Fractures

Sacral and coccygeal fractures are usually caused by direct injuries most often resulting from falls.

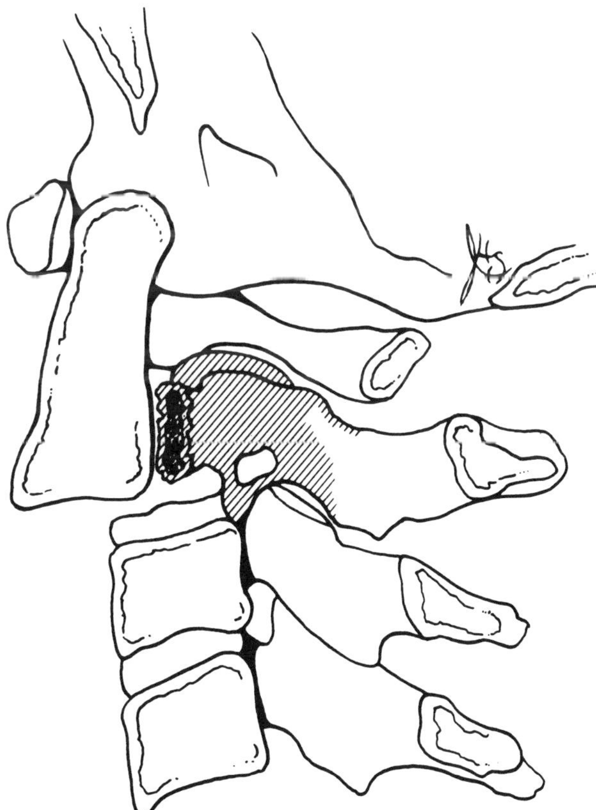

Fig. 8–6—Hangman's fracture with anterior subluxation of C-2 on C-3 and bilateral pedicle fractures of C-2.

Source: Reprinted from *Emergency Medicine: A Comprehensive Review* (p 621) by TC Kravis and CG Warner (eds), Aspen Systems Corporation, © 1983.

Vertebral Dislocation

Injury to supporting ligaments can cause unilateral or bilateral facet dislocation (Figure 8–7). Subluxation, or partial dislocation of one vertebra on another, occurs. Since alignment of the vertebral column is disrupted, there may be injury to the spinal cord.

Trauma that causes hyperflexion of the head may result in tearing of the posterior longitudinal ligament resulting in instability of the cervical vertebral column. Forces causing hyperextension can damage the anterior longitudinal ligament resulting in one vertebra being pushed backward. The cord can become compressed by the vertebra or an intervertebral disk. Fractures of the vertebrae may or may not occur.[13]

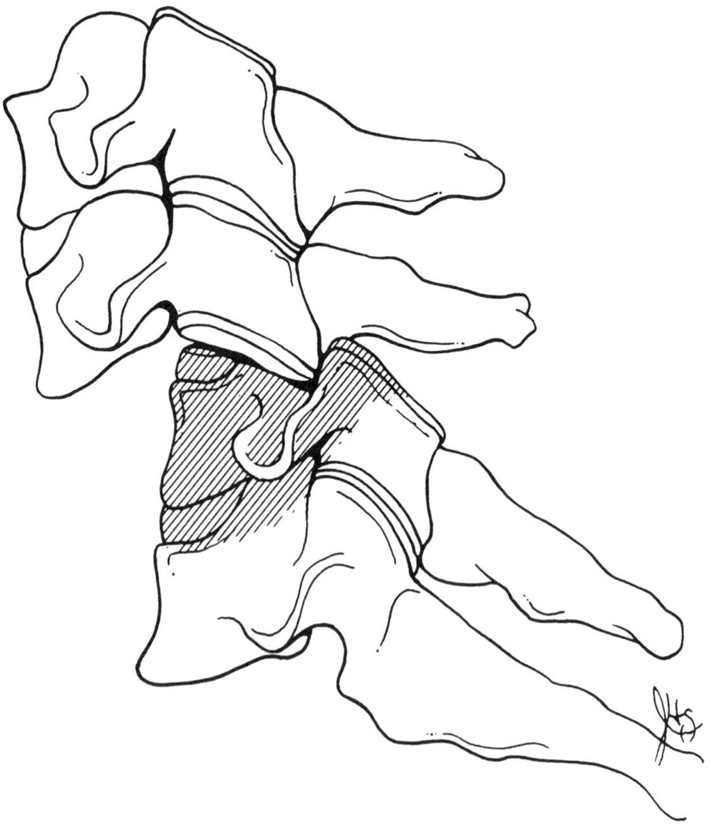

Fig. 8–7—Interlocking articular facets.
Source: Reprinted from *Emergency Medicine: A Comprehensive Review* (p 618) by TC Kravis and CG Warner (eds), Aspen Systems Corporation, © 1983.

Pathophysiology of Spinal Cord Injury

The spinal cord may be concussed, compressed, stretched, or contused. Cord laceration can occur from bony vertebral fragments and from penetrating injuries (Figure 8–8). Interruption of blood supply to the cord from bony angulations can further enhance the severity of cord injury.

Pathophysiological events occurring after spinal cord injury are varied. When the spinal cord is compressed there may be small hemorrhages into the gray matter. Blood flow to the cord may become compromised, leading to cord hypoxia. Autoregulation of blood supply is lost and cord edema occurs. Concurrently there is a localized release of catecholamines and other vasoactive substances such as dopamine and serotonin, leading to further ischemia, hypoxia, and tissue necrosis.[38]

Cord contusion leads to hemorrhage and edema with demyelination and degeneration of tissue. Cord laceration causes actual transection of nerve tracts with loss of function, and no regeneration.[13]

The degree and type of injury influences the permanence of neurological deficit. With spinal cord concussion, there may be only a momentary loss of function. In patients with cord compression, surgical decompression can sometimes restore cord function.

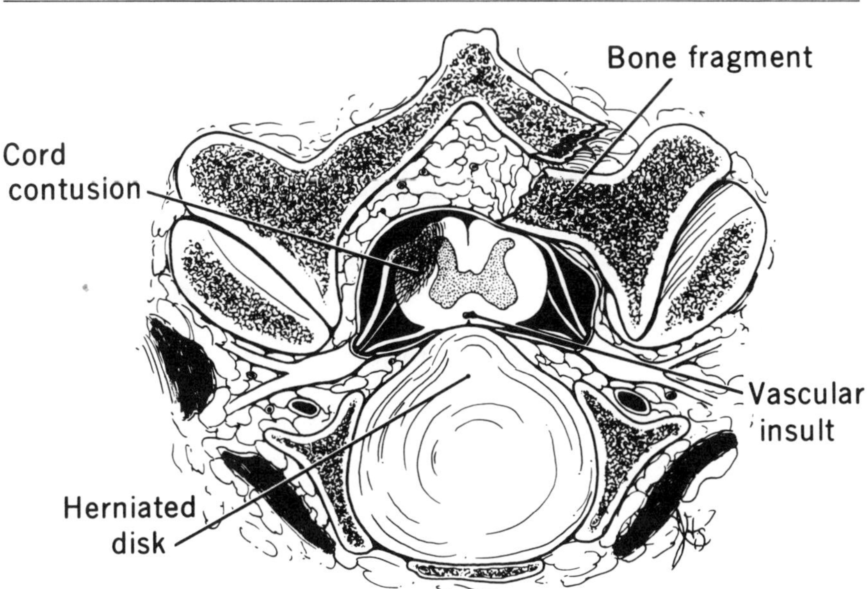

Fig. 8–8—Mechanisms of cord injury associated with trauma.
Source: Reprinted from *Emergency Medicine: A Comprehensive Review* (p 622) by TC Kravis and CG Warner (eds), Aspen Systems Corporation, © 1983.

Hemorrhage into the cord in the first few hours after injury and cord edema can extend the level of damage both above and below the initial injury site. Both of these events lead to increased degrees of functional loss. In some cases of cord edema where no irreversible damage has occurred, there is return of function as the edema resolves.[17(p258)]

Clinical Features

There are various types of spinal cord injury causing various degrees of neurological deficit. Spinal cord injury can be classified by the level of injury (see Table 8–1). It is important to remember that the phrenic nerves that supply the diaphragm, the major muscle of respiration, arise from the spinal cord above the C-4 level. Innervation of the intercostal muscles that also affect respirations arise from the upper half of the thoracic spine. The lower tip of the spinal cord, the conus, is at the L-1 level. Lesions here or lower will interrupt sympathetic and parasympathetic control of bladder function.

A brief review of the concepts of upper motor neuron versus lower motor neuron injury is appropriate for an understanding of the clinical manifestations of various levels of spinal cord injury. A lesion which damages or destroys an upper motor neuron (UMN) and its influence over the lower motor neuron is termed an UMN lesion. UMNs run from the motor cortex of the brain, through the internal capsule and brainstem, and down the spinal cord to the areas where individual UMNs synapse with lower motor neurons arising in the spinal cord. UMN lesions ultimately result in muscle spasticity with increased tendon reflexes. Patients with UMN spinal cord lesions will have initial flaccid paralysis, followed by spastic paralysis, which can lead to contractures, and contribute to difficult motor control during rehabilitation. UMN lesions occurring above the lumbar area spare the bowel and bladder reflexes, and with proper training and medications patients with these lesions can learn bowel and bladder control.[12(p408)]

The lower motor neurons (LMNs) are located in the anterior gray matter throughout the entire length of the spinal cord. These LMNs have long axons that extend out from the spinal roots and peripheral nerves and eventually synapse with peripheral muscle fibers. Damage to an LMN causes a flaccid type paralysis. These injuries often occur lower in the cord and can result in a permanent loss of bowel and bladder control.[12(p408)]

Spinal cord injury is also classified according to the degree of cord involvement.

Complete Spinal Cord Transection

While injuries do not usually cause an actual anatomical separation (transection) of the spinal cord, there can exist a functional transection because of the interruption of motor and sensory tracts. Three major syndromes that occur as a

Table 8–1 Functional Loss from Spinal Cord Injury

Segmental Level of Injury	Functional Loss	Rehabilitative Potential
Above C-3	Quadriplegia and total loss of respiratory function Risk of hypotension, hypothermia, ileus, and atonic bladder Sensory loss from neck down	Will be ventilator dependent unless phrenic nerve stimulator used Probably unable to survive with less than skilled nursing care
C-3 to C-4	Quadriplegia and may have loss of respiratory function due to edema involving phrenic nerves; may resolve with return of diaphragmatic breathing Risk of hypotension, hypothermia, ileus, and atonic bladder Sensory loss below clavicles	Can live in community with attendant; operate electric wheelchair with tongue switch; use adaptive tools held in mouth; may require intermittent ventilator; return of bowel and bladder reflexes can "trigger" bladder emptying
C-5 to C-6	Quadriplegia with partial function of shoulders and forearms Phrenic nerves intact, but not intercostals; will have diaphragmatic breathing Risk of hypotension, hypothermia, ileus, and atonic bladder Sensory loss below clavicles, but some arm sensation	Can operate electric wheelchair; needs assistance to transfer; return of bowel and bladder reflexes
C-6 to C-7	Quadriplegia (incomplete) with intact biceps but not triceps, partial wrist function Diaphragmatic breathing Risk of hypotension, hypothermia, ileus, and atonic bladder Sensory loss below clavicles and parts of arms	May be able to propel wheelchair; can drive car with quad controls; return of bowel and bladder reflexes
C-7 to C-8	Quadriplegia (incomplete) with biceps and triceps intact; limited function of hands Diaphragmatic breathing Risk of hypotension, hypothermia, ileus, and atonic bladder Sensory loss upper chest down and part of hands	Independent in transfers; can propel wheelchair; can drive car with quad controls; return of bowel and bladder reflexes

Table 8–1 continued

Segmental Level of Injury	Functional Loss	Rehabilitative Potential
T-1 to L-2	Paraplegia with various amounts of intercostal and abdominal muscle function Risk of hypotension, hypothermia, ileus, and atonic bladder if injury above T-6 level Sensory loss depends on level: T-4 supplies nipple line T-10 supplies umbilicus T-12 supplies groin area L-2 supplies upper thighs	Completely independent in wheelchair; return of bladder and bowel reflexes; limited, difficult ambulation, with long leg braces, corset, and underarm crutches
Below L-2	Paraplegia (incomplete) Various bowel and bladder dysfunctions Sensory loss depends on level: Lumbar: loss of sensation to upper legs, part of lower legs, feet, and ankles Sacral: loss of sensation from lower legs, feet, and perineum	Completely independent in wheelchair; varying ability to walk with braces; bladder remains areflexive if sacral segments involved

result of complete spinal cord transection are motor loss (paralysis), sensory loss, and spinal shock.

Paralysis. Initially there is a flaccid paralysis with loss of all voluntary motor activity below the level of injury. Quadriplegia refers to the loss of leg function accompanied by various degrees of paralysis of the arms caused by injury to the cervical cord. Paraplegia, or paralysis of the legs, results from spinal cord lesions below the cervical spine.

With complete spinal cord transection, paralysis is usually permanent. Several months after spinal cord transection there is a return of exaggerated spinal reflex arcs below the level of injury, which may lead to spasticity of various muscle groups. This spasticity is due to the loss of moderating or inhibitory UMN influence from the central cortex on those LMNs located below the level of injury. This hyperactivity includes exaggerated withdrawal reflexes and may also spread to include visceral and autonomic outflow. This phenomenon is called mass reflex and may be evoked unintentionally or occur spontaneously without obvious stimulation.[39] See ''autonomic dysreflexia'' later in this chapter.

Sensory Loss. All sensory impulses that depend on intact ascending spinal pathways are lost. There is loss of the sensations of pain, temperature, proprioception, pressure, and touch, and an absence of somatic and visceral sensations below the level of injury. There may be pain at the site of the injury because of a zone of heightened sensitivity just above the level of the lesion. [17(p258)]

Occasionally sacral reflexes may be present immediately following complete spinal cord transection, but this is often transient, and these reflexes usually disappear within one to two days. It is theorized that these reflexes are due to the electrical charge remaining in the isolated cord which finally dissipates. [12(p411)]

Spinal Shock. Following spinal cord transection there is a state of transient reflex loss below the level of the lesion known as spinal shock. This syndrome begins within 30–60 minutes following injury and usually lasts for three to six weeks, but may extend over a period of several months. Spinal shock includes the flaccid motor paralysis and sensory losses mentioned previously and also includes signs and symptoms manifested by the interruption of sympathetic outflow if the injury is above the T-6 level. As a result, the following signs and symptoms may be seen: [38]

- loss of vasomotor tone and decreased venous return resulting in hypotension
- loss of ability to perspire below the level of injury
- bradycardia, because of a loss of sympathetic control
- bladder and bowel dysfunctions with initial retention of urine and feces (anal sphincter tone may or may not be lost)
- loss of temperature control because of sympathetic interruption. The patient's body temperature tends to move toward the ambient temperature of the environment
- priapism, an abnormal, prolonged penile erection in the male patient

The return of any reflex that had initially been absent below the level of injury is a sign of recovery from spinal shock. Often, the return of sphincter tone signals the resolution of spinal shock.

Incomplete Spinal Cord Transections

Depending on the location of the spinal cord lesion, various degrees of motor and sensory losses can occur (Figure 8–9). Concurrently there may be evidence of sparing of some of the spinal cord tracts. While the patient may exhibit a flaccid paralysis, the presence of rectal sphincter tone and an intact bulbocavernosus reflex indicates that some of the sensory tracts lying more peripheral in the cord are still intact. This phenomenon is known as sacral sparing and indicates an incomplete spinal cord lesion. The patient might retain saddle area sensation in the presence of paralysis and loss of other sensations below the level of injury. [12(p410)]

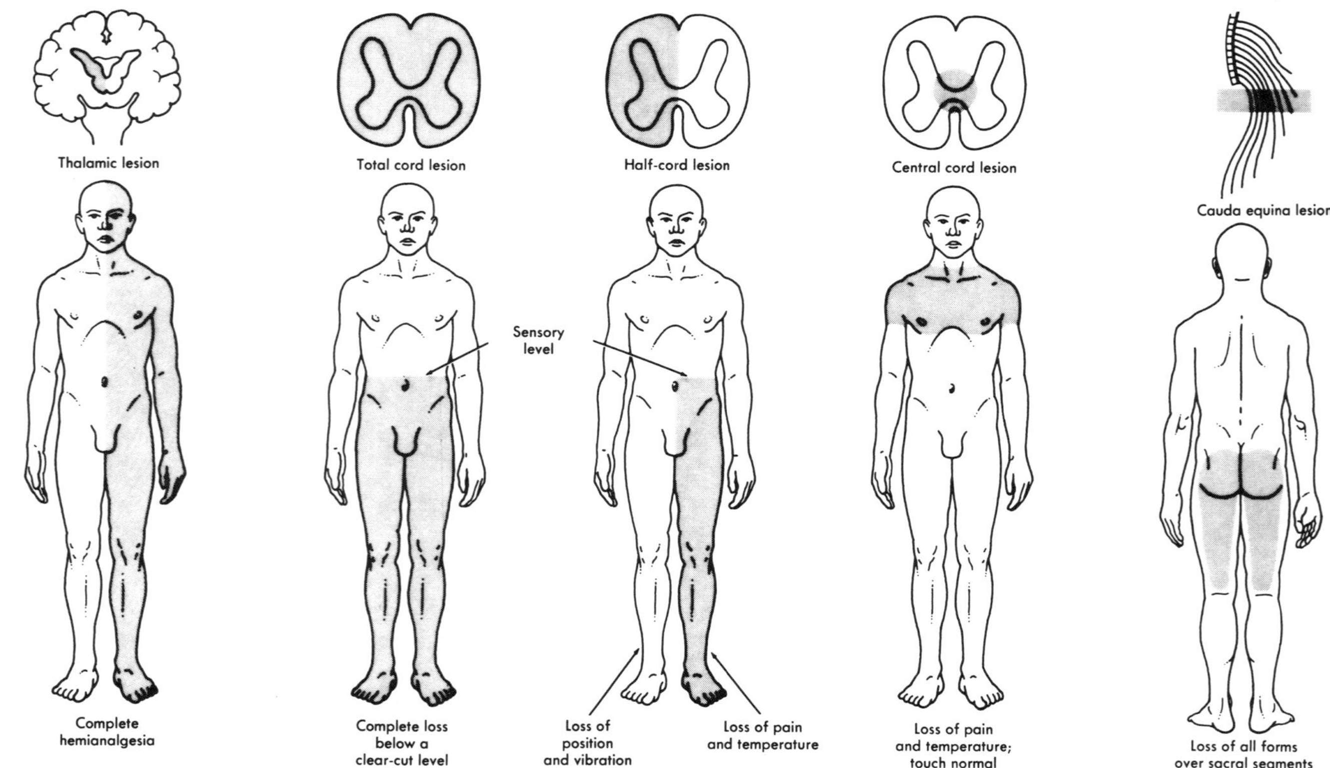

Fig. 8–9—Common patterns of sensory abnormality. Upper diagrams show site of lesion; lower diagrams show distribution of corresponding sensory loss.

Source: Reprinted from *Emergency Nursing: Principles and Practice* (p 314) by Susan A Budassi and Janet M Barber with permission of the CV Mosby Company, © 1981.

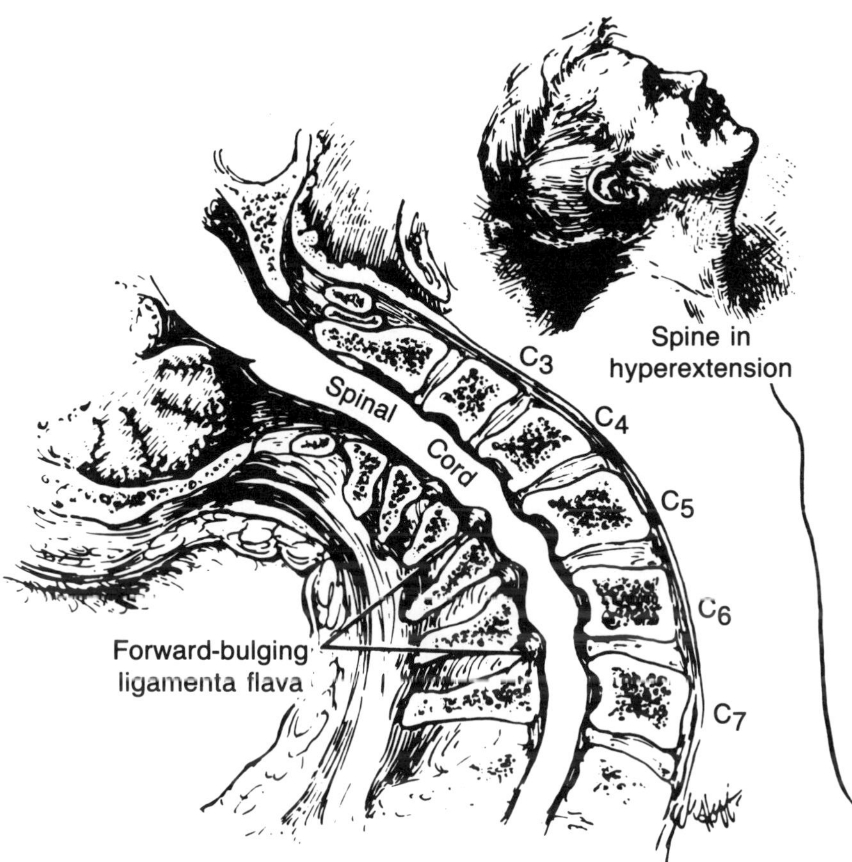

Fig. 8–10—Mechanism of cord compression in hyperextension injuries of the cervical spine.
Source: Reprinted from *Emergency Medicine: A Comprehensive Review* (p 620) by TC Kravis and CG Warner (eds), Aspen Systems Corporation, © 1983.

Central Cord Syndrome.   A central cord syndrome may be caused by hemorrhage, edema, and vascular insufficiency within the central gray matter of the spinal cord. Fibers of the corticospinal tracts supplying the upper extremities lie more centrally and are more vulnerable to this type of injury than those supplying the lower extremities, which lie more peripherally. Hyperextension injuries (Figure 8–10), with or without vertebral fracture, or interruption of the blood supply to the central cord can cause the following clinical manifestations:

- motor weakness greater in the upper extremities than in the lower extremities. The arm paralysis may be of the LMN type

- varying degrees of bladder dysfunction
- various sensory losses

Aggressive control of cord edema may, in some cases, result in partial or complete return of function.[17(p259)]

Brown-Sequard Syndrome. The Brown-Sequard syndrome results from hemitransection of the cord, usually as a result of penetrating injuries, unilateral articular process fractures, or spinal cord tumors. Injury to one-half of the cord may result in the following clinical manifestations, but often the signs and symptoms are not so clearly defined[40]:

- ipsilateral motor paralysis below the level of injury (corticospinal tract injury)
- ipsilateral loss of position and vibration sense below the level of injury (posterior column injury)
- contralateral loss of pain and temperature sensation below the level of injury (lateral spinothalamic tract injury).

Anterior Cord Syndrome. Anterior cord syndrome results from interruption of blood supply from the anterior spinal artery, compression of the anterior portion of the cord by bony fragments in cervical compression and hyperflexion injuries, or acute herniated disk. The following clinical manifestations are characteristic of anterior cord syndrome:

- paralysis below the level of injury
- loss of pain and temperature below the level of injury
- preservation of sensations of touch, motion, position, and vibration due to intact posterior columns.

Surgical decompression and control of cord edema may afford some patients improvement in function.[17(p259)]

Posterior Cord Syndrome. Posterior cord syndrome is a rare injury to the posterior columns. It is caused by hyperextension injuries of the cervical spine. Motor function remains intact while there is loss of the senses of touch, position, and vibration.

Cauda Equina Lesions. Cauda equina lesions often result from direct trauma of fracture dislocations. Nerve roots may be involved either unilaterally or bilaterally with unpredictable neurological sparing. Sensory and motor losses may occur in sacral segments. Recovery from these losses by nerve root regrowth is possible if the nerve roots are not severed.[12(p410)]

Other Incomplete Lesions. Involvement of specific nerve tracts causes dysfunctions that fit no specific pattern, unlike those previously mentioned.[38]

Medical and Nursing Management

It is important to remember that most damage to the spinal cord occurs at the time of injury, but secondary spinal cord injury can result from improper handling and stabilization of the patient's spine.

Prehospital Management

The immediate care rendered at the scene of the accident can have a profound effect on the patient's outcome. Spinal cord injuries (SCIs) often accompany head injuries. Recognition of possible SCI is one of the primary responsibilities of prehospital medical personnel. While spinal fractures may not initially cause SCI, improper stabilization and handling can result in neurological damage. Prehospital medical personnel are taught the importance of safe extrication and are skilled at maintaining airway and respiratory function while protecting the spine from unnecessary movement.

Following the assurance of the ABCs of resuscitation, a rapid assessment for multisystem trauma is carried out. External bleeding is controlled with direct pressure. Large bore intravenous (IV) lines are established and MAST suit is placed to treat potential hypovolemia or spinal shock. The patient is assessed for only gross neurological dysfunction, with the spine being gently palpated before the patient is moved.

The patient is transported with full C-spine precautions (see Chapter 1). These include placement of the patient in a neutral supine position on a long backboard, the application of a stiff immobilization cervical collar (unless neck swelling is evident), sandbags to each side of the head, and a wide strip of adhesive tape placed across the forehead and secured to the sides of the backboard. The goals of treatment in the emergency department are to suspect and confirm SCI and prevent further injury.

Signs of Spinal Cord Injury

Spinal cord injury is suspected by the mechanism of injury and in patients with head injury. In addition, any of the following signs and symptoms should be considered due to SCI until proved otherwise[41]:

Pain. The conscious patient will be able to complain of pain in the neck or back. This important clue will of course be absent in the unconscious patient and in patients who may be lying in a position of comfort or distracted by more intense pain from other injuries.

Tenderness. Local tenderness over any area of the spinal column warrants spinal cord precautions. Careful palpation down the entire length of the spine is carried out without disturbing the alignment of the spine.

Painful Movement. The patient may experience increased pain on attempts to move. The patient must be allowed to move unassisted, very carefully, and without disturbing spinal alignment. The patient should not be encouraged to move if pain is experienced.

Deformity. Infrequently spinal deformities can be observed or palpated. The spinal processes may be prominent at an area of fracture. Absence of deformity does not rule out SCI.

Lacerations and Contusions. Lacerations and contusions on various parts of the body give clues to the mechanism of injury and the possibility of associated SCI. Facial cuts and bruises frequently accompany cervical spine injuries. The absence of associated lacerations and contusions does not rule out SCI.

Paralysis and Anesthesia. If the conscious patient is unable to voluntarily move the extremities or has loss of sensation in some areas, SCI is suspected.

If the patient is unconscious, the mechanism of injury (motor vehicle accident, fall) may suggest associated SCI. The following signs suggest cervical SCI in the unconscious patient[20]:

- flaccid extremities, loss of reflexes, including loss of rectal sphincter tone
- diaphragmatic breathing
- arms that may flex, but will not extend (may assume ''hold-up'' position)
- facial grimaces to painful stimulus applied above, but not below, the clavicles
- hypotension without other evidence of shock (patient has warm extremities and slow pulse)
- priapism

Assessment

Priorities in assessment include evaluations of the respiratory, circulatory, neurological, and general medical status, followed by diagnostic evaluation.

Respiratory Status. Assessment of respiratory status is carried out while maintaining full C-spine precautions. The jaw thrust maneuver is used initially to maintain an open airway in unconscious patients (see Chapter 1). There is a possibility of aspiration with the patient lying supine and immobilized. Associated head injury predisposes the patient to vomiting. If vomiting occurs, the patient and the backboard, as a unit, are turned to the side and the airway is suctioned as needed. Supplemental oxygen is applied and arterial blood gases are monitored.

Respiratory effort is assessed and abnormal respirations such as diaphragmatic breathing are noted. If indicated, intubation (nasotracheal, or endotracheal using a fiberoptic bronchoscope) is carried out. It may be necessary to perform an emergency tracheotomy (or cricothyrotomy) to assure an adequate airway. Mechanical ventilation is instituted if indicated by clinical status or arterial blood gas analysis.

Circulatory Status. Circulatory status is assessed and any external bleeding controlled. Frequent assessment of vital signs and continuous ECG monitoring are carried out. Intravenous fluids are usually limited to maintenance levels unless volume replacement is needed to treat hemorrhagic shock, or to improve cardiac output and spinal cord perfusion in spinal shock.[20] The insertion of a central line will facilitate rapid IV fluid administration.

Neurological Status. Assessment of neurological status includes establishing the level of consciousness using the Glasgow Coma Scale (see Chapters 1 and 3), and identifying the level of any neurological deficits. This includes assessing movement and muscle strength, sensation, and reflexes (see Chapter 3).

SCI is usually described relative to the neurological lesion and not the bony lesion. For example, in a C5-6 vertebral fracture dislocation, the neurological lesion would be at the C6-7 level because the C6 neurons arise above the area of dislocation. Below the C8 nerve root, the LMNs originate just opposite or above the vertebral body of the same number, although the nerves exit the spine by way of the foramina immediately below the corresponding vertebra. Below T-6 the neurons of the same root level concentrate at levels higher than the same numbered vertebral body (see Figure 2–21). A T11-12 vertebral fracture dislocation may destroy the L3-5 neurons.[42]

The assessment of motor function and strength of all major muscle groups tests the integrity of the corticospinal tracts. Some of the simple tests that can be performed to rapidly assess and approximate the patient's best level of functioning include the following:

C4-5   can shrug shoulders
C5-6   can flex arms at elbows (biceps)
C6   can wiggle thumbs
C7   can wiggle index finger
C7-8   can extend arms at elbows (triceps)
C8   can wiggle fifth fingers
T1-7   can use intercostal muscles
T6-12 can tense abdominal muscles
L1-3   can flex hips
S1-2   can plantar flex feet
S3-5   can tense perianal muscles

The sensory examination includes having the patient identify areas stimulated by pinprick while keeping the eyes closed. This assesses the spinothalamic tracts. The ability to differentiate between sharp and dull pain may indicate an incomplete lesion with some preservation of the lateral columns.[20] Some simple tests that can be performed to rapidly test the patient's level of sensory loss include:[20]

C2	two inches behind the tip of the ear
C4	top of the shoulder
C6	tip of the thumb
C7	tip of the middle finger
C8	tip of the fifth finger
T4	the nipple line
T6	the lower tip of the sternum
T10	the level of the umbilicus
L1	just below the iliac crest
L3	just above the kneecap
L5	anterior lower leg and anterior foot
S1	top of the fifth toe
S3	medial thigh
S4-5	perianal area (sacral sparing)

The function of the posterior columns is assessed by testing position sense, vibratory sense, or deep pain sensation. The sensation of light touch tests the anterior columns. Reflexes that are tested include deep tendon (DTRs), superficial abdominal, and the cremasteric in the male patient (see Chapter 3).

To test for the presence of sacral sparing, the patient is assessed for the presence of the bulbocavernous reflex. To perform this, the patient's leg is gently raised and the examiner observes for contraction of the anal sphincter in response to glans penis or clitoris compression, or gentle traction applied to an indwelling urinary catheter. This reflex can also be assessed by inserting a finger into the anus and checking for palpable contraction of the sphincter in response to these same stimuli.[5(p51)] This reflex will be absent in spinal shock, but may be the first reflex to return when spinal shock resolves.

General Medical Status. Assessment of the general medical status of the patient includes a description of the accident to determine the mechanism of injury, the patient's medical history, including any drug therapies, and a general physical examination to search for associated injuries (see Chapter 1).

In the presence of hypotension, evaluation must proceed for ruling out hemothorax or intraabdominal bleeding. The paralyzed patient with intraabdominal trauma will not complain of abdominal discomfort, and guarding will not be present.

Diagnostic Studies. Diagnostic studies include cross-table lateral cervical spine x-rays obtained as soon as life-threatening problems are identified and controlled. All seven cervical vertebrae must be seen. It may be necessary to pull the patient's shoulders down to accomplish visualization of C-7. A lateral swimmer's view may also be needed. If these x-rays are normal, anterior/posterior and open-mouth odontoid x-rays may be indicated. Under the direct supervision of the neurosurgeon, flexion and extension views of the cervical spine may also be obtained.

If thoracic SCI is suspected, lateral and anterior/posterior x-rays that include all 12 thoracic vertebrae are obtained. Lateral and anterior/posterior lumbar x-rays that visualize all five lumbar vertebrae may also be needed.

Spinal x-rays are examined for contour and alignment of the vertebral bodies, displacement of bone fragments into the spinal canals, linear or comminuted fractures of the laminae, pedicles, or neural arches, and soft tissue swelling.[20]

Skull, chest, extremity, and abdominal x-rays may also be done if the need is indicated by clinical examination or mechanism of injury. CT scanning may demonstrate the anatomy of spinal trauma and possible spinal canal compromise more clearly than plain x-rays. Sometimes emergency myelograms are indicated. Spinal cord angiography is used when vascular injury is suspected. Somatosensory evoked potentials may be assessed in treatment centers equipped to perform such tests.

Treatment

Following the immediate resuscitation phase, priorities in the immediate treatment of SCI patients include immobilization of the spinal column, the administration of medications to reduce spinal cord edema, intravenous fluids, bladder catheterization, and nasogastric intubation.

Immobilization. Patients with spinal instability from C1 to T1 are placed in cervical traction. Cervical traction should never be applied in the prehospital phase or emergency department until cervical spine x-rays are viewed. The insertion of Gardner-Wells skull tongs (see Chapter 1) is the easiest and quickest way to institute cervical traction. Generally five pounds of weight per cervical level involved are applied. An additional ten pounds of weight for the head may be added. The concurrent administration of muscle relaxants such as diazepam may help in the reduction and realignment of the spinal column.[2(p261)] Follow-up x-rays and sometimes myelograms are done to assess the correction of alignment. The patient in skull tongs must be placed on a turning frame such as a Stryker frame, Foster frame, CircOlectric bed, or a kinetic bed that provides automated movement. All of these beds serve to reduce the complications of immobilization.

Trippi-Wells Dual Purpose Cranial Tongs may be used to facilitate the progression of the patient from cervical traction to a halo vest. Once satisfactory alignment is achieved (often in two to eight weeks), the four skull pins act as the halo, with metal struts connecting the halo to a rigid plastic vest. This immobilizes the neck, allowing no flexion, extension, or rotation. The purpose of the halo brace is to expedite early mobilization and ambulation. Some patients with vertebral fractures, but without SCI will have the halo brace applied in the emergency department. This should be done only on patients in stable condition, since the jacket prevents the placement of a central line or the performance of cardiac massage should an emergency arise.

Occasionally, dislocations involving locked facets of the vertebrae (Figure 8–7) can be reduced manually under general anesthesia with fluoroscopic monitoring. Once closed reduction is carried out, the position is maintained with traction.[2(p260)]

Stable injuries to the thoracic or lumbar spine are usually managed with bed rest. All lifting and turning of the patient must be done with a minimum of three nursing personnel. One nurse ensures cervical alignment, one assures thoracolumbar alignment, while the third nurse watches leg alignment.

Surgical intervention is indicated in patients showing increasing neurological deficits and to stabilize grossly unstable fractures in which cord transection is not complete. Laminectomy and fusion, anterior fusion, or placement of Harrington rods may be carried out. Surgical debridement and dural repair is indicated for penetrating injuries to the cord.[12(p403)]

Control of Spinal Cord Edema. If neurological deficits are present, the patient is often given corticosteroids such as dexamethasone or methylprednisolone in an effort to reduce or minimize cord edema, stabilize cellular membranes, increase spinal cord perfusion, and to minimize the effects of ischemia. Corticosteroid use in SCI remains controversial.[2(p255)]

Some treatment centers administer osmotic agents such as mannitol to combat cord edema. They need to be given cautiously, if at all, in the presence of shock. Concurrent monitoring of pulmonary artery pressures is indicated in hemodynamically unstable patients.[2(p255)] Blood glucose levels require periodic monitoring in steroid and mannitol therapy. Urine should be tested for glucose and acetone every six hours.[2(p265)] Oxygen administration is also used to treat cord ischemia that can result from edema, circulatory impairment, or hemorrhage.

Intravenous Fluids. SCI patients are not maintained in a dehydrated state as are head injury patients. Often IV fluids are run at a rate of 125 ml per hour in adults. Intravenous antibiotics may be administered, especially in cases of penetrating injury.[2(p256)]

Bladder Catheterization. The insertion of an indwelling urinary catheter is required in the early stages of SCI, especially if mannitol has been administered. Spinal shock or lumbosacral SCIs will cause flaccidity of the bladder. With interruption of autonomic control of bladder tone and the reflexes for bladder emptying, the flaccid bladder distends with large amounts of urine. Any voiding that may take place represents overflow.[13]

Nasogastric Intubation. Nasogastric intubation and suction is frequently necessary to prevent gastric distention and aspiration due to paralytic ileus and to control vomiting that may result from swallowing blood from head or mouth trauma.

Experimental Treatment. Increasing interest in the role that neurotransmitters and endogenous opioids play in SCI has resulted in research in the use of opiate antagonists such as naloxone and the endogenous antagonist thyrotropic-releasing hormone. There is some evidence that these substances may have beneficial effect in reversing the circulatory collapse in spinal shock and may possibly help reduce the extent of an acute spinal cord lesion.[43]

Research done with dimethyl sulfoxide (DMSO) has indicated that it may be useful in improving cerebral circulation. Consequently, researchers are evaluating its usefulness in improving microcirculation in the spinal cord.

There are conflicting reports about the value of using spinal cord cooling measures such as local normal saline perfusion of the injured cord.[44,45]

The media have presented some of the testing being done with computerized muscle stimulation.

Complications

SCI can induce pathology in most of the body's systems. Neglect in the early management of these dysfunctions can lead to life-threatening emergencies and can also create long-term disabilities. While some of the complications discussed do not occur in the acute setting, an informed nurse is better prepared to answer the patient's questions, and to anticipate and prevent these complications when possible. Complications associated with SCI include:

- Respiratory system alterations
- Cardiovascular complications
- Temperature control changes
- Elimination problems
- Integumentary problems
- Sexual dysfunctions
- Autonomic dysreflexia

Respiratory System Alterations. Respiratory complications can include hypoventilation when diaphragmatic breathing is all that the patient can effect.

There is decreased tidal volume and vital capacity, with ineffective cough due to the loss of intercostal muscle function.[38]

Retained secretions, immobility, and aspiration can all lead to the development of pneumonia. The intubated patient is at risk because of the easy access afforded the infectious agent. Pulmonary edema can result from overzealous administration of IV fluids.[38]

Prevention is the best treatment for these pulmonary complications. Frequent assessment of vital capacity and tidal volume combined with arterial blood gas analysis is needed. Intubation and mechanical ventilation, as previously mentioned, may be necessary.

Nonintubated patients should be instructed in deep breathing and diaphragmatic coughing exercises. These exercises may initially be required as often as hourly. Periodic cultures of sputum should be obtained. Adequate hydration as well as adequate humidification of the airways is essential for effective sputum removal.

Pulmonary edema can be prevented by guiding fluid therapy on the basis of hemodynamic monitoring. Frequent assessment of lung sounds and periodic chest x-rays are indicated.

Cardiovascular Complications. Cardiovascular complications result from alterations in cardiovascular reflexes caused by spinal shock. Hypotension results from vasodilation and decreased venous return when there is interruption of sympathetic outflow in spinal cord transections above the T-6 level. Hypotension may require treatment with fluid administration, although it is often self-limiting. Colloid administration may be needed as well. Hemodynamic monitoring can assess the adequacy of fluid volume replacement.[38] Infrequently, symptomatic hypotension may require the administration of vasopressors.

Following the resolution of spinal shock the patient may still experience orthostatic hypotension, which can interfere with the rehabilitative process. Vasopressor and cardiac reflexes remain inadequate, with a profound drop in blood pressure experienced when the patient is taken from a reclining to an upright position. This most often occurs in patients who have been confined to bed for a prolonged period.[17(p273)]

Vasopressor drugs may be required to treat orthostatic hypotension. Ace wraps, elastic stockings, and an abdominal binder all help to improve venous return. The patient should be elevated to a sitting position very gradually, with frequent checks of blood pressure and pulse. A tilt table is often used to accustom the patient to gradually assuming an upright position.[17(p273)]

Bradycardia occurs as a result of interrupted sympathetic stimulation, and intact parasympathetic stimulation. Bradycardia may be aggravated by hypothermia or hypoxia. Symptomatic bradycardia may require treatment with atropine in addition to eliminating those aggravating factors.[38]

The patient is at risk for developing a vasovagal reflex (see Chapter 11). This reflex may be so severe as to cause cardiac arrest. A vasovagal reflex can be induced by suctioning, which causes hypoxia and vagal stimulation. Preoxygenation and limited suctioning time are carried out under continuous ECG monitoring.[38]

Immobility, decreased rate of blood flow, and lack of muscle tone all contribute to the risk of the development of venous thrombosis in the legs or pelvic veins. Pulmonary embolus can result. Clinically, venous thrombosis in the legs is difficult to detect because the patient will not complain of pain or calf tenderness. The legs must be periodically assessed for areas of warmth, localized swelling, or a red streak running up the extremity. Venous thrombosis in the pelvic veins may be essentially undetectable. In preventing venous thrombosis, support stockings may help, as well as low dose prophylactic anticoagulation.[17(p272)] Some centers utilize the Rotorest bed to help reduce the complications of immobilization.

Temperature Control Changes. Spinal shock also results in the loss of body temperature regulation. The loss of sympathetic influences causes inability to sweat below the lesion and vasodilation. The body temperature cannot automatically adjust to environmental temperature changes. The patient's temperature tends to move toward the ambient temperature of the environment, increasing the risk for the development of hypothermia. Treatment consists of preventing excessive loss of body heat and controlling the environmental temperature. Cautious use of a warming mattress may be required.[38]

Elimination Problems. Elimination problems involving the gastrointestinal and urinary systems are common. The most serious gastrointestinal complication in the acute phase is paralytic ileus. Although peristaltic activities are mediated by the parasympathetic nervous system, sudden interruption of spinal cord pathways seems to interfere with the control of gastrointestinal motility. Cervical SCI patients often have a more prolonged and severe ileus.[12(p419)]

Untreated ileus with abdominal distention can lead to vomiting and aspiration, respiratory distress, dehydration as a result of third-spacing or pooling of fluids in the gut, electrolyte imbalance, and sepsis. Treatment consists of nasogastric intubation and aspiration until gastrointestinal motility returns (usually in 3 to 5 days); correction of electrolyte imbalance; and appropriate antibiotic therapy.[12(p419)] Prolonged ileus could be due to retroperitoneal hematoma in thoracolumbar fracture.

Once paralytic ileus is resolved and feeding begins, the patient must begin bowel training. While most of the bowel is controlled by the parasympathetic nervous system, the lower one-third of the colon is mostly autonomous. A few days following injury it will begin to function more normally. Normal emptying will not occur, however, because the rectum may be more inactive. Constipation becomes a problem because of decreased emptying and a lack of food and fluid. Because voluntary control of bowel evacuation may be lost, regulation of bowel movements is accomplished by assuring adequate fecal bulk through a high fiber diet, increased fluid intake, and stool softeners. The rectal emptying reflex is stimulated with suppositories and digital stimulation optimally timed to occur after a meal in order to take advantage of the gastrocolic reflex.[42]

During this period there is also increased risk for the development of GI stress ulcers. Stress ulcers are thought to be caused by increased levels of circulating catecholamines and steroids following injury. Prophylactic administration of drugs that inhibit the secretion of gastric acid and antacids may be administered.[12(p419)]

Urinary retention increases the risk of infection. Strict aseptic technique, frequent peri care, careful I & O, and maintaining acidic urine will all help to prevent the occurrence of urinary tract infections.[17(p277)]

Following the resolution of spinal shock, bladder training should begin with the goal of removing the indwelling catheter as soon as possible and instituting an intermittent catheterization program. In patients with injury above the conus medullaris, bladder tone will return and the patient will be left with a spastic or UMN bladder. The patient can be trained to apply certain tactile stimuli that will ''trigger'' the bladder to empty. Patients with sacral SCI on the other hand will be left with a permanently flaccid or LMN bladder. These patients will learn to crede the bladder to empty it as well as perform intermittent catheterizations.[42]

Integumentary Problems. The prevention of integumentary problems begins in the emergency department and must be continued for the rest of the patient's life. Denervated tissues break down faster and heal more slowly than tissues with normal nerve supply. Poor circulation may add to the patient's risk. Pressure sores are the most dreaded complication and are very costly in terms of time and money spent in treatment. Extra care is required on the part of all care givers to protect the patient's skin and avoid injuries that can easily occur because of decreased or absent sensation.

Some measures that can be taken to prevent pressure sores include frequent (every one to two hours) repositioning of the patient to relieve pressure on any one body part, padding all pressure points, keeping the skin in areas of pressure dry, and increasing circulation to pressure areas by frequent cleaning and gentle rubbing. Patients are taught to change position every one to two hours while in the wheelchair, and to inspect their entire body daily (using a hand mirror) for early signs of pressure sores. The importance of adequate nutrition is also stressed.[12(p420)]

Sexual Dysfunction. Sexuality and sexual activities are subjects that are of great concern to the SCI patient. Nurses are cautioned to listen for clues that the patient is ready to discuss these concerns, and to not approach the subject prematurely. To offer too much information at once may prove overwhelming for the patient.[12(p422)] Specially trained counselors and rehabilitation health care workers can assist the nursing staff in discussing this subject in depth with the patient.

In brief, most quadriplegic and paraplegic males are capable of having reflex erections from physical stimulation and psychic erections secondary to cerebral arousal. Emission or ejaculation may occur in a reflex manner, but not in a coordinated manner. Sensation of course will be absent. Female patients will have menstrual periods, be able to become pregnant, and some are capable of vaginal delivery. Again, sensation will be lacking. Labor can be precipitous in quadriplegics and can lead to dysreflexia. This necessitates a higher incidence of caesarean section.[42]

The presence of a caring partner is perhaps the most important factor leading to satisfying sexual activity following SCI.

Autonomic Dysreflexia. Autonomic dysreflexia (hyperreflexia) is a condition that may affect any patient with a cervical or high thoracic (above T-6) SCI. It can occur at any time after the acute phase of SCI. Any noxious stimulus such as a distended bladder, urinary calculus, fecal impaction, or pressure sore can initiate a reflex action causing excessive sympathetic or parasympathetic discharges. Increased sympathetic tone causes a sustained constriction of the splanchnic arterioles which increases the resistance to blood flow. Severe hypertension, which cannot be relieved by action of the vasomotor center, results. The parasympathetics are unable to inhibit the action of the sympathetics because of the level of the spinal cord lesion. The hypertension, if not controlled, can reach blood pressures of 300/160. The vagus nerve inhibits cardiac rate causing a slowing of the pulse. The hypertension results in a pounding headache. Superficial vasodilation occurs in areas above the cord injury, resulting in flushing of the head and neck, engorgement of temporal and neck vessels, and nasal congestion. Sweating occurs above the level of cord injury and goose bumps appear. Chills without fever may occur. If this excessive hypertension is not relieved, myocardial failure, intracranial, or retinal hemorrhage can occur.[12(pp411–415),17(pp273–274)]

This is a medical emergency and the patient should not be left alone. One nurse monitors the blood pressure and patient status while another provides treatment. Treatment consists of placing the patient in an upright sitting position and immediately removing the offending cause. If a catheter is not in place, the patient is immediately catheterized. The catheter should first be lubricated with lidocaine hydrochloride jelly. Five hundred cc of urine are drained and the blood pressure is checked. If it is still elevated, then another 500 cc are drained. If the blood pressure declines after the bladder is empty, it should still be watched closely as the bladder can go into severe contractions causing hypertension to recur. Thirty cc of tetracaine can be instilled through the catheter to stop the flow of impulses from the bladder.[128(pp414–415)]

If a catheter is in place, it and the closed drainage system are checked for kinks or obstructions. If it is suspected that the catheter is plugged it is irrigated slowly with no more than 30 cc of irrigating solution. If the bladder is in tetany, the fluid will go in but will not come out. If the catheter cannot be irrigated, it should be changed immediately.

If the bladder is not the cause of the dysreflexia, the rectum is checked for impaction. If impaction is detected, an anesthetic ointment is inserted into the rectum ten minutes before removal of the impaction. This prevents excessive stimuli from being transmitted to the spinal cord from digital stimulation.[12(p414)]

If the bladder and rectum findings are negative, the skin is checked for cuts, pimples, boils, pressure sores, ingrown toenails, etc. If symptoms do not subside, have available IV solutions and antihypertensive drugs of the physician's choice. The physician may choose to use phentolamine (Regitine), diazoxide (Hyperstat), hydralazine hydrochloride (Apresoline), or others. Atropine may be administered to relieve bladder tetany by acting on the parasympathetic system.[12(pp411–415),17(pp273–274)] A low spinal anesthesia may be utilized when medications are ineffective.

To control frequent episodes of autonomic dysreflexia, the patient may be placed on oral ganglionic blocking agents such as pentolinium (Ansolysen), mecamylamine (Inversine), phenoxybenzamine (Dibenzyline), or guanethidine sulfate (Ismelin).[17(p274),46]

Patients with SCI above the T-6 level are taught about autonomic dysreflexia, its causes, symptoms, and management. Some patients carry informational cards that they present to medical personnel if they feel that they may be developing dysreflexia.

Emotional Support

Throughout their hospital stay, patients with SCI will require emotional support from the nursing staff. Often the return of reflexes or muscle spasticity is misinterpreted by the patient or the family as a return of voluntary movement. Tact and honesty are required in responding to such situations and to the patient's many questions. The best attitude to convey to the family may be to hope for the best but prepare for the worst.

Nursing plays a major role in teaching patients and families about the condition of SCI so that they can understand its signs, symptoms, and anticipated prognosis. Emotional support and appropriate professional referrals can help these patients deal with the many lifestyle changes they face.

Conclusion

Following emergency diagnosis and stabilization, it is desirable, when appropriate, to transfer the SCI patient to a designated SCI center, of which there are several located in various regions of the United States. The multidisciplinary team of physicians and allied health personnel who staff such centers are committed to comprehensive, optimal care in all phases of SCI, from acute through rehabilitation and home training.

REFERENCES

1. McGuffin JF: Basic cerebral trauma care. *J Neurosurg Nurs* 1983:15:189–193.

2. Green BA, Marshal LF, Gallagher TJ: *Intensive Care for Neurological Trauma and Disease.* Orlando, Fla, Academic Press, 1982.

3. Dudas S, Stevens KA: Central cord injury: Implications for nursing. *J Neurosurg Nurs* 1984;16:84–88.

4. Stanton GM: A needs assessment of significant others following the patient's spinal cord injury. *J Neurosurg Nurs* 1984;16:253–256.

5. Trunkey DD, Lewis FR: *Current Therapy of Trauma 1984–1985.* Philadelphia, BC Decker, 1984.

6. Campbell E, Kuhlenbeck H: Mortal brain wounds: A pathological study. *J Neuropath Exp Neurol* 1950;9:139–149.

7. Perdue P: Life-threatening head and spinal injuries. *RN* June 1981, pp 37–41, 102.

8. Parkinson J: The ballistics of craniocerebral gunshot wounds. *J Neurosurg Nurs* 1982; 14:232–238.

9. Yanko J: Head injuries. *J Neurosurg Nurs* 1984;16:173–180.

10. Thygerson AL. Motor vehicle accidents. *Emergency* 1984;16:66–71.

11. Price SA, Wilson LM: *Pathophysiology: Clinical Concepts of Disease Processes.* New York, McGraw-Hill, 1978, pp 626–629.

12. Rudy EB: *Advanced Neurological and Neurosurgical Nursing.* St Louis, Mosby, 1984.

13. Synder M, Jackle M: *Neurological Problems: A Critical Care Nursing Focus.* Bowie, Md, Brady, 1981.

14. Roberts JR: Pathophysiology, diagnosis and treatment of head trauma. *Top Emerg Med* 1979;1:41–61.

15. Stephenson HE, Jr: *Immediate Care of the Acutely Ill and Injured,* ed 2. St Louis, Mosby, 1978, pp 204.

16. Budassi SA, Barber JM: *Emergency Nursing: Principles and Practice.* St Louis, Mosby, 1981, pp 270-317.

17. Hickey JV: *The Clinical Practice of Neurological and Neurosurgical Nursing.* Philadelphia, Lippincott, 1981.

18. Jennett B, Teasdale G: *Management of Head Injuries.* Philadelphia, FA Davis Co, 1981.

19. Troupin RH: *Diagnostic Radiology in Clinical Medicine,* ed 2. Chicago, Year Book, 1980, pp 146–150.

20. American College of Surgeons Committee on Trauma: *Advanced Trauma Life Support, Instructor's Manual,* Chicago, 1982, pp 87–112.

21. Ward JD: Emergency treatment of major head trauma. *Hosp Med,* March 1980, pp 58–65.

22. Franco LM: Cerebral contusion: A prototype for head injury. *J Neurosurg Nurs* 1984;16:45–49.

23. Gennarelli TA, Spielman GM, Langfitt TW, et al: Influence of the type of intracranial lesion on outcome from severe head injury. *J Neurosurg* 1982;56:26–32.

24. Mahoney BD, Rockswold GL, Ruiz E, et al: Emergency twist drill trephination. *Neurosurgery* 1981;8:551–554.

25. Weir BKA: Results of burr hole and open or closed suction drainage for chronic subdural hematomas in adults. *Can J Neurol Sci* 1983;10:22–26.

26. Gennarelli TA: Cerebral concussion and diffuse brain injuries, in Cooper PR (ed): *Head Injury*. Baltimore, Williams & Wilkins, 1982, pp 83–96.

27. Adams JH, Graham MR, Murray LS, et al: Diffuse axonal injury due to nonmissile head injury in humans: An analysis of 45 cases. *Ann Neurol* 1982;12:557–563.

28. Adams JH, Mitchell DE, Graham DI, et al: Diffuse brain damage of immediate impact type. *Brain* 1977;100:489–502.

29. Teasdale G, Mendelow D: Pathophysiology of head injury, in Brooks N (ed): *Closed Head Injury: Psychological, Social and Family Consequences*. Oxford, Oxford University Press, 1984, pp 4–34.

30. Doczi T, Tarjanyi J, Huszka E, et al: Syndrome of inappropriate secretion of antidiurectic hormone (SIADH) after head injury. *Neurosurgery* 1982;10:685–688.

31. Smith J, Geist BL: Evaluation and care of the acute craniotomy patient. *J Neurosurg Nurs* 1978;10:102–111.

32. Safar P, Bleyaert A, Nemoto E, et al: Resuscitation after global brain ischemia-anoxia. *Crit Care Med* 1978;6:215–225.

33. Abramson N: Brain function in resuscitology. *Curr Top Emerg Med* 1981;1(no 5).

34. Eilers M: Pharmacologic therapeutic modalities: Osmotic and diuretic agents. *Crit Care Q* 1983;5:63–69.

35. Hoffman JR, Orban DJ, Podolsky S: Pharmacologic therapeutic modalities: Corticosteroids. *Crit Care Q* 1983;5:52–59.

36. Bowers SA, Marshall LF: Severe head injury: Current treatment and research. *J Neurosurg Nurs* 1982;14:210–218.

37. Roberts JR: Trauma of the cervical spine. *Top Emerg Med* 1979;1:63–77.

38. Nikas DL: The nervous system, in Borg N, Nikas DL, Stark J, et al (eds): *Core Curriculum for Critical Care Nursing*, ed 2. Philadelphia, WB Saunders, 1981, pp 177–254.

39. Chusid JG: *Correlative Neuroanatomy and Functional Neurology*, ed 15. Los Altos, Ca, Lange Medical Publications, 1973, pp 73.

40. Taylor JW, Ballenger S: *Neurological Dysfunctions and Nursing Intervention*. New York, McGraw-Hill, 1980, pp 407.

41. The Committee on Allied Health, American Academy of Orthopedic Surgeons: *Emergency Care and Transportation of the Sick and Injured*, ed 2. Menasha, Wis, George Banta, 1977, pp 171–173.

42. Williamson-Kirkland TE, Berni R: Neurological aspects of rehabilitation: Part 2, Spinal cord injury. *ARN Journal*, July-August 1980, pp 8–13.

43. Mathias CJ, Frankel HL: Autonomic failure in tetraplegia, in Bannister R (ed): *Autonomic Failure*. Oxford, Oxford University Press, 1983, pp 453–488.

44. Wells JD, Hansebout RR: Local hypothermia in experimental spinal cord trauma. *Surg Neurol* 1978;10:200–204.

45. Tator CH, Deecke L: Value of normothermic perfusion, hypothermic perfusion and durotomy in the treatment of experimental acute spinal cord trauma. *J Neurosurg* 1973;36:52–63.

46. Conway-Rutkowski BL: *Carini and Owens' Neurological and Neurosurgical Nursing*, ed 8. St Louis, Mosby, 1982, pp 640.

Chapter 9

Neurovascular Emergencies

Intracranial vascular lesions are the third leading cause of death in developed countries.[1] Neurovascular disease may be due to lesions of the veins, capillaries, and most commonly, arteries. Impairment of cerebral circulation in one or more blood vessels supplying the brain results in a stroke or cerebral vascular accident (CVA).

In any one year, approximately one-half million persons in the United States will suffer a stroke. Less than half of these people will survive beyond a month. Of those surviving, only ten percent will recover fully. At any one time, roughly 2.5 million people in the United States are living with disabilities common to stroke, creating a heavy demand on health care resources. Disabilities can range from mild neurological deficits to severe motor, speech, sensory, and perceptual impairment, with ten percent of the survivors requiring long-term institutional care.[1]

The anatomy of the cerebral blood supply and various extrinsic and intrinsic factors that regulate and/or affect cerebral blood flow are discussed in Chapter 2. It is important to recall that the vascular network comprising the circle of Willis at the base of the brain allows for the direction and redirection of blood flow to all areas of the brain. The collateral vascular connections can provide adequate perfusion to areas of the brain if occlusion occurs in a smaller supply artery. This feature accounts for the recovery of many stroke victims.[2]

In discussing neurovascular emergencies, five major pathological processes contribute to the development of a stroke: atherosclerosis (thrombosis), embolism, hypertensive intracerebral hemorrhage, ruptured saccular (berry) aneurysm, and ruptured arteriovenous malformation. Each is described in detail later. While ruptured aneurysm most often results in subarachnoid hemorrhage, which usually presents with headache and altered mentation, other vascular lesions can result in characteristic neurological signs based on the level of involvement within the brain. Initial evaluation of the patient includes delineation of the level of involvement within the brain followed by determination of the etiology of the stroke.

SUPRATENTORIAL LESIONS

Supratentorial vascular lesions affect the cerebral cortex or the subcortical structures such as the internal capsule and the thalamus.

Cortical Lesions

Characteristic motor deficits associated with cortical lesions include paresis or paralysis of the lower half of the face, arm, and leg on the side opposite the lesion. Initial flaccid paralysis will be followed within weeks by spastic paralysis which can result in contractures. Spastic paralysis results from the restoration of muscle tone by spinal reflex nerves. Spastic paralysis as seen in stroke represents an upper motor neuron disorder and is characterized by hyperreflexia in the affected extremities and an extensor plantar response (Babinski reflex). Eventually some motor improvement may be seen, and is usually more complete in the lower extremity than in the upper extremity.[3]

Middle Cerebral Artery Syndrome

Middle cerebral artery syndrome is the most common of all cerebral occlusions. Figure 9–1 depicts some of the more common motor, sensory, and perceptual deficits associated with destructive lesions of the right and left hemispheric cortices caused by occlusion of the main stem of the middle cerebral artery. There may be vomiting and a rapid onset of coma which lasts a few weeks. A massive infarction can cause extensive cerebral edema.[4]

Lesions of the Right Hemisphere. Patients with injury to the right cerebral hemisphere may exhibit some or all of the following dysfunctions: left hemiparesis or hemiplegia, left hemihypesthesia (decreased sensation on the left side of the body), deviation of the head and eyes to the right, inattention to objects in the left visual field and to left auditory stimuli, left homonymous hemianopsia (hemianopia), a blindness in the left half of both visual fields. (See Figure 9–2.)

Various sensory agnosia or comprehension losses may occur. Astereognosia refers to the inability to recognize objects placed in the hand without the aid of visual clues. Astatoagnosia is the inability to determine the position of body parts. Tactile inattention is the lack of attention to simultaneous stimuli. Anosognosia denotes the patient's unawareness of neurological deficits.

Apraxia is the inability to carry out, on command, complex or skilled movements when the motor systems for these movements are intact. Construction apraxia is demonstrated when patients do not complete the left half of figures they are asked to draw. In addition, patients with right cerebral hemisphere injuries may display an inability to dress themselves properly (dressing apraxia).

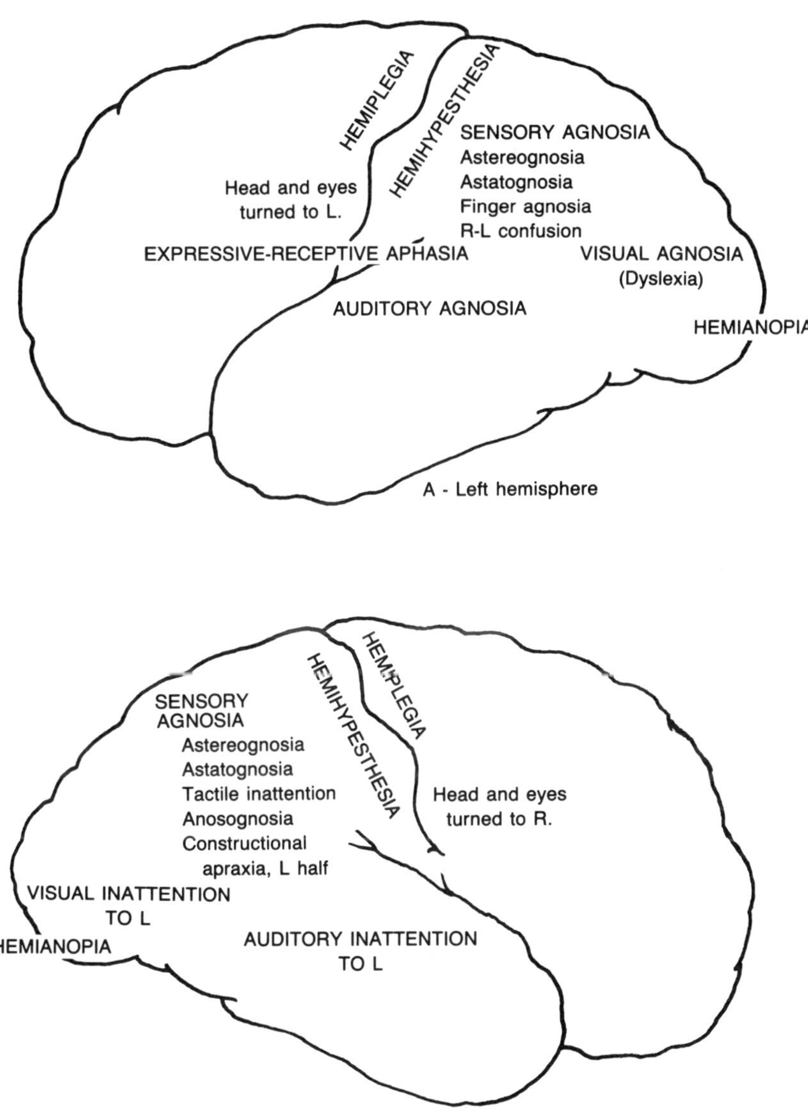

Fig. 9–1—Signs and symptoms that occur with focal destructive lesions in the right or left cerebral hemisphere.

Source: Reprinted from *Technique of the Neurologic Examination* ed 3 (p 354) by William DeMyer with permission of the McGraw-Hill Book Company, © 1980.

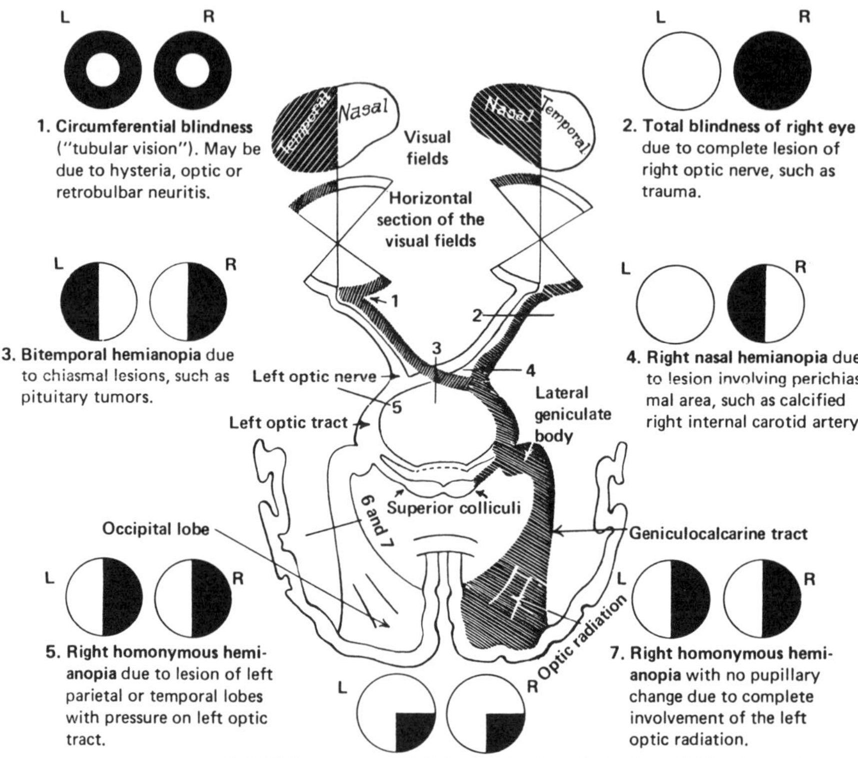

Fig. 9–2—Visual field defects associated with lesions of visual system.
Source: Reprinted from *Correlative Neuroanatomy and Functional Neurology* ed 19 (p 114) by Joseph Chusid with permission of Lange Medical Publications, © 1985.

Lesions of the Left Hemisphere. Patients with injury to the left cerebral hemisphere may exhibit right hemiparesis or hemiplegia, right hemihypesthesia, right homonymous hemianopsia, and deviation of the head and eyes to the left. Additional sensory agnosias seen with left hemisphere lesions include finger agnosia (an inability to identify the finger touched), and right-to-left confusion.

Various degrees of aphasia may also result if the speech centers in the left cerebral hemisphere are affected. Explanations for the various complexities of speech disorders are beyond the scope of this book. In brief, expressive aphasia (Broca's aphasia) refers to the inability to transform sounds into articulated speech. The deficit ranges from a slight difficulty with articulation to an almost complete loss of the power of speech. In addition, the patient is also unable to express written thoughts, so handwriting cannot be used as a means of communication. Receptive aphasia (Wernicke's aphasia) refers to the inability to understand spoken or written words. The patient may still be able to talk, but cannot comprehend spoken words. Such patients also have difficulty naming objects. Mixed or global aphasia involves both expressive and receptive language disorders. All language modalities may be affected, and the impairment may be so severe that the patient is unable to communicate on any level. The global aphasic generally has an accompanying severe hemiplegia. Conduction aphasia occurs when a lesion disrupts the connection between Broca's and Wernicke's areas. The patient may produce words, but speech conveys little meaning. Many errors of syntax and grammar are made. Some of these patients may be aware of their deficits and can comprehend what is said to them, but are incapable of self-initiated speech or repetition of words.[1(pp118–120)]

Auditory agnosia refers to difficulty in recognizing not only words, but also other sounds such as bells or whistles. Visual agnosia is the inability to recognize objects or people. In addition, the patient may see only part of an image, rather than the whole.

Anterior Cerebral Artery Syndrome

This syndrome is uncommon because the anterior cerebral artery is the least often occluded. If the occlusion occurs distal to the anterior communicating artery, infarction of the medial aspect of one frontal lobe will occur. Symptoms include contralateral leg and foot paralysis, impaired gait, paresis of the contralateral arm, mental impairment with flat affect, slowness, perseveration, and amnesia. Urinary incontinence is common. Hemianopsia and aphasia are not seen with anterior cerebral artery syndromes.[4]

Posterior Cerebral Artery Syndrome

The most prominent neurological deficit associated with posterior cerebral artery occlusion is contralateral homonymous hemianopsia. There may also be visual hallucinations, color blindness, and lack of depth perception. Memory deficits and perseveration may also be present.[4]

Internal Carotid Artery Syndrome

In most cases, occlusion of an internal carotid artery results in stroke of the middle cerebral artery with similar signs and symptoms. The internal carotid artery also supplies the optic nerve and retina, and approximately 25 percent of the patients with progressive occlusion of the internal carotid will report transient warning attacks of blindness in one eye (amaurosis fugax).[1(p14)]

Subcortical Lesions

Significant subcortical supratentorial structures involved in stroke include the internal capsule and the thalamus. Clinical symptoms associated with subcortical lesions are similar to those involving cortical structures, although hemorrhage into the internal capsule causes motor paralysis that is more pronounced than accompanying sensory losses. Thalamic lesions, on the other hand, cause sensory losses greater than motor losses.[2] Unlike cortical lesions which cause conjugate eye deviation toward the side of the lesion (away from the paralyzed side), thalamic strokes cause deviation of the eyes downward to "look" at the nose. The pupils may be unreactive to light.[3]

SUBTENTORIAL LESIONS

Subtentorial vascular lesions affecting the brainstem or cerebellum may produce a wide assortment of signs and symptoms. Brainstem lesions are characterized by a sudden loss of consciousness and a "crossed paralysis," i.e., ipsilateral involvement of one or more cranial nerves and contralateral hemiplegia. Sensory deficits are also crossed. In brainstem lesions, there may be a dysconjugate gaze, or the eyes may deviate away from the side of the lesion. Abnormalities of the cranial nerves allow one to more easily identify at which level in the brainstem the lesion is located. For instance, midbrain lesions cause oculomotor nerve paralysis and pupillary dilation, while pontine lesions cause pupillary constriction. Complete paralysis, coma, and decerebrate rigidity usually precede death from pontine hemorrhage.[3]

Cerebellar hemorrhage is characterized by severe occipital headache, vertigo, vomiting, nystagmus, and ataxia. The eyes are usually conjugately deviated away from the side of the lesion.[3]

DIAGNOSTIC PROCEDURES

Accurate diagnosis of the etiology of stroke will determine the medical and nursing care required. It is vital that the distinction be made between an ischemic and a hemorrhagic stroke. Ischemic strokes are usually of thrombotic or embolic etiology. Hemorrhagic strokes are most often caused by hypertensive vascular disease, a ruptured cerebral aneurysm, or hemorrhage from an arteriovenous malformation (AVM).

The most frequently used diagnostic procedures are CT scanning and cerebral angiography. See Chapter 1 for descriptions of and nursing responsibilities associated with common neurological diagnostic procedures.

Computerized Tomography

Computerized tomography (CT scanning) makes it possible to differentiate between cerebral infarction and intracerebral hemorrhage. The use of contrast media with CT scanning helps differentiate an AVM from a clot or tumor, but the definitive diagnosis of an AVM or an aneurysm still requires angiography. Hydrocephalus can be identified on a CT scan. Necrotic areas of brain tissue caused by thrombosis may not be evident until a few days after infarction. Lacunar infarctions (small cavities formed by brain softening as a result of occlusions of penetrating arteries) also appear on the CT scan later in the patient's course.[4]

Cerebral Angiography

Cerebral angiography probably represents the most definitive diagnostic study in determining the location and etiology of a stroke. It is important that four-vessel visualization be done to adequately evaluate the extracranial vessels, the carotids and vertebrals, as well as the intracranial vessels.[2] If bleeding has destroyed an AVM, the arteriogram may appear normal. Also, cerebral vasospasm, while visible on angiography, may prevent adequate visualization of some vascular abnormalities.[4]

Certain risk factors are associated with cerebral angiography and include rebleeding following subarachnoid hemorrhage, vasospasm, and stroke as a consequence of vessel occlusion or embolization.

Digital Subtraction Angiography

An image of cerebral and extracerebral arteries is made before and after intravenous injection of contrast material and a computer subtracts the original image from the later image. While not as consistently accurate as conventional angiography, digital subtraction angiography has the advantage of intravenous injection, as well as intraarterial, and sometimes does not require hospitalization. A smaller concentration of contrast media is required for visualization of vessels.

Lumbar Puncture

Lumbar puncture (LP) is being performed less since the increased availability of CT scanning. In thrombotic stroke, the cerebrospinal fluid (CSF) is clear, but may show an elevated protein content. Bloody CSF and elevated white blood cell (WBC) and protein levels are seen in hemorrhagic strokes in which bleeding occurs into the subarachnoid space or ventricles.[5] CSF pressure may also be elevated in hemorrhagic stroke. An LP must be performed with caution in patients suspected of having elevated intracranial pressure. As CSF is withdrawn from the lumbar space, there may be a downward displacement of the brain (herniation).

Positive Emission Tomography

Positive emission tomography (PET scanning) provides information on brain cell metabolism as well as cerebral blood flow and cerebral blood volume. Cerebral infarction size and location can be defined by this extremely expensive new technology.[2]

Nuclear Magnetic Resonance Imaging

Nuclear magnetic resonance imaging (NMR or MRI) provides detailed images similar to those made by CT scanners, but without the use of x-ray radiation. Arteries may be seen as tubular structures. Altered blood flow patterns may be detected. Cerebral infarction with its accompanying edema formation will demonstrate localized increased water content. Hemorrhage into the soft tissue of the brain can be readily visualized.

Noninvasive Blood Flow Studies

Noninvasive blood flow studies such as carotid Doppler sonography, Doppler ultrasound, thermography, and ophthalmodynamometry assess the adequacy of extracranial vessel circulation. Stenotic lesions can often be identified. While these studies are painless, of no risk to the patient, and help monitor therapy, their use mainly just complements other more definitive diagnostic studies.[2]

Skull Films

While skull x-rays do not offer definitive diagnoses, they demonstrate abnormal areas of calcification that require further investigation. Certain tumors and some vessels may contain areas of increased calcification.[4] Severe swelling of cerebral tissue or an intracerebral hemorrhage may cause a shift of the calcified pineal body away from midline toward the side opposite the lesion.

Electroencephalogram

An electroencephalogram (EEG) can be helpful in localizing areas of cerebral dysfunction and can sometimes help localize AVM lesions.[4]

Consideration must also be given to the differential diagnosis as many other pathological processes can mimic stroke. Metastatic or primary brain tumors may present with strokelike signs and symptoms. Tumors can also precipitate a hemorrhagic stroke. Seizures followed by Todd's postictal paralysis (see Chapter 10) can simulate stroke, as can disorders such as hypoglycemia, hyper- and hyposmolar states, hepatic and uremic encephalopathy.[6]

In addition to the above diagnostic procedures, laboratory studies including complete blood cell count (CBC), urinalysis, arterial blood gases, coagulation panel, serum osmolality, electrolytes, blood sugar, triglycerides, blood urea nitrogen (BUN), and creatinine are obtained.

A baseline electrocardiogram (ECG) should also be obtained because the neurological system has a profound effect on cardiac function. Likewise, cardiovascular function directly affects the neurological system.

ETIOLOGY OF STROKE

Strokes are usually classified according to their etiologic bases. They can be subdivided into ischemic and hemorrhagic varieties.

Ischemic Strokes

Nearly two-thirds of patients with stroke will have the ischemic variety in which the blood vessel lumen becomes occluded as a result of thrombosis or embolism.

Thrombotic Strokes

Atherosclerotic cerebral infarction from thrombus formation represents the most common cause of stroke. Inflammatory disease of the arterial wall and mechanical constriction of arteries can also contribute to cerebral artery thrombosis. Prolonged cerebral vasoconstriction, inadequate cerebral perfusion, hematological disorders, and hypercoagulability are additional causes of thrombotic stroke.[2] Vessel occlusion often occurs within the cerebral arteries or in the extracranial vessels such as the carotid or vertebral arteries.

Thrombotic strokes often occur during periods of inactivity. Sixty percent of thrombotic strokes occur during sleep.[4] There may be an abrupt onset of signs and symptoms, or progressive levels of neurological deficit may be evident. The stroke may be preceded by a localized headache or a seizure. The location of the headache and manifestations of the seizure may help in determining the location of the cerebral infarction, as will the nature of the neurological deficits.[2]

Embolic Strokes

Embolism is the second most common pathological process causing stroke and is primarily caused by heart and carotid artery disease. Blood clots and other substances such as plaques and vegetations can form in the heart and be expelled into the circulatory system. Contributing cardiac diseases include rheumatic endocarditis, postrheumatic valvular disease, bacterial endocarditis, myocardial infarction with mural thrombus formation, congenital heart disease, and atrial fibrillation and other dysrhythmias.[1]

Emboli can also arise from atheromatous plaques lining the carotid, basilar, and vertebral artery systems. Additional causes of cerebral emboli include foreign substances such as air, tumor, fat, or foreign bodies.[2]

When an embolus travels to the brain, a stroke results. Clinical signs and symptoms vary with the size and location of the vessel that is occluded. Unlike thrombosis, the symptoms of cerebral embolus develop rapidly. A large embolus may initially produce severe neurological deficits that clear somewhat as the clot breaks up and passes, in many small pieces, into smaller vessels.[1] In some cases an embolic occlusion of a vessel produces a hemorrhagic infarction. Patients with untreated underlying conditions that can cause cerebral embolism are at great risk for developing subsequent episodes of stroke.

Clinical Features

Cerebral arterial occlusive disorders can be further classified according to their temporal profile.

Transient Ischemic Attacks. Transient ischemic attacks (TIAs) are focal neurological deficits caused by localized cerebral ischemia. They are characterized by a rapid onset (no symptoms to maximal symptoms in less than 5 minutes) and brief duration (usually less than 15 minutes, but less than 24 hours by definition). The term reversible ischemic neurological deficit (RIND) is sometimes used to describe TIAs in which symptoms persist longer than 24 hours.

Signs and symptoms of TIA vary with the arteries involved. Carotid and cerebral artery disease may lead to transient blindness in one eye, contralateral hemiparesis or hemiplegia and hemianesthesia, speech disturbances, and confusion. Signs and symptoms associated with TIA caused by vertebral artery disease may include dizziness, diplopia, numbness, visual defects in one or both visual fields, and dysarthria (difficult and defective speech).[4] Drop attacks, the sudden loss of postural tone without loss of consciousness, may also be seen in vertebrobasilar or brainstem ischemia.[2]

Many patients are symptom-free by the time they reach the emergency department (ED). Carotid or vertebral artery disease should be investigated in any patient with a history suspicious of TIA.[3] Approximately one-third of the patients who experience TIAs will develop cerebral infarction.[2]

Progressive (Stroke in Evolution). Stroke in evolution leads to motor and sensory deficits that develop and worsen over a period of hours or days, culminating in a cerebral infarction.[1]

Completed Stroke. In completed stroke, a cerebral infarction has occurred and the resulting neurological deficits are maximal.[1] The onset is gradual in thrombosis but may be sudden when caused by embolism.[2]

Medical and Nursing Management

Intensive nursing management of stroke is described later in this chapter. More emphasis is placed here on the medical and surgical management of ischemic stroke. The following medical therapies remain controversial and are probably of most benefit to patients who have experienced TIAs and have not yet suffered cerebral infarction.

Anticoagulation Therapy. Anticoagulation therapy with intravenous heparin followed by oral anticoagulants has been beneficial in some cases in halting the progression of stroke. Additional nursing responsibilities include teaching the patient and family about the drug, its dosage and administration, and side effects to watch for and report, such as bleeding. Instruct the patient about proper diet and what drugs to avoid, such as aspirin. Stress the importance of regular follow-up visits for required laboratory tests.[2]

Antiplatelet Aggregation Therapy. Antiplatelet aggregation therapy is used to prevent emboli formation in patients with cerebrovascular disease, particularly those who have experienced TIAs. The drugs most often used are aspirin, dypyridamole (Persantine), and sulfinpyrazone (Anturane). Again, instruct the patient in the dosage and administration of the drug and the possible side effects to watch for and report, which include gastrointestinal upset and gastrointestinal bleeding.[2]

Patients with acute cerebral infarction are sometimes treated with intravenous infusions of low molecular weight dextran in an attempt to prevent further platelet aggregation and clot formation. This treatment is considered of questionable benefit.[2] Antiplatelet aggregation therapy is also used following extracranial-to-intracranial bypass surgery.

Vasodilation Therapy. Vasodilation therapy has been used to improve cerebral blood flow (CBF) and promote the use of collateral circulation channels. Such drugs as papaverine hydrochloride and acetazolamide (Diamox) have all been shown to increase CBF, but have not been shown to improve the outcome of patients with TIAs or completed strokes.[2]

Surgical Management. Surgical procedures such as clot removal and endarterectomy with bypass graft may reduce the incidence of further ischemic stroke in patients with extracranial vascular disease.

Microsurgery techniques now allow for surgical intervention for some intracranial arterial obstructions. Extracranial to intracranial vessel bypass surgery may be especially useful when the occluded pathways are not surgically accessible. Such bypass techniques include anastomosing the superficial temporal artery to a branch of the middle cerebral artery. The occipital, middle meningeal, and subclavian arteries also serve as donor arteries. Microvascular surgery is not indicated for embolic strokes.[2]

Surgical techniques for extracranial vertebrobasilar ischemic disease include anastomosis of the vertebral artery to the ipsilateral common carotid artery. In cases of subclavian steal syndrome, transposition of the subclavian artery to the common carotid artery is just one approach that has been taken. Removal of atherosclerotic plaques and saphenous vein bypass grafts of vertebral arteries have also been successfully performed.[7]

Hemorrhagic Strokes

Intracranial hemorrhage is the third most common cause of stroke. Of the many causes of intracranial bleeding, the most common are hypertensive vascular disease, ruptured cerebral aneurysm, or AVM hemorrhage. Hypertension results in hemorrhage within the brain tissue while rupture of a cerebral aneurysm usually results in bleeding into the subarachnoid space. Rupture of an AVM can result in subarachnoid hemorrhage, intracerebral hemorrhage, or both.[2]

Intracranial hemorrhage usually occurs during some form of physical exertion, affecting most frequently those in middle age and the elderly. Signs and symptoms occur suddenly and vary depending on the size and location of the bleed, involvement of the surrounding brain tissue, degree of ischemia resulting from interruption of blood supply and vasospasm, and brain compression caused by cerebral edema. Regardless of the cause, intracranial hemorrhage is associated with a high mortality rate.[1]

Hypertensive Intracranial Hemorrhage

Hypertension and arteriosclerosis of the cerebral arteries predispose the patient to develop a hypertensive intracranial hemorrhage.[1] The incidence of hypertensive intracranial hemorrhage is higher in blacks than in whites.[8]

Pathophysiology. Rupture of an intracranial vessel resulting from hypertension usually occurs in arteries that penetrate the brain itself rather than in those of the circle of Willis. The putamen and adjacent internal capsule, various parts of the central white matter, the thalamus, a cerebellar hemisphere, and the pons represent the most common sites of hemorrhage. Extravasated blood acts as a mass lesion, causing tearing, compression, and displacement of adjacent brain tissue.[1]

Clinical Features. In addition to lateralizing neurological deficits, signs and symptoms include severe headache and hypertension. Vomiting and focal seizures are not uncommon.[1] There is usually an abrupt onset and rapid evolution of symptoms, occuring over minutes, hours, or occasionally, days.[8]

If the bleeding is confined to a restricted area, as brain swelling and cerebral edema resolve and the extravasated blood is absorbed, improvement in local cerebral blood flow leads to improvement in the patient's level of consciousness and responses.[1]

Prolonged bleeding may cause blood to leak into the ventricles leading to increased intracranial pressure, bloody CSF, and pyrexia. As the mass increases in size, brain shifts may occur leading to brain herniation with compression of vital centers (see Chapter 4). Coma and death can result.[1]

In pontine hemorrhage, the patient rapidly becomes comatose, may exhibit decerebrate rigidity, and will have small (1 mm) reactive pupils. Death usually occurs, but some patients with small tegmental hemorrhages have been known to survive. They may exhibit disturbances of lateral eye movements, crossed sensory or motor disturbances, small pupils, and cranial nerve palsies.[8]

Cerebellar hemorrhage is characterized by repeated vomiting, occipital headache, vertigo, dysarthria and dysphagia, and an inability to stand or walk. There may be deviation of the eyes to the side opposite the lesion or other abnormal eye movements. The patient may become comatose as a result of brainstem compression.[8]

Medical and Nursing Management. The general medical treatment for the patient with hypertensive intracranial hemorrhage is essentially supportive. This includes maintaining adequate oxygenation and ventilation (may include hyperventilation therapy), control of systemic hypertension, control of intracranial hypertension with dehydration therapy such as fluid restriction and the administration of diuretics and osmotic agents, and corticosteroid administration.

Surgical evacuation of a clot by aspiration or evacuation is sometimes lifesaving, but massive intracerebral hemorrhage carries a poor prognosis. An encapsulated hematoma is more amenable to successful surgical resection. In cerebellar hemorrhage, surgical evacuation of the clot may be necessary to prevent herniation.[1] Often for small lesions, conservative methods of treatment are as beneficial as surgical intervention.[1]

Ruptured Cerebral Aneurysm

Ruptured cerebral aneurysms represent the fourth most frequent cerebrovascular disorder.[8]

Pathophysiology. Aneurysms are localized dilations of blood vessels caused by congenital defects or acquired weaknesses in vessel walls. Aneurysms may be saccular (berry shaped) or fusiform (circumferential dilation). Mycotic aneurysms can occur from a septic embolus causing an infectious process in a vessel. Eighty-five percent of cerebral aneurysms form on vessels of the anterior portion of the circle of Willis, often at areas of bifurcation (Figure 9–3).[5] The average size of an aneurysm is 8–10 mm, but the size may vary from 2 mm to as large as 3 cm in diameter. Aneurysms smaller than 6 mm in diameter rarely rupture. Aneurysms are often multiple.[1]

The rupture of a cerebral aneurysm causes a subarachnoid hemorrhage, and represents the most common cause of death from cerebrovascular lesions in people under 45 years of age. Women are affected more often than men. About 50 percent of these patients die or become permanently disabled as a result of the initial hemorrhage. Approximately 20 percent of these deaths occur before patients reach the hospital. Some of these deaths may be caused by cardiac dysrhythmias (see Chapter 11). Of those reaching the hospital, about 30 percent die during the next several days to months as a result of the initial hemorrhage and its complications. Of those surviving the initial bleed in whom the aneurysm is left untreated, one-third will die as a consequence of rebleeding, most often occurring within the first two weeks.[9]

The high mortality is caused by rebleeding, or by the acute effects of the hemorrhage which include intracranial hypertension, destruction of brain tissue by hematoma, cerebral edema, acute hydrocephalus, and cerebral ischemia. Hypothalamic compression produces excessive sympathetic discharge which can lead to lethal cardiac dysrhythmias. Vasospasm caused by extravasated blood leads to increased cerebral ischemia and can lead to cerebral infarction.[5] Acute, severe hydrocephalus can develop if hemorrhage occurs into the ventricles.[9]

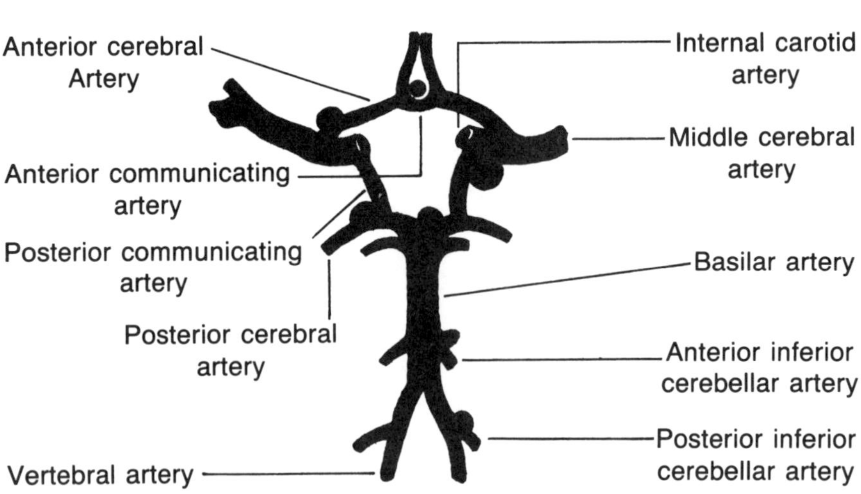

Fig. 9–3—Common locations for cerebral aneurysms.

Later complications can include communicating hydrocephalus from blockage of the reabsorption of CSF by blood in the subarachnoid space, and rebleeding which occurs as the result of the lysis of the fibrin-platelet clot that was formed to seal the original bleeding point.[9]

Clinical Features. In most cases, cerebral aneurysms cause no symptoms until the time of rupture, although almost 40 percent of patients with major aneurysmal rupture do have warning symptoms caused by expansion of the aneurysm. Focal signs such as localized head pain, diplopia, and a dilated pupil resulting from compression of the oculomotor nerve may occasionally be seen prior to aneurysmal rupture. Nonfocal signs such as generalized headaches, nausea, neck pain, back pain, malaise, and occasional photophobia may be seen in patients who have experienced a ''minor leak'' in the aneurysm.[9]

Rupture of an aneurysm occurs most often when the patient is active and engaging in physical activity. Rupture leads to hemorrhage under pressure into the subarachnoid space. Most often the attack begins with a sudden severe headache or a transient loss of consciousness followed by a headache. If bleeding is minimal, consciousness may never be lost. The headache may initially be localized to the suboccipital or frontal region, but soon becomes generalized and is often described as ''explosive.'' The blood acts as a foreign substance causing irritation of blood vessels, brain surface, and meninges. Meningeal signs such as photophobia, nuchal rigidity, and Kernig's sign develop several hours later, so may be initially absent on physical exam. Headache and nuchal rigidity may persist up to ten days. This meningitis may be so severe as to interfere with CSF reabsorption leading to hydrocephalus.[2]

Funduscopic examination often reveals subhyaloid hemorrhages on the retina. These appear as irregular blots of blood on the most superficial layer of the retina.[9]

There are no lateralizing neurological signs if the bleeding is confined to the subarachnoid space, although occasionally an aneurysm ruptures into brain substance and produces lateralizing neurological deficits. Lateralizing signs may also develop after subarachnoid hemorrhage because of surrounding vasospasm that interferes with blood supply to certain areas of the brain.[1] A transient paraparesis (weakness of the legs) suggests rupture of an anterior cerebral artery—anterior communicating artery aneurysm. Hemiparesis or aphasia may be seen with rupture of a middle cerebral artery aneurysm, while an oculomotor nerve palsy and pain around the orbit may result from rupture of an internal carotid artery–posterior communicating artery aneurysm.[5]

ECG changes, gastrointestinal (GI) disturbances, chest pain, back pain, leg pain, and vertigo may also occur, further confusing the diagnosis of subarachnoid hemorrhage.[5]

With massive hemorrhage, the patient may be stuporous or comatose, may exhibit focal neurological deficits such as hemiplegia or display extensor (decerebrate) rigidity. Death may ensue within minutes or following several days.[1]

Aneurysms are often categorized according to the severity of symptoms[2]:

grade I   minimal bleeding: alert, minimal headache, no neurological deficit

grade II   mild bleeding: alert, headache, minimal nuchal rigidity, no neurological deficit other than cranial nerve palsy

grade III moderate bleeding: lethargic, severe headache, nuchal rigidity, but may be alert, with focal neurological deficit such as hemiparesis or dysphasia

grade IV   moderate to severe bleeding: decreased level of consciousness with or without neurological deficit, nuchal rigidity

grade V   severe bleeding; comatose, moribund, with pathological responses such as decerebrate posturing

Medical and Nursing Management. The goals of management during the acute stage of ruptured cerebral aneurysm are to maintain adequate cerebral perfusion, prevent rebleeding, and prevent or minimize the effects of vasospasm.

Prevention of rebleeding. The cause of recurrent bleeding is not understood, but may be related to naturally occurring mechanisms of clot formation and lysis.[8] Rebleeding is characterized by deterioration in neurological function with an alteration in level of consciousness and an increase in severity of headache.

These signs and symptoms are similar to those associated with vasospasm. CT scanning and/or angiography is needed to determine the etiology of the deterioration.

Early medical therapy to prevent rebleeding (subarachnoid precautions) includes: bed rest in a quiet environment; a darkened room to lessen the symptoms of photophobia; restriction of visitors; sedation; analgesics; a soft, high-fiber diet; and stool softeners.[5]

Antihypertensive medications and diuretics are used to control systemic hypertension. Generally the blood pressure is maintained high enough to ensure adequate cerebral perfusion pressure and lessen vasospasm, yet not so high as to induce rebleeding. Each patient requires individualization of this therapy. Concurrent measures to reduce intracranial pressure (ICP) may be needed if elevated.

Antifibrinolytic therapy may also be used to prevent rebleeding. The formation of a fibrin clot and vasospasm are responsible for the initial cessation of bleeding following rupture of an intracranial aneurysm. Fibrinolysis, or the dissolving of the fibrin clot, occurs approximately seven days after hemorrhage. This accounts for the high incidence of rebleeding experienced within the first two weeks following subarachnoid hemorrhage.[2]

Aminocaproic acid (Amicar) prevents fibrinolysis by inhibiting the conversion of plasminogen to plasmin. Aminocaproic acid is most effective when started as soon as possible after an accurate diagnosis of subarachnoid hemorrhage has been established. The usual daily dosage is 24–36 g administered by constant intravenous infusion. Major complications of aminocaproic acid therapy are rare and include psychiatric disturbances, restlessness, nausea, abdominal cramps, and dizziness. Oral administration has resulted in complaints of diarrhea. Too rapid intravenous administration can result in hypotension.[2]

Antifibrinolytic therapy remains controversial. There have been reports of a higher incidence of delayed hydrocephalus in patients given aminocaproic acid. Some claim that antifibrinolytic agents are associated with an increased incidence of vasospasm, deep vein thrombosis, and pulmonary embolism. The beneficial effects are generally thought to outweigh these remote risks.[9]

Nursing actions include frequent assessment of peripheral circulation, noting any signs or symptoms of thrombophlebitis.

Treatment of vasospasm. Cerebral vasospasm is a serious and common complication that begins shortly after the initial bleed, and is again exacerbated following surgical repair of a vascular lesion. Vessels adjacent to the bleeding vessel are affected first, but vasospasm may spread throughout the major vessels at the base of the brain, resulting in widespread areas of cerebral ischemia and possible infarction.[4] Symptoms are variable and depend on the vessels involved. Usually a deterioration in the patient's mental status occurs and the appearance of, or worsening of, lateralizing neurological deficits appear over a period of hours to several days.

Various forms of therapy such as vasodilators, alpha and beta blockers, papaverine hydrochloride, and prostaglandin inhibitors have all been tried with inconsistent beneficial effects. Calcium channel blockers (nifedipine, nimodipine) are receiving increased interest as agents that promote vascular smooth muscle relaxation. The use of kanamycin has been tried in an effort to reduce circulating serotonin levels. Continuous infusions of isoproterenol and aminophylline are being used in some centers to induce vascular relaxation.[4,6,10]

Augmentation of cerebral perfusion pressure (CPP) by expansion of intravascular volume with regular infusions of colloid, vasopressors, cardiac stimulants, and measures to reduce ICP are also being used to treat vasospasm.[9] These vigorous measures aimed at improving cerebral perfusion are facilitated by the continuous monitoring of the patient's arterial blood pressure, pulmonary capillary wedge pressure, and ICP.[6] Monitoring ICP by intraventricular catheter will allow the removal of CSF to further improve CPP.

Surgical Management. Surgery is performed for ruptured cerebral aneurysm to prevent recurrence of bleeding. Controversy still exists on whether to operate early after subarachnoid hemorrhage or to wait until vasospasm has been minimized. Early surgical intervention may be required for evacuation of an intracerebral clot associated with aneurysmal rupture. Early surgery (within the first 24 to 48 hours) is often advocated for patients with grades I to III aneurysms.[10]

A number of lesions can be treated by clipping or ligation of the parent artery, sometimes combined with a microsurgical bypass graft to bring blood to the distal portion of the ligated artery.[9] Intracranial resection of some aneurysms can be carried out. Inaccessible lesions may require ligation of the common carotid artery. Ventricular shunting may be required in the presence of hydrocephalus.[1]

Ruptured Arteriovenous Malformation

AVMs are anomalous blood vessels in which arterial blood moves directly into veins without intervening capillaries.

AVMs appear as coiled masses of dilated blood vessels (Figure 9–4).

Pathophysiology. They are thought to be congenital in origin, the result of a birth injury, or to develop later as a result of head injury in which a shunt for blood

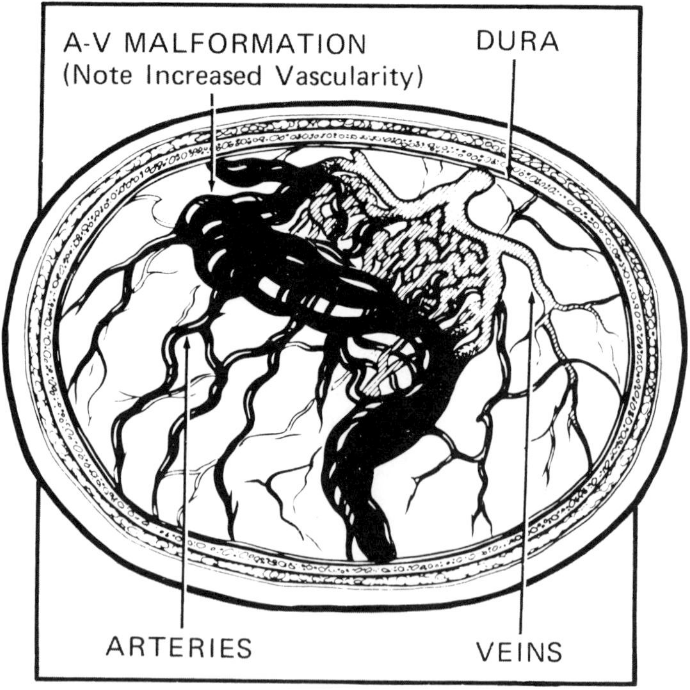

Fig. 9–4—Ateriovenous malformation.

> *Source:* Reprinted from *Neurological Problems: A Critical Care Nursing Focus* (p 100) by Mariah Snyder and Mary Jackle with permission of the Robert J Brady Company, © 1981.

develops around a clot. Acquired dural sinus AVMs have been reported in which a clot in the dural sinus causes recanalization or revascularization.[11] AVMs can range in size from tiny to large enough to cover a large cerebral area. They may involve only meningeal tissue or may extend into brain parenchymal tissue. The vessel walls are thin and subject to leaking, or worse, rupture, with a resultant subarachnoid hemorrhage, intracerebral hemorrhage, or both.[2]

Unlike ruptured cerebral aneurysms, AVM bleeding usually occurs in younger patients, often between the ages of 20 and 40 years.[12]

Clinical Features. Clinical features associated with AVMs include the development of seizures, focal or generalized, and vascular-type headaches resulting from increasing AVM size as the vessels continue to dilate. Intracranial pressure may rise as the AVM produces a mass effect. Focal neurological signs may also develop from localized brain tissue hypoxia that is caused by the AVM stealing blood away from brain tissue.[11] Patients with dural AVMs often report a pulsatile tinnitus. Others report a murmur within their skull. Sometimes a bruit can be auscultated over the eyes or skull.[2]

There have been reports of cardiac hypertrophy and congestive heart failure in infants and young children who have large vein of Galen anomalies. Large volumes of blood can pass through such a defect, overloading the capacity of the heart.[4]

Rupture of an AVM often produces symptoms of subarachnoid hemorrhage, including severe headache, other signs of meningeal irritation, and a decrease in consciousness. Bleeding can also extend into the ventricles leading to increased intracranial pressure. The appearance of focal neurological signs such as hemiparesis, hemisensory deficits, and hemianopsia indicate that bleeding has occurred into brain tissue.[2]

Rupture of AVMs, while not as explosive as the rupture of an intracerebral aneurysm, have the potential for being life threatening. The risk of rupture does not appear to be related to the size of the lesion.[11]

Medical and Nursing Management. The patient with a ruptured AVM is treated as a candidate for rebleeding with similar subarachnoid precautions as previously described. It is important that the reasons for these precautions be explained and reinforced so that patient cooperation is optimal. The patient may also be managed on the same drug regimens used for patients with ruptured cerebral aneurysm.[4]

The decision for surgical treatment of an AVM depends on the location and surgical accessibility of the lesion, the anatomy of the lesion, the age and condition of the patient, the presence of neurological deficit, and previous history of hemorrhage.[4] If the AVM and its feeder vessels are surgically accessible, complete surgical excision is the treatment of choice. About 50 percent of AVMs are successfully treated by this block dissection.[8] When this is not possible, obliteration of the lesion by ligation of feeder vessels may be carried out.

Inaccessible AVMs are sometimes treated with embolization. Embolization techniques usually involve a femoral puncture, with a catheter guided radiographically into the carotid artery, and from there to the feeder artery of the AVM. Small silastic beads (3 mm in diameter) are introduced via the feeder arteries into the lesion to block the flow of blood into the AVM. This may not be a permanent solution because there is a high incidence of rebleeding. It may shrink the AVM until definitive surgery can be performed.[2]

Polymerizing agents (rapidly setting plastics) which thrombose the AVM are also being introduced via small balloon catheters placed into the feeder arteries. AVMs supplied by the middle cerebral artery are the most effectively treated by this technique.[2]

The use of a low-dose focused proton beam has been shown to be capable of shrinking some AVMs and obliterating small ones.[8]

Postprocedural management of patients undergoing embolization procedures includes the frequent monitoring of vital signs, neurological function, and observations of the femoral site for hematoma formation and assessment of distal leg perfusion.[4]

COMPLICATIONS OF ACUTE STROKE

It is not practical to cover all of the many complications that are associated with stroke. Several of the complications that can occur in the acute phase of stroke are the same as those that can accompany severe head injury. More detailed discussions of these complications have been covered in other parts of the text and will only briefly be mentioned here. The reader will be referred to appropriate chapters for additional information.

Early recognition of the potential complications of acute stroke depends, in part, on the anticipation of such complications.

Hypothalamic Syndromes

Functional or structural abnormalities in the hypothalamus can result from subarachnoid hemorrhage, cerebral infarction, hydrocephalus, trauma, and numerous other lesions. The following syndromes are all related to disease of the hypothalamus.

Inappropriate Antidiuretic Hormone Secretion

The syndrome of inappropriate antidiuretic hormone secretion (SIADH) with its resulting water retention and hyponatremia can lead to neurological deterioration in the form of irritability, confusion, stupor, muscle weakness, loss of tendon reflexes and Babinski signs, and in some cases, seizures. See Chapter 8 for descriptions of treatment for SIADH.[8(p413),12]

Diabetes Insipidus

A deficient secretion of ADH results in diabetes insipidus with the passage of large quantities of dilute urine. This can lead to intense thirst and can result in dehydration and electrolyte imbalance. See Chapter 8 for further description of this disorder and its treatment.[8(p413),12]

Disturbances of Temperature Regulation

Lesions in the anterior hypothalamus contribute to hyperthermia while more posterior lesions result in loss of body heat or hypothermia.[8(p413)] Hyperthermia greatly increases oxygen consumption by the brain and can contribute to secondary brain ischemia. Hyperthermia also causes weakness, lethargy, and seizures, especially in children, and can contribute to dehydration through salt and water loss.

Somnolence and hypotension are associated with hypothermia. Refer to Chapter 11 for detailed descriptions of the disorders of temperature regulation and their treatment.

Gastric Bleeding

Severe stroke, especially from massive brain hemorrhage, can impair the function of the hypothalamus which contributes to the development of superficial erosions or ulcerations of the gastric mucosa (Cushing ulcer). Combined with the body's stress response, gastric bleeding can result.[8(p413)] Steroid administration is also linked to the development of gastric ulceration.[4]

The best treatment is prevention with the use of medications such as cimetidine to reduce gastric acid secretions, and the administration of antacids. Stools should be assessed daily for the presence of occult blood.

Cardiovascular Complications

Hypothalamic compression produces massive autonomic nervous system discharges resulting in increased levels of circulating catecholamines. Ischemic ECG changes and potentially lethal cardiac dysrhythmias can result. Stroke patients warrant continuous ECG monitoring. In addition to assuring normal fluid and electrolyte balance, antiarrhythmic agents are administered when serious cardiac dysrhythmias are evident. Low cardiac output states must be corrected since they can potentiate cerebral ischemia.

Other cardiovascular complications can occur as a result of hemodynamic changes and include the Cushing response, vasovagal reflex, and neurogenic pulmonary edema. These are covered in detail in Chapter 11.

Hydrocephalus

As in severe head injury, hydrocephalus can occur in the stroke patient as a result of obstruction of CSF circulation or impairment of CSF reabsorption.

Vascular abnormalities, aqueductal stenosis, and blood can obstruct the circulation of CSF through the aqueducts or through the foramina into the subarachnoid space. This results in a noncommunicating or obstructive hydrocephalus in which the CSF is under great pressure. Signs of increased ICP will be evident.[8(p464)]

A communicating hydrocephalus can develop following subarachnoid hemorrhage from an aneurysm or an AVM. Presumably there is plugging of the arachnoid villi by blood and debris. Less tension or pressure exists with this type of hydrocephalus which may manifest itself as a deterioration in mental status, confusion, drowsiness, and intermittent headache.[4(p170)]

Emergency treatment for hydrocephalus may include a ventriculostomy, but an emergency shunting procedure may need to be performed if acute obstructive hydrocephalus develops.

ACUTE STROKE: CRITICAL CARE CONSIDERATIONS

Priorities in the medical and nursing management of the stroke patient are to preserve the patient's life and vital functions, and prevent further neurological damage. In patients with hemorrhagic stroke, especially those caused by rupture of a cerebral aneurysm or AVM, these efforts include the prevention of recurrent bleeding.

The etiology of the underlying disorder must be established and primary medical problems and their complications must be identified and treated. Since medical and nursing care will be based on an understanding of the underlying pathological process, a thorough history and physical assessment are essential (see Chapter 3).

History and Physical Assessment

As part of the patient's history, the practioner should establish the presence of risk factors for stroke that have been identified by the American Heart Association. These include hypertension, history of TIA, atherosclerosis, especially of coronary arteries and vessels of the neck and legs, diabetes mellitus, elevated blood cholesterol and fat levels, gout, high red blood cell (RBC) level, and heavy smoking.[13] While the incidence of stroke increases with age, the development of stroke in women of child-bearing age has been linked to the use of oral contraceptives.[2]

In addition to the identification of neurological signs and symptoms, the mode of onset should be investigated. Here, a family member may be able to provide valuable information on events they have witnessed. For example, if the symptoms occurred suddenly and/or during activity, the stroke may have been caused by embolism or infarction. Symptoms that have appeared gradually or intermittently or during sleep are most often the result of thrombosis. Symptoms consisting of neurological deficits that have resolved within minutes or hours are attributed to TIA. A complaint of severe headache accompanying other symptoms probably represents a hemorrhage rather than an ischemic event. The absence of a history of head injury assists in ruling out epidural or subdural hematoma as a cause of signs and symptoms.[13]

Neurological assessment was covered in detail in Chapter 3 and will not be repeated here. In addition to performing a thorough neurological assessment, the practitioner also assesses for other findings that may be related to cerebrovascular disease.

An evaluation of extracranial arteries should be included as part of the neurological assessment. This includes the techniques of arterial palpation and auscultation. The carotid arteries are palpated and any inequality is noted. Occlusion of a carotid artery may be manifested by a lack of pulsations. A decreased or absent superficial temporal artery pulsation may indicate ipsilateral carotid artery disease. The presence of a thrill (palpable vibration) indicates increased blood turbulence and a probable pathological lesion at that location. Inequality of radial artery pulsations or a significant difference in blood pressures in the arms may indicate subclavian steal syndrome. Subclavian steal syndrome is a vascular disorder in which a subclavian artery is occluded, causing blood destined for the brain to be shunted from one vertebral artery across and down the vertebral artery on the side of the occlusion. There is reversed blood flow in the vertebral artery which steals blood from the brain. Signs and symptoms of vertebrobasilar insufficiency appear during activity involving the ipsilateral arm.[13]

The carotid, vertebral, and subclavian arteries, orbits, and skull should be auscultated for the presence of a bruit, an abnormally turbulent blood flow sound caused by aneurysms, AVMs or fistulae, or occlusive vascular disease. The bell of the stethoscope should be used. Figure 9–5 demonstrates sites for auscultation of the head and neck. The presence or absence of a bruit is not always clinically significant. Bruits are sometimes heard in normal individuals, while they may be absent in others with significant vascular occlusions.[13] A small percentage of patients with AVMs will have a bruit, with its presence more likely in children due to their thinner skull.[4]

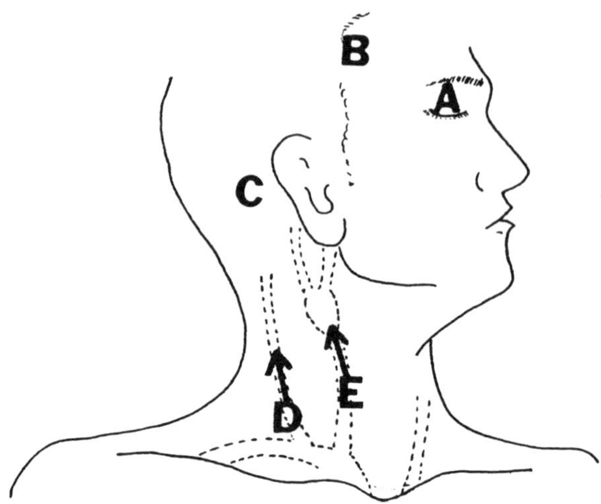

Fig. 9–5—Sites for auscultation of head and neck. Using the bell of the stethoscope, auscultate over: (A) Each eye, (B) frontal-parietal regions, (C) each mastoid process, (D) each vertebral artery, and (E) each carotid artery. Arrows represent the course of the vertebral and carotid arteries.

General Management of Acute Stroke

Intensive management of acute stroke centers on preventing, reversing, and minimizing the progression of the ischemic state. Chapters 4 and 5 presented in detail the nursing and medical interventions for intracranial hypertension and brain resuscitation. Most of these treatment modalities can be applied to the acute stroke patient. In brief, the goals and interventions are summarized below:

1. frequent neurological assessments to identify any progression or regression of neurological deficits; use of a neurological flow sheet will expedite documentation
2. maintenance of an adequate airway and respiratory function with the prevention of hypoxemia, carbon dioxide retention, and aspiration
3. facilitation of venous return by elevation of the head to 30–40 degrees unless contraindicated by shock. Some clinicians keep the ischemic stroke patient flat for two to three days in hopes of avoiding further cerebral ischemia. Avoid neck flexion, extension, and rotation; prevent hip flexion; prevent straining and Valsalva maneuver.

4. control of pain and hyperactivity by administration of mild analgesics and sedatives, and reduction of environmental stimuli
5. prevention and control of seizures by administration of anticonvulsant medications
6. maintenance of adequate cerebral perfusion pressure by control of systemic blood pressure, and reduction of intracranial pressure
7. treatment of brain edema by administration of osmotic agents and diuretics, and the possible administration of corticosteroids, barbiturates, and hyperventilation therapy[6]
8. control of temperature and prevention of fever
9. maintenance of an accurate intake and output record (I&O), with probable fluid restriction
10. protection of integumentary and musculoskeletal integrity through frequent inspection, proper positioning, range of motion exercises, protection of skin, corneas, etc. (see Chapter 15)
11. prevention of gastric aspiration in absence of protective airway reflexes by nasogastric intubation and suction
12. control of bowel and bladder dysfunctions by insertion of indwelling urinary catheter only if absolutely necessary, and institution of bowel program once GI motility is ensured and feeding program commenced. Constipation is to be prevented.

While corticosteroids have not been proven to be beneficial in stroke, they may help reduce the cerebral edema accompanying cerebral infarction.[6] Hyperventilation therapy is also controversial in stroke. It may not be beneficial if cerebral autoregulation is lost and vasomotor paralysis is present.

Experimental evidence supports a beneficial effect of the opiate antagonist naloxone at high doses (2–5 mg/kg). The mechanism of its therapeutic effect in stroke is yet unclear. It has been suggested that it may act on nonopiate receptors, may effect lipid peroxidation or calcium flux, or may have direct effects on cerebral microcirculation. Improvement in functional recovery following acute cerebral ischemia has been reported following the administration of naloxone.[14]

Sensitivity is required on the part of medical personnel in caring for those stroke patients who experience language, intellectual, and/or emotional deficits. Dealing with language disorders begins by evaluating what language skills are intact. Speak clearly and in simple sentences, using gestures as necessary. Allow ample time for the patient to grasp what is being said and to respond. Assist family members to understand and accept the patient's speech limitations, and stress that the patient is now neither mentally ill nor retarded.[4]

There may be intellectual deficits such as memory loss, short attention span and easy distractability, poor judgment, and decreased reasoning ability. Facilitate the patient's comfort by controlling excessive environmental distractions, setting realistic expectations for the patient, and dividing activities for reaching these expectations into short, simple steps. Constant supervision may initially be necessary to protect the patient from injury.[4]

Emotional lability may be seen with loss of self-control and social inhibitions. There may be outbursts of frustration, anger, hostility, and fear. With a change in body image, many stroke patients experience withdrawal and depression. Nurses can be supportive by accepting the patient and disregarding the outbursts. Explain to the patient and family that emotional lability is common in stroke. Allow the patient and family to verbalize and clarify any misconceptions. Involve the patient is his/her own activities of daily living as much as is possible. Provide a supportive environment and preserve the patient's dignity at all times.[4]

The aggressive management of the stroke patient also includes the early implementation of physical therapy, occupational therapy, and speech therapy to promote maximal level of functioning.

REFERENCES

1. O'Brien MT, Pallett PJ: *Total Care of the Stroke Patient*. Boston, Little, Brown, 1978.

2. Rudy EB: *Advanced Neurological and Neurosurgical Nursing*. St Louis, Mosby, 1984, pp 200–241.

3. Neighbor ML: Localized weakness. *Top Emerg Med* 1982;4:1–4.

4. Hickey J: *The Clinical Practice of Neurological and Neurosurgical Nursing*. Philadelphia, Lippincott, 1981, pp 376–494.

5. Adams HP, Sahs AL: Aneurysmal subarachnoid hemorrhage. *Mod Concepts Cardiovasc Dis* 1981;50:49–54.

6. Green BA, Marshall LF, Gallagher TJ: *Intensive Care for Neurological Trauma and Disease*. Orlando, Fla, Academic Press, 1982.

7. Diaz FG, Ausman JI: Surgical reconstruction of vascular lesions of the vertebral basilar circulation. *Curr Concepts Cerebrovasc Dis: Stroke* 1984;19:19–23.

8. Adams RD, Victor M: *Principles of Neurology*, ed 3. New York, McGraw-Hill, 1985, pp 569–637.

9. Heros RC, Kistler JP: Intracranial arterial aneurysm, an update. *Curr Concepts Cerebrovasc Dis: Stroke* 1983;18:1–5.

10. Chase M, Whelan-Decker E: Nursing management of a patient with a subarachnoid hemorrhage. *J Neurosurg Nurs* 1984;16:23–29.

11. Fode NC: Cerebral arteriovenous malformations: Update for neuroscience nurses. *J Neurosurg Nurs* 1984;16:319–321.

12. Zucker AR, Chernow B: Diabetes insipidus and the syndrome of inappropriate antidiuretic hormone release. *Crit Care Q* 1983;6:63–74.

13. Conway-Rutkowski BL: *Carini and Owen's Neurological and Neurosurgical Nursing*, ed 8. St Louis, Mosby, 1982; pp 600–621.

14. Faden AI: Opiate antagonists in the treatment of stroke. *Curr Concepts Cerebrovasc Dis: Stroke* 1983;18:27–31.

Chapter 10

Seizures

A seizure has been described as "a sudden, recurrent, transient disturbance in mental function, or movements, or both, which results from excessive discharging of populations of brain cells."[1]

PATHOPHYSIOLOGY

Neurons and groups of neurons are intrinsically excitable and there is normally a balance of excitation and inhibition allowing smooth and orderly electrical discharges.[2] It is not known whether seizures arise from increased excitability or decreased inhibition.[1] It is known, however, that denervated neurons become hypersensitive, remaining in a state of partial depolarization with increased permeability, so that they are more easily excited than normal cells.[2,3] Localized groups of denervated neurons, resulting from injury or disease, may form a seizure focus which will emit excessively large numbers of disorganized, paroxysmal discharges even in the absence of clinical seizures.[4]

Why the seizure focus suddenly erupts, and what causes the seizure to end is not fully understood. It is assumed that, in susceptible individuals, the seizure threshold is lowered, so that there is a progressive increase in the amplitude and frequency of neuronal discharges. When the intensity of the discharges reaches a certain level, adjacent neurons are affected. These discharges may spread to the opposite hemisphere, basal ganglia, thalamus, and brainstem. It is at this point that the clinical manifestations of the seizure become apparent. The particular signs and symptoms accompanying the seizure depend on the portion of the brain from which the seizure originated (the seizure focus).[3]

Termination of the seizure is associated with a major hyperpolarization and suppression of the seizure focus. Inhibitory influences and neuronal exhaustion may result in postictal paralysis (Todd's palsy), aphasia, or hemianopsia.[3]

269

ETIOLOGY

Not all cortical lesions result in the formation of a seizure focus. It has been postulated that those lesions that result in seizures have caused certain neurons to be disconnected from the surrounding areas, the opposite hemisphere, or other structures. Inhibiting neurons may have been destroyed so that the interneural relationships have become disorganized.[3] Furthermore, seizures can occur when no lesion is present, as in febrile seizures and those related to the use of drugs and alcohol. It is known that, given the right circumstances, anyone can have a seizure. Some individuals appear to have a genetic predisposition to seizures so that the seizure threshold is lowered. For such individuals, stimuli that are benign for most people may trigger a seizure.[4] The seizure threshold may also be lowered by fever, changes in electrolyte or water balance, fatigue, stress, menstruation, pregnancy, metabolic abnormalities, and other factors.[5]

Epilepsy or ideopathic epilepsy are terms that have been used to describe recurrent seizures in which there is no identifiable cause. As more is known about the pathophysiology of seizures, the term epilepsy is becoming obsolete. Since the term continues to carry a degree of social stigma, it is probably preferable to use the more generic term ''seizure'' or ''seizure disorder'' which lends itself to qualification and classification.[3]

It must be pointed out that a seizure disorder is a symptom, not a disease. The specific pathology that can cause seizures varies, but includes the following:

- congenital defects
- birth injuries
- metabolic disorders such as hypocalcemia or phenylketonuria
- trauma
- infectious processes such as brain abscess or encephalitis
- alcohol, drug use, or poisoning
- brain tumors
- vascular disorders such as stroke, vascular malformations, aneurysms, or degenerative disorders

Even when no specific cause for the seizure(s) can be found, the assumption is that cells have been damaged at some time, either before birth or later. The onset of seizures in childhood is more likely to be ideopathic or congenital, while initial onset in the adult is more likely to be due to an identifiable lesion, such as an injury, tumor, or disease state.

CLINICAL FEATURES

Virtually any activity of the cerebral cortex, voluntary or involuntary, can be duplicated by a seizure. As stated earlier, the focus of the seizure and the spread of abnormal discharges determine the initial signs manifested, the course of the seizure, and the postictal behavior. The clinical events can usually be correlated with changes in the electroencephalogram (EEG), although the EEG may occasionally be normal, particularly during partial or partial, complex seizures (described later). Because seizure activity is so variable, classification systems have been difficult to develop. The most widely used system at present is based on the correlation of clinical and EEG findings and is derived from an earlier system developed in 1969 by the International League Against Epilepsy.[6] The newer classification system, published in 1981,[7] will be used in the discussion that follows.

Seizures are broadly classified as partial (focal, local) and generalized. Partial seizures are so categorized because initial activation of neurons occurs in only one part of one hemisphere. Generalized seizures are those in which both hemispheres are involved from the beginning. Within each of the broad categories there is wide diversity with subcategorization.

Partial Seizures

Partial seizures are further subdivided into simple partial or complex partial depending on whether or not consciousness is altered.

Simple Partial Seizures

Simple partial seizures do not result in the loss of consciousness. Subcategorization of simple partial seizures is necessary because of the diversity of signs that can occur.

Simple Partial Seizures with Focal Motor Signs. Simple partial seizures with focal motor signs may involve any part of the body on the contralateral side such as the face, hand, arm, or leg. The movements may remain localized (without march) or may spread to adjoining areas (with march). The term Jacksonian seizure is used to designate the simple partial seizure with spread or march.

Simple Partial Seizures with Focal Sensory Signs. Simple partial seizures with focal sensory signs may produce tingling, pins and needles, buzzing, or numbness in similar parts of the contralateral side of the body, with or without spread to adjoining areas.

Simple Partial Seizures with Focal Somatosensory Signs. Simple partial seizures with focal somatosensory signs may produce signs that are visual in nature, varying from simple phenomena such as flashing lights to formed visual hallucinations. Similarly, there may be simple auditory phenomena such as ringing or buzzing sounds, or complex auditory hallucination such as musical sounds or undifferentiated voices.

The seizure may also take the form of a recurrent, usually unpleasant and unidentifiable odor, or a strange, often metallic taste. There may be vertiginous signs such as a sensation of falling, floating, or rotatory vertigo. The hallucinations produced by seizures can be differentiated from psychiatric symptoms by their episodic appearance, with normal mental status between episodes. In addition, the patient often is aware that the phenomena are unreal, even though distressing.[3]

Simple Partial Seizures with Autonomic Signs. Simple partial seizures with autonomic signs can cause such things as epigastric sensations, pallor, sweating, flushing, or pupil dilation.

Simple Partial Seizures with Psychic Symptoms. Simple partial seizures with psychic symptoms may include dysmesic experiences such as distorted memories, déjà vu, jamais vu, dreamy states, or panoramic vision. There may be cognitive disturbances such as a feeling of time distortion, or size distortion, with head or limbs feeling abnormally large or small. The symptoms may be affective, including feelings of unprovoked anger, fear, or joy. While these phenomena may occur as a simple partial seizure, they are most often associated with complex partial seizures.

Complex Partial Seizures

Complex partial seizures are often referred to as psychomotor, or less accurately, as temporal lobe seizures. Such seizures may begin with a disturbance of consciousness or may begin as a simple partial seizure with spread and loss of consciousness. Further spread may occur with evolution into a generalized seizure. Complex partial seizures may appear with or without automatisms or the psychic phenomena described earlier. Automatisms are defined as coordinated, adaptive, involuntary motor activity occurring with clouded consciousness either during or after a seizure, often followed by a period of amnesia.[6] Automatisms may consist of eating movements such as chewing and swallowing; mimicry including expressions of emotional states such as crying or laughing; gestures such as picking, tapping, rubbing, or even complex movements such as unbuttoning or removing clothing or taking off coverings; ambulation as when the patient continues to walk, run, or even drive, but in a random manner; or verbalization with repetitive vocalization of a word or phrase. It should be pointed out that while automatisms can vary significantly from patient to patient, they tend to be fairly consistent for a particular patient. The psychic symptoms described earlier may be part of the seizure itself or may appear as the aura prior to the alteration of consciousness.

Generalized Seizures

Generalized seizures may be either convulsive or nonconvulsive, but are usually accompanied by loss of consciousness. When motor activity occurs, it is always bilateral. There are numerous subcategories of generalized seizures.

Absence Seizures

Again, subcategorization is required because of the variety of clinical manifestations that have been documented. Absence seizures originate in the diencephalon with discharges from the thalamic reticular system.[8]

Petit Mal Absence Seizures. Typical petit mal absence seizures are characterized by a loss of consciousness of sudden onset and brief duration. There is a momentary interruption of activity accompanied by a blank stare. This type of seizure is most commonly seen in children. While each seizure lasts only a moment, there may be many episodes following one another in close succession. The child appears dull and inattentive, and has difficulty learning in school. These seizures may stop spontaneously during the teens, but are often replaced by tonic-clonic seizures at adolescence.

Absence with Mild Clonic Movements. Absence with mild clonic movements is similar to the typical absence attacks as described, but with jerking of the eyelids, mouth, or other muscle groups.

Absence with Mild Tonic Movements. Absence with mild tonic movements is characterized by an increase in muscle tone. The head may extend and the back arch, or the head may turn to one side.

Absence with an Atonic Component. Absence with an atonic component is a momentary loss of consciousness with loss of muscle tone. The head may droop or the patient may suddenly fall.

Absence with Automatisms. Absence with automatisms may include movements such as chewing, smacking, walking, or fumbling with clothing or other articles. Such patients may respond to being touched or spoken to by rubbing the part touched or turning to the speaker.

Atypical Absence. Atypical absence is usually of longer duration with a more gradual recovery, but is otherwise similar to the more typical absence seizure.

Myoclonic Seizures

Myoclonic seizures are brief, shocklike contractions (jerks) that may be generalized or confined to the face, trunk, or extremities. They may be single or multiple. People with myoclonic seizures can injure themselves if they fall to the ground. Such seizures must be differentiated from nonseizure myoclonus resulting from noncerebral conditions.

Tonic-Clonic Seizures

A tonic-clonic seizure is the typical grand mal seizure of older classifications. The seizure may begin with an aura, or the initial event may be a sudden, involuntary movement such as turning the head, staring into space, or standing up. As consciousness is lost, the patient falls, the body becomes rigid, the back may arch, the arms adduct, elbows flex, hands pronate, and legs hyperextend. Air is forced out of the lungs, often resulting in a loud cry. The jaws lock, often with the tongue caught between the teeth. The pupils dilate and may be nonreactive. Respirations are suspended and the color becomes dusky. The bladder may empty. This is the tonic phase and lasts for about 10–20 seconds. The clonic phase begins with a mild trembling, which develops into violent, rhythmic contractions occurring bilaterally. Blood from the bitten tongue, mixed with saliva, produces frothing from the mouth. The patient perspires profusely, the pulse is rapid, there is facial grimacing, and the color becomes cyanotic as apnea continues. Gradually the movements subside, the patient takes a deep breath, and the color returns to normal. The pupils begin to react, but coma may persist for some time. Eventually the eyes open, but the patient will appear sluggish and confused. Left alone, the patient will often sink into a deep sleep, awakening several hours later with a severe headache and no memory of the preceding events.[5]

Tonic Seizures

A tonic seizure is a generalized seizure, but with a tonic phase only.

Clonic Seizures

A clonic seizure is also a generalized seizure, but with a clonic phase only.

Atonic Seizures

Atonic seizures are characterized by a sudden loss of muscle tone with slackening of the jaw, dropping of a limb, or falling to the ground. These seizures must be distinguished from other forms of ''drop'' attacks such as those caused by heart block or fainting.

Some patients have seizures that do not fit into any of the categories described. Seizure activity may be mixed, combining features of several classifications. Furthermore, seizures may evolve from one type into another. Present knowledge is inadequate to explain all of the various electrical and biochemical activities of the brain, so that the manifestations produced by abnormal impulses remain mysterious.

Seizures, particularly those labeled partial complex, may produce behavior that is so bizarre that it may be mistaken for psychiatric, hysterical, or behavioral phenomena. Even expert observers may disagree as to whether a particular episode is a real seizure. In all such cases, the safest course is to assume that the patient has had a seizure and await further evidence, rather than to risk inappropriate interventions.

Consideration of the following characteristics of seizures may assist in differentiating seizures from other conditions.

- Seizure activity is episodic, with normal or near normal behavior between seizures.

- Seizure behavior tends to be repetitive. While seizure phenomena vary widely from individual to individual and may be of mixed forms, a given patient is likely to show the same pattern with each seizure. Behavior, however bizarre, that recurs with each episode and does not appear between episodes is probably a real seizure.

- Seizures are generally unprovoked, although a loss of sleep, emotional and physical stress, use of drugs or alcohol, onset of menses, or other life events may lower the seizure threshold and precipitate a seizure or a series of seizures. Furthermore, there is a phenomenon known as reflex epilepsy in which a seizure is produced in a susceptible individual by a specific physiological or psychological stimulus. The stimulus may be a flashing or flickering light, change from darkness to light, sounds of a certain frequency, eating a large meal, certain movements, or a sudden fright or similar event. Conversely, certain individuals may be able to avert a seizure by force of will or change to a different activity. Sometimes the seizure can be averted in its early stages by application of a very strong stimulus such as a loud clap.[3]

- An abnormal EEG favors the diagnosis of a seizure disorder, but the absence of such abnormalities does not rule out the diagnosis.[3]

MEDICAL AND NURSING MANAGEMENT

The management of seizure disorders is determined by the underlying condition. Every patient having a first seizure requires a thorough workup to exclude a treatable cause. Drug or alcohol related seizures rarely require long-term therapy and seldom recur. Post-traumatic seizures occur in a substantial number of patients within the first two years following head injury. Such seizures are usually responsive to anticonvulsant drug therapy, and often decrease in frequency over time. Post-traumatic seizures may be either partial or generalized.

Seizures may be an early symptom of an acute infectious condition of the central nervous system and are treated as part of the overall management of the patient's disease. A cerebrovascular condition or tumor may precipitate seizures. In such cases, removal of the cause is the obvious treatment.

For those patients eventually diagnosed as having recurrent seizures of unknown cause (ideopathic epilepsy), adequate treatment with anticonvulsant drugs along with attention to physical and mental hygiene will usually be effective in controlling the seizure activity. It should be kept in mind that there are a number of drugs available for control of seizures, and some experimentation may be required to find the most effective drug or combination of drugs for any given patient. Before concluding that a particular regime is not effective, it is important to establish that the prescribed drugs have in fact been taken as directed. Young people in particular tend to be noncompliant. Since seizure control depends on the maintenance of therapeutic blood levels of anticonvulsant drugs, irregular or missed doses may be the precipitating cause of increased seizures.

Since seizure thresholds may be lowered by biochemical alterations, fatigue, stress, drugs, alcohol, and sometimes specific stimuli, patients should be assisted to identify possible situations or events that may have preceded a seizure or series of seizures.

Any patient with recurrent seizures should be instructed to carry identification and wear a medical alert tag or card so that should a seizure occur, appropriate treatment can be provided promptly and inappropriate treatment avoided. Such patients should also be warned about engaging in potentially dangerous activities. Patients with uncontrolled, irregular, or unpredictable seizures should avoid unsupervised swimming, boating, operating machinery, heights, and other situations that could result in disaster for themselves or others should a seizure occur. At the same time, those with well-controlled seizures should not be precluded from school, work, or other activities that would provide a satisfying life.

A few states require medical personnel to report ''epileptics'' to the department of motor vehicles. However, whether or not state laws are in effect, patients who might represent a hazard to themselves or others should be strongly advised not to drive. Data indicate that drivers with seizure disorders in general have only a slightly higher accident rate than individuals with diabetes or cerebrovascular disease.[9] Thus, for any given individual, the relative risks of driving should be weighed, based on the likelihood that a seizure will occur while the individual is driving.

For patients with intractable seizures after adequate trials of medication, surgical intervention may be considered. Surgery is potentially effective only when a clearly identifiable focus can be found in an area that is surgically accessible and, if removed, will not leave serious neurological deficits. Recent advances in EEG technology with videotape recordings and the use of positron emission tomography have greatly improved the selection process of surgical candidates. Consequently, successful surgical intervention for seizure control is being more frequently reported.

The advent of a single generalized convulsive (grand mal seizure), although dramatic, rarely requires emergency care. The major goal during the seizure is to prevent injury and provide supportive care during a period of vulnerability. If possible, the patient should be prevented from falling, and should be moved to a place of safety, away from radiators, obstructions, or other sources of injury. The head and limbs should be protected as the patient flails about, but the movements should not be restrained. If possible, the head may be turned to the side to allow for drainage of saliva or vomitus. In the hospital setting, suction equipment should be kept on standby.

The seizure should be carefully observed from beginning to end, since the onset, course, and sequence of events are useful in establishing the location of the seizure focus. Preceding events, evidence of an aura or warning, where the movements began, whether there was both a tonic and clonic phase, length of each phase, incontinence, vomiting, changes in vital signs or pupils, whether the patient responded to stimuli, and postictal behavior should all be observed and recorded.

When the tonic-clonic movements have ended, the patient should be carefully examined for postictal symptoms such as Todd's palsy, aphasia, confusion, headache, and drowsiness. Vital signs should be checked and pupils examined. If the vital signs are normal, pupils reactive, and the patient can be aroused, the patient may be left in peace to ''sleep it off.'' Follow-up care can usually be provided by the patient's regular physician.

Complex partial seizures with automatisms (psychomotor seizures) may sometimes result in disruptive or combative behavior. If possible, without danger to the patient or harm to others, the patient should be carefully observed, but no effort should be made to stop the automatisms. Like the patient with generalized convulsive seizures, the patient may be drowsy following the seizure and should be allowed to rest with supervision until the mental status has returned to normal.

STATUS EPILEPTICUS

Status epilepticus refers to a state in which seizures recur so frequently that there is no recovery between attacks. The patient is in danger of respiratory arrest or circulatory collapse and must be treated as a medical emergency. The goals of care are to prevent injury and support vital functions while the seizures are brought under control. Large doses of anticonvulsant drugs may be required to stop the seizures, thus causing additional respiratory and circulatory compromise.

The patient will need intensive monitoring and aggressive management until the seizures have ended and mental status has returned to normal. Respiratory support may be indicated and would require nasotracheal intubation to avoid having the patient bite the tube. Fluid and electrolyte balance also needs to be maintained. Nasogastric suctioning may be advisable to prevent vomiting and aspiration. Meticulous pulmonary hygiene is essential. In addition skin care and other routine measures are needed as in the care of any comatose patient. Specific aspects of the nursing management of patients with seizures are discussed in detail in Chapter 16.

REFERENCES

1. Goldensohn ES, Ward AA: Pathogenesis of epileptic seizures, in Tower DB (ed): *The Nervous System: Volume II, The Clinical Neurosciences.* New York, Raven, 1975.

2. Livingston RB: Neural integration, in Frohlich ED (ed): *Pathophysiology,* ed 2. Philadelphia, Lippincott, 1976.

3. Adams R, Victor M: *Principles of Neurology,* ed 3. New York, McGraw-Hill, 1985.

4. Hickey J: *The Clinical Practice of Neurological and Neurosurgical Nursing.* Philadelphia, Lippincott, 1981.

5. Taylor JW, Ballenger S: *Neurological Dysfunctions and Nursing Interventions.* New York, McGraw-Hill, 1980.

6. Gastaut H: Clinical and electroencephalographic classification of epileptic seizures. *Epilepsia* 1970;11:102.

7. Proposal for the Revised Clinical and Electroencephalographic Classification of Epileptic Seizures, Commission on the Classification for Terminology of the International League Against Epilepsy. *Epilepsia* 1981;8:489.

8. Cline BA, Fisher ML: The patient with a seizure disorder, in Rudy EB: *Advanced Neurological and Neurosurgical Nursing.* St Louis, Mosby, 1984.

9. Mausland RL: The physician's responsibility for epileptic drivers. *Ann Neurol* 1978;4:485–486.

Chapter 11

Medical Emergencies Related to Neurological Disease

The nervous system regulates and controls vital body functions. In this chapter a number of conditions will be discussed that may bring patients to the emergency room in acute distress because of failure of the mechanisms controlling respiratory function, cardiovascular stability, or temperature regulation.

RESPIRATORY FAILURE

The effects of disease of the brainstem structures on the central control of respirations was discussed in Chapters 3 and 4. In this section the discussion will focus on a group of neurological conditions that may result in actual or potential respiratory failure due to disruption of the mechanics of breathing.[1]

The major force of inspiration is the contraction of the diaphragm and intercostal muscles which are innervated by nerves exiting the spinal canal in the upper cervical region. Accessory muscles including the sternocleidomastoid, trapezius, and those of the face, tongue, and pharynx are innervated by cranial nerves and upper cervical spinal nerves.[1] Respiratory failure may be precipitated by weakness of the respiratory muscles with inadequate chest expansion and suppressed cough and sneeze reflexes. Difficulties in swallowing with impaired gag reflex may produce both upper and lower airway obstruction, which makes the work of breathing more difficult. With little reserve inspiratory power, respiratory failure may occur with surprising suddenness in susceptible patients who develop an otherwise mild upper respiratory infection, fever, or other illness. Stress or a strong emotional response (including anxiety and fear) can also increase respiratory distress. Thus for all of the conditions described in this section, anticipation of problems and careful monitoring of respiratory function form the basis of care.

The specific conditions to be described include examples of diseases affecting the motor end plate (myoneural junction), the peripheral nerves and roots, and the motor neurons in the cerebral cortex, brainstem, and spinal cord.

Neuromuscular Junction (Motor End Plate) Disorders

Transmission of motor impulses from nerves to muscles occurs at the myoneural junction. The neurotransmitter, acetylcholine (Ach), is released from the distal fiber of the nerve (axon) to facilitate depolarization of the muscle fiber. Acetylcholinesterase, produced by the postsynaptic muscle fiber, causes hydrolysis of the Ach, thus restoring polarization and preparing the end plate for the next impulse.[2] Muscle weakness, including the muscles of respiration, can result from abnormalities of impulse transmission even when both nerve and muscle are otherwise intact.[2]

Myasthenia Gravis

Myasthenia gravis is a disorder of the postsynaptic membrane. It is believed to be an autoimmune disease characterized by abnormal fatigue of striated muscles during activity, with some recovery of function after rest. This fatigue is related to the reduction in the number of Ach receptor sites and the presence of anti-acetylcholine antibodies, which block the remaining receptors. Receptor antibodies are found in the circulating blood of 50–85 percent of myasthenic patients.[3]

Myasthenia gravis may be found in every age group but is most common in young females and older males. Infants of myasthenic mothers may have a transient form of myasthenia, and a congenital form has been identified. Many myasthenic patients have either a thymoma or hyperplasia of the thymus gland, which is known to be involved with the development of autoimmune bodies.[4] Myasthenia is known to be associated with lupus and thyroiditis, as well as other autoimmune diseases.

Clinical Features.   The most striking clinical feature of myasthenia is fluctuating weakness and easy fatigability of affected muscles and muscle groups. Patients have difficulty sustaining muscle activity, but strength improves after periods of rest.[5] Thus, activities that the patient may be able to perform at one time may be impossible at other times. This characteristic, along with the frequency with which symptoms increase with stress or emotional events has led to the mistaken diagnosis of hysteria or hypochondriasis. Exacerbations may be precipitated by pregnancy, onset of menstruation, and minor illnesses such as a cold or the flu.

Since any muscle or group of muscles may be affected, the particular dysfunction varies widely from patient to patient and over time in the same patient. In general, the onset is usually gradual, although occasionally a patient will present with a rapid fulminating course with early involvement of bulbar and respiratory muscles.

The initial symptoms may be weakness of the muscles of the eyes with diplopia, ptosis, and difficulty in closing the eyelids. As the weakness spreads, the limbs, trunk, throat, and neck muscles are involved. Bulbar weakness causes difficulty in chewing, swallowing, and talking. The patient may complain of difficulty rising from a chair, climbing steps, or lifting the arms to shave or comb the hair.[6] When the muscles of respiration are affected, respiratory failure is a serious threat. During severe exacerbations (myasthenic crisis) the patient may be acutely paralyzed in all muscle groups. These are the patients most likely to appear in the emergency room.

Tentative diagnosis can usually be made on the basis of the history and physical findings. Muscles are tested for weakness after sustained activity. The patient may be told to hold an upward gaze, to blink, to hold the eyes closed against resistance, to hold the arms outstretched as long as possible, or to count out loud.[3] Grips may be tested by asking the patient to squeeze the examiner's hands and to hold against resistance for a few seconds. Ambulatory patients may be asked to raise themselves from a sitting position several times.

Several diagnostic tests are commonly used to help confirm the diagnosis. Electromyography (EMG) will show decremental decreases in responses to repetitive stimulation of selected muscles in 95 percent of the patients.[6]

The Tensilon test (edrophonium chloride), along with other evidence, may help confirm the diagnosis and may help in differentiating myasthenic crisis (worsening of the disease) from cholinergic crisis (overmedication with cholinergic drugs) in patients whose condition has rapidly worsened. Edrophonium is a very rapid acting cholinergic (anticholinesterase) drug, with effects lasting 30 seconds to four or five minutes. Preselected muscles are tested prior to injection and again while the drug is in effect. If muscle strength improves with the injection, myasthenia (or myasthenic crisis) is suspected. If no improvement occurs or the weakness is increased, cholinergic crisis may be present. Results of the test are helpful but not definitive since there is evidence that other neurological conditions may also respond temporarily to cholinergic drugs. Since edrophonium may produce both increased weakness and side effects including excessive salivation, atropine and respiratory resuscitation equipment should be immediately available during the test.[2]

Antibody titers for Ach receptor antibodies are useful both for helping to establish the diagnosis and for following the results of therapy, since there is fairly good correlation between titer levels and severity of the disease.

Respiratory effort may be measured by observing for chest expansion, listening for breath sounds, and asking the patient to blow out a match or count out loud as long as possible without taking a breath.[3] Vital capacity may be monitored with a spirometer at regular intervals or at any time a question arises about the effectiveness of breathing. It should be kept in mind that the signs of incipient respiratory failure in the myasthenic patient are subtle. Vital signs usually remain normal. Respiratory rate may not increase. Arterial blood gases remain normal until actual respiratory failure occurs. Patients who have had myasthenia for some time or who have previously experienced myasthenic or cholinergic crises are often the best monitors of their conditions. Their complaints should never be ignored.[3] Anxiety, restlessness, difficulty speaking or swallowing, and the use of accessory muscle are all precursors of respiratory failure.

Medical and Nursing Management. Medical and nursing management has reversed the assumption that myasthenia gravis is a fatal disease for most patients. Many patients are diagnosed and treated as outpatients, remaining in the community and leading fairly normal lives. Hospitalization may result from either a sudden or gradual worsening of the disease or because treatment has become ineffective in controlling the symptoms.[2]

With greater understanding of the pathogenesis of the disease, several new treatment modalities have been introduced in recent years. However, treatment usually begins with carefully titrated dosages of cholinergic medication such as neostigmine bromide (Prostigmin), pyridostigmine bromide (Mestinon), or ambenonium chloride (Mytelase). While these drugs may be very useful in improving strength and muscle function, they also produce side effects including excessive salivation, diaphoresis, cramping and diarrhea, and muscle cramps.[3] Furthermore, overdosage may produce weakness (cholinergic crisis) which may be mistaken for underdosage or worsening of the disease (myasthenic crisis). The patient (or physician) may then increase the dosage of medication to counteract the weakness, thus compounding the problem. Such patients often appear in the emergency room in actual or incipient respiratory failure.

Immunosuppression with corticosteroids is often prescribed as an adjunct to other therapy. Many patients initially become severely worse when steroid therapy is begun and may require hospitalization for close observation. To counteract this effect, many neurologists recommend beginning with small doses and gradually increasing the doses until maximal benefits are achieved. Doses of up to 40–45 mg of prednisone every day or twice this dose every other day are common. Complications of long-term steroid therapy are common, so careful follow-up is essential.[6]

Cytotoxic drugs such as azathioprine (Imuran) are often used along with other therapies to suppress immune bodies. As with steroids, side effects can be serious, so the patient must be carefully monitored and protected from exposure to infections.[3]

Thymectomy is often recommended for patients who do not respond satisfactorily to more conservative treatment. Once thought to be effective only in young women early in the disease, the procedure is much more widely used in recent years. Improvement in the myasthenia may be noted immediately after the surgery or may not appear for weeks or months.[5] The patient's condition following surgery may be extremely labile, so expert care and observations are crucial. Ventilatory support may be required, and all medication dosages will need to be readjusted.[3]

Plasmapheresis has been used extensively in recent years, often in conjunction with thymectomy, steroids, and other immunosuppressive drugs. Total remissions have been reported in some patients and dramatic improvements are not uncommon. Whether these improvements are permanent is still not known since these treatments are all still relatively new.

Priorities for nursing management include providing a supportive, stress-free environment, considerations to reducing unnecessary muscle activity, and prevention of respiratory failure.

Patients with known myasthenia gravis or those with the onset of fluctuating muscle weakness suggestive of myasthenia require careful assessment and monitoring. The history should include information about medications, recent upper respiratory infections, or other mild illnesses. Patients treated with cholinergic drugs tend to be very dose dependent. That is, a missed dose of medication or even a dose delayed more than a few minutes may result in weakness of the bulbar muscles, making it impossible for the patient to swallow the medication. Thus, even in the emergency department (ED), every effort should be made to obtain and administer regular doses of medication. Should it be necessary, due to swallowing difficulties, to substitute intramuscular medication for oral doses, keep in mind that the parenteral dose of most cholinergic drugs is about one-thirtieth the size of the oral dose.

It is of course essential that myasthenic crisis requiring cholinergic therapy be differentiated from cholinergic crisis (overdosage). A Tensilon test may help. In addition, the presence of cholinergic side effects is indicative of overdosage. When doubt still remains, the best procedure may be to withold medications to see if the symptoms improve. Be prepared, however, to initiate respiratory resuscitation.

In any case, intubation and the initiation of ventilatory assistance should be instituted before respiratory failure occurs. A vital capacity below 1000 ml, use of accessory muscles, or a minimal increase in $Paco_2$ are all adequate reasons for intubation.

Eaton-Lambert Syndrome

Eaton-Lambert syndrome is a myasthenic-like disease associated with carcinoma, usually oat cell carcinoma of the lung. Signs and symptoms are similar, but the pathology is related to a decrease in the amount of acetylcholine secreted at the axonal nerve endings. The receptor sites in the muscle fibers are normal.[6]

Usually only the trunk and shoulder girdle muscles are affected, and respiratory complications are rare except as they relate to the underlying diagnosis. The condition is slowly progressive, and the patients respond poorly to the treatments used for myasthenia gravis.[6]

Botulism

Botulism results from food poisoning, and is caused by the exotoxin of *Clostridium botulinum.*[6] This organism is found widely in the soil and in the intestinal tract of domestic animals. Botulism is rare but highly fatal; death usually occurs as a result of respiratory failure. The toxin acts primarily at the myoneural junction, blocking release of acetylcholine at the synaptic nerve endings.

Clinical features. Symptoms of botulism usually appear within 24–48 hours after ingestion of the spoiled food. The patient complains of nausea and vomiting, followed by diplopia, visual blurring, ptosis, and ocular palsies. The pupils may be dilated and nonreactive but the patient remains awake and alert. As other bulbar muscles become involved there may be hoarseness and difficulty with speaking and swallowing. The patient may also complain of vertigo and deafness. There is progressive weakness of the neck, trunk, and limbs with loss of deep tendon reflexes. When the respiratory muscles become weak, respiratory failure can occur.[6]

Diagnosis is by history and the presence of the clinical signs. The condition may appear as part of an epidemic if others ate the same spoiled food. Recovery for those patients who survive is very slow. Strength may return first in the eye muscles and other bulbar muscles. Functional recovery of the trunk and limbs may take several months.

Medical and Nursing Management. Medical and nursing management consists of the administration of trivalent antiserum (toxin types A, B, and C), and appropriate antibiotics.[6] Survival and recovery, however, depend totally on prompt and aggressive management of respiratory paralysis and general supportive care during the long course of the disease.

Neuromuscular Blocking Agents

Curareform drugs (*d*-tubocurarine, decamethonium) act at the myoneural junction, preserving sensation and consciousness while effecting complete and generalized paralysis. Obviously, such drugs are normally used only under conditions where respiratory support is available.

Other more benign drugs may result in neuromuscular transmission blockage in some individuals. Certain antibiotics such as neomycin, gentamycin, streptomycin, tetracycline, and others are known to produce a myastheniclike weakness, and will exacerbate the symptoms of patients with myasthenia gravis or Eaton-Lambert syndrome.[2]

A drug history is important for any patient with the onset of unexplained weakness whether or not there is any indication of respiratory failure.

Peripheral Nerve and Root Disease

There are an almost infinite number of peripheral nerve diseases that cause paralysis and sensory loss. Few of these conditions are like to result in respiratory failure except as a complication of immobility or aspiration pneumonia. Those that may present with incipient respiratory failure will be discussed in this section.

Guillain-Barré Syndrome (Landry-Guillain-Barré; Acute Ideopathic Polyneuritis; Acute Polyradiculopathy; Infectious Polyneuritis)

Guillain-Barré syndrome is a disease that affects the peripheral nerves (axons) with involvement of the nerve roots and segmental demyelination of the axons. Both sensory and motor nerves are affected, so that the patient has sensory abnormalities as well as paresis. As part of the peripheral nervous system, the autonomic nerves (sympathetic and parasympathetic) may also be involved, resulting in associated fluctuations of blood pressure and pulse, sometimes with cardiac dysrhythmias. The primary dangers in this disease are cardiovascular collapse and respiratory failure. The disease is, however, self-limiting, and for those who survive the acute phase, recovery is usually complete with little or no residual deficit.[2]

The disease strikes one in every 75,000 persons annually. It affects both men and women, although it may be slightly more common in men. While those over 40 years of age are the most frequent victims, no age group is immune. At least half of the patients who develop the disease report an antecedent upper respiratory infection, gastrointestinal (GI) disturbance, or a febrile illness one to three weeks prior to onset.[6] There is some evidence that there is a higher than normal incidence in patients who received swine flu vaccine.[4]

The mortality rate has been reported as high as 20–50 percent, but has decreased to 2 percent since aggressive supportive care and respiratory assistance has been generally available.[6] Mortality at present is usually associated with complications such as pneumonia and other infections. Full recovery of function may take from 3 to 12 months, but is usually complete. An occasional patient suffers a relapse of the disease months or years later, but for most persons this is a single episode.

Pathophysiology. The pathophysiology of Guillain-Barré initially involves an inflammation and swelling in the perivascular spaces around the nerve roots. Later, inflammatory demyelination occurs, followed by segmental demyelination with destruction of the axon itself. The cause is unknown, but has been related to an autoimmune process perhaps triggered by a viral invasion.

Clinical Features. Typically, the patient reports the gradual onset of flaccid weakness in the lower extremities, which over hours or days ascends to include the hands, arms, trunk, and cranial nerves. The weakness is often accompanied by muscle tenderness and myalgialike pain. Reflexes in the affected extremities are diminished to absent. There may be sensory loss, particularly loss of proprioception. Muscle atrophy is mild to moderate. With involvement of the autonomic nerves, there may be fluctuations of blood pressure (particularly orthostatic hypotension) and cardiac dysrhythmias.[6]

As the cranial nerves are affected, the patient develops difficulty swallowing and talking, and may be unable to open and close the eyes. Paralysis of the vagus nerves results in an inability of the bronchi to constrict and dilate normally, so the patient is prone to atelectasis and pneumonia. Paresis of the muscles of breathing leads to respiratory failure.

The patient is usually afebrile, unless there is a concurrent infection, and other vital signs may be normal. The patient remains awake and alert. Rarely, there may be urinary retention and bowel incontinence.

Diagnosis is based on the history, the progressive nature of the illness, and on the results of cerebrospinal fluid (CSF) analysis. The CSF usually shows an albuminocytologic dissociation, an elevation of the protein without a corresponding elevation of white blood cells.[7] The CSF protein level may be normal early in the disease, with a gradual rise as the disease progresses. While there is no exact correlation between the protein level and the severity of the symptoms, the protein level does return to normal as the patient recovers, so it may give some indication of when the disease has reached a peak and is beginning to recede.

While an ascending paralysis is the most common presentation, occasionally symptoms begin in the hands and arms. There is also a variant that presents with cranial nerve signs and ataxia.[6] The disease does not always progress to the point of total paralysis and respiratory failure. Mild forms of the disease may consist of transient weakness in the extremities with rapid recovery. However, since at onset there is no way to predict either the extent or rapidity of progression, each patient must be closely monitored until the disease has peaked and begins to recede.

Medical and Nursing Management. There is no specific medical treatment for Guillain-Barré syndrome. Some neurologists believe that the use of steroids early in the course of the disease may reduce or retard progression, but this remains controversial. Symptomatic care remains the basis of treatment.

Mechanical ventilation and vasopressor drugs may be needed early in the disease. Infections, atelectasis, and pneumonia need to be prevented and treated aggressively when they occur. Nutrition often becomes a major complicating factor because of the lengthy course of the disease and the patient's inability to swallow. Nasogastric feedings may be initiated unless there is a paralytic ileus. Precautions to prevent aspiration are essential. Parenteral nutrition may be required for some patients.

Aggressive nursing care is the key to survival for the paralyzed patient. The nurse must anticipate and recognize early critical events so that treatment is not delayed. Like the patient with myasthenia gravis described earlier, respiratory failure may give little warning. Inadequate chest expansion may allow a buildup of carbon dioxide, which may cause drowsiness and lethargy, so that the patient does not exhibit anxiety. The paralyzed patient cannot call for help or complain of dyspnea. Vital signs, including respiratory rate, may not change until respiratory failure has already occurred. Frequent assessment of vital capacity is essential. Intubation or tracheostomy should be done as an elective procedure whenever difficulties in swallowing with accumulation of secretions is evident, when vital capacity falls below 1000 ml, or when $Paco_2$ levels begin to rise.

Rigorous lung hygiene, including frequent position change and chest physical therapy, is essential throughout the course of the disease. Attention to skin, bladder, and bowel function and prevention of foot drop and other deformities is also critical. In view of the inflammatory nature of the disease, rest and limited activity may be important during the acute phase of the illness, with active rehabilitation delayed until the recovery period.

The fact that the patient is fully awake and alert throughout the illness places unusual responsibility on the nurse for addressing the psychological problems faced by the patient. The patient who is totally paralyzed and whose life is completely dependent on machines and on the willingness and skill of others may find it difficult to believe that recovery will, in fact, occur. A trusting relationship with care givers needs to be developed early and carefully sustained. The patient should be warned early in the disease process that progression of symptoms can occur and that respiratory support may be needed. It should be stressed from the beginning that while the disease may be progressive and lengthy, recovery is almost certain. Thus, when predicted events happen, the patient is likely to give more credence to the predictions of recovery. Trust is developed, and despair may be minimized.

Porphyric Polyneuropathy

Porphyria is an inherited, autosomal recessive condition, marked by intermittent episodes of generalized or localized abdominal pain and variable neurological symptoms including psychoses, delirium, confusion, and convulsions. Some forms of the disease may have an associated polyneuropathy resembling Guillain-Barré syndrome. There is rapidly advancing symmetrical weakness with involvement of sensory and autonomic nerves. There may be tachycardia, fever, leukocytosis, and in severe cases, respiratory paralysis.[6]

Pathologically, there is a metabolic defect of the liver, with increased production of the urinary excretion of porphyrins. Attacks may be precipitated by the ingestion of drugs such as barbiturates, sulfonamides, or estrogens. The neuropathic changes include degeneration of both the axons and myelin sheaths. There is an inflammatory reaction similar to that found in other forms of neuropathy.

For those patients who survive, recovery of function is usually complete, with symptoms subsiding over a period of weeks to months. Recurrence is common.

Medical and nursing care is largely supportive as in Guillain-Barré. There is no specific treatment. Ventilatory and nutritional support may be needed. Uremia is a common complication, so dialysis may be necessary.

Motor Neuron Disease

The term motor neuron disease is used to describe a number of conditions affecting the motor neurons of the spinal cord, brainstem, and motor cortex.[6] While there are a number of variants, all are characterized by progressive muscle weakness, atrophy, and upper motor neuron signs such as hyperreflexia and spasticity.

Amyotrophic Lateral Sclerosis

Amyotrophic lateral sclerosis (ALS) is the most common form of motor neuron disease and is the basis for the discussion in this section. This disease occurs most frequently in middle to older age groups and is universally fatal, usually within a period of two to six years.[6]

Pathophysiology. The pathophysiology of ALS is better understood than the etiology. The cause of the disease is unknown, although the possibilities of a slow-growing virus or an autoimmune process have been considered. Initially in the course of the disease there is gradual loss of nerve cells in the anterior horns of the spinal cord and in the motor nuclei of the brainstem controlling the cranial nerves. Remaining motor neurons are abnormally small, shrunken, and filled with lipid material. As nerve cells are lost they tend to be replaced by astrocytic cells. Eventually the nerve roots and axons leading from the motor neurons degenerate. Similar changes occur in the motor neurons of the cerebral cortex with degeneration of the pyramidal tracts in the brain and spinal cord. Sensory pathways remain intact so that only motor function is impaired.

Clinical Features. Diagnosis of ALS is based primarily on the clinical findings. Onset is usually gradual, often beginning with clumsiness and cramping of the hands or feet. The patient may notice twitching of the muscles. As the disease progresses, spasticity develops in the legs. There is usually severe atrophy, often first evident in the hand and shoulder muscles. Eventually all muscles show severe atrophy so that the patient develops a cadaveric appearance.[6]

Reflexes in the affected muscles are often active or hyperactive even though there is severe atrophy and fasciculations (both upper and lower motor neuron signs). Bowel and bladder function is usually normal, although the patient may become constipated because of weakness of the abdominal muscles and immobility. There are no sensory findings (an important diagnostic distinction) and the mental status remains normal virtually until death.

Bulbar and respiratory involvement may occur early or late in the process. Whenever it appears it is usually predictive of a terminal phase of the disease. Patients have little or no discomfort other than that associated with immobility and increasing difficulty swallowing and breathing. These patients, awake and alert to the very end, literally witness their own deaths.

Laboratory tests are generally normal. EMG shows denervation fibrillations and fasciculations, and reduced motor conduction velocities.[6]

Medical and Nursing Management. Since there is no definitive therapy for patients with ALS, management is essentially supportive in nature. The use of guanidine hydrochloride is sometimes prescribed, but with little evidence that it is beneficial. Similarly, the use of steroids, snake venom, plasmapheresis, interferons, thyrotropin-releasing hormone, and other remedies have been tried without success. High-dose vitamins are sometimes given, along with dietary supplements and muscle relaxants, which may make the patient more comfortable but do not effect the progress of the disease.

The inevitability of death as the outcome for this more or less rapidly progressive, disabling disease raises certain legal, moral, and ethical questions not applicable to the other diseases discussed. Patients and families faced with this diagnosis will need to make crucial decisions about the desirability of using life support systems in the terminal stages of the disease. Discontinuance of ventilatory support, even when requested by an alert and mentally competent patient, is problematical. Thus, should the patient and family elect not to prolong the patient's life artificially, plans must be made before respiratory failure is imminent.

Both patient and family should understand the nature of the disease and its prognosis, and should have adequate counseling and a strong support system with opportunities to discuss all of the alternatives before a crisis develops and the decisions are taken out of their hands. When a patient appears in the ED in acute respiratory distress it is virtually too late for such decisions to take place.

The goal of nursing care for patients with ALS is to contribute to the supportive efforts of the entire health care team, to assist the patient to retain independence for as long as possible, and to achieve a peaceful death according to the expressed wishes of the patient and family.

CARDIOVASCULAR COMPLICATIONS

Cardiovascular changes can occur secondary to central nervous system (CNS) injury and disease. The hemodynamic effects of spinal cord injury are discussed in other chapters. This section will concentrate on the cardiovascular changes associated with intracerebral insult. These changes often include electrocardiographic (ECG) abnormalities, altered hemodynamics, and pulmonary edema. A brief review of local, humoral, and nervous control of the cardiovascular system provides a basis for better understanding the nature of these changes.

Regulation of Cardiovascular Performance

The major forces regulating cardiovascular performance can be divided into intrinsic and extrinsic factors.

Intrinsic Factors

Intrinsic regulators of cardiovascular performance include the inherent ability of the heart to initiate its own beat in the absence of any nervous or hormonal control, and the heart's capacity to adapt to changing hemodynamic states through alteration of the contractile force of cardiac muscle itself.

Peripheral circulation is influenced intrinsically by the metabolic demands of the tissues, and by autoregulation, the ability of vessels to maintain blood flow in various organ systems in the face of marked changes in systemic arterial blood pressure.

Extrinsic Factors

Extrinsic factors that can alter cardiovascular performance include humoral factors (catecholamines and various hormones), baroreceptors located in the aortic arch and carotid bodies that sense stretch exerted by blood pressure, and chemoreceptors located in those same areas that sense Pao_2, $Paco_2$ and pH changes. Baroreceptors and chemoreceptors influence the vasomotor regions in the medulla (see Figure 11-1). Decreased blood pressure and moderately decreased Pao_2 stimulate vasoconstrictor regions in the vasomotor center causing systemic vasoconstriction of resistance and capacitance vessels resulting in the elevation of the blood pressure. Cardiac acceleration also occurs as a result of these stimuli. Elevated $Paco_2$ and decreased Pao_2 in the brain directly stimulate the vasomotor regions. A severe decrease in Pao_2 actually depresses the vasomotor region. Increased blood pressure inhibits vasoconstriction, stimulates the vagus nerve, and causes a decrease in the blood pressure and a slowing of the heart rate.[8]

The autonomic nervous system is the major extrinsic factor that accounts for most of the cardiovascular changes observed in patients with various intracranial pathologies. The sympathetic and parasympathetic divisions of the autonomic nervous system normally exert tremendous control on cardiovascular performance. There is autonomic representation at all levels of the brain, with a network of pathways between the cerebrum, diencephalon, and brainstem structures, which are all capable of exerting some degree of influence on the peripheral autonomic nervous system.[9]

Sympathetic Influences. The sympathetic nervous system has a profound facilitory effect on the cardiovascular system. Sympathetic fibers to peripheral resistance vessels, the arterioles, and capacitance vessels, the veins, secrete norepinephrine when stimulated, leading to vasoconstriction. Sympathetic inner-

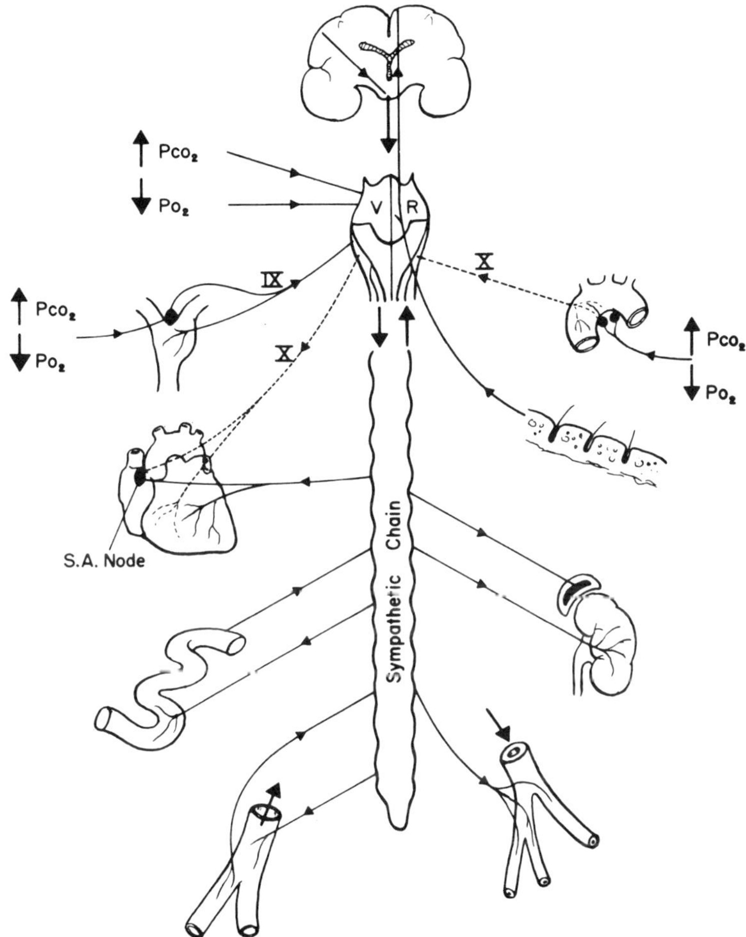

Fig. 11–1—Neural input and output of the vasomotor region (VR); IX, glossopharyngeal nerve; X, vagus nerve.

Source: Reprinted from *Cardiovascular Physiology* ed 4 (p 143) by RM Berne and MN Levy with permission of the CV Mosby Company, © 1981.

---

vation of the heart results in increased contractility, rate, and atrioventricular (A-V) conduction.

Parasympathetic Influences. Parasympathetic vagus nerves exert profound depressant effects on cardiac pacemaker function, A-V conduction, and atrial and ventricular contractility. Only a small proportion of the resistance vessels of the body receive parasympathetic fibers, therefore parasympathetic effect on total vascular resistance is small.[8]

Systemic Cardiovascular Effects of Intracranial Disorders

Dramatic changes in heart rate, rhythm, and contractility have been demonstrated experimentally by stimulation of various areas of the cerebral cortex, diencephalon, and brainstem.[8] These experiments demonstrate the influence of various regions of the brain on the autonomic nervous system.

Several intracranial disorders have been implicated in producing systemic cardiovascular changes; these include severe brain trauma with brain edema and intracranial hypertension, meningitis, ischemia and infarcts, subarachnoid and intracerebral hemorrhages following strokes or ruptured aneurysms, and postcraniotomy disorders. Cardiac dysrhythmias, conduction disturbances, myocardial damage, the Cushing response, and neurogenic pulmonary edema are among the cardiovascular effects that are triggered by the brain.[9]

Cardiac Hemodynamic Changes

Cardiac and hemodynamic changes include variables in heart rate and contractility, and peripheral vascular resistance.

Cushing Response. The Cushing response results when intracranial hypertension and ischemia stimulate the vasomotor centers in the medulla. Stimulation of the sympathetic nervous system leads to an elevation of the systolic blood pressure in an attempt to maintain cerebral perfusion pressure. This leads to a widening of the pulse pressure. The increased blood pressure causes a reflex slowing of the heart rate via vagal reflexes. Associated respiratory irregularities also occur. The Cushing response is a late clinical sign and signifies brain decompensation.

Vasovagal Reflex. A vasovagal reflex can occur in response to parasympathetic stimulation and is manifested by reduced heart rate and blood pressure, leading to a fall in cardiac output and peripheral perfusion.[10] The autonomic instability observed in patients with intracranial pathology puts these patients at risk for developing a vasovagal reflex in response to such nursing actions as airway suctioning, although suctioning most often stimulates the sympathetic nervous system. In its extreme form, the vasovagal reflex can lead to asystole. Preoxygenation and limited suctioning may reduce the chance of triggering a vasovagal reflex in the brain injured patient. Atropine should be available at the bedside of these patients.

Neurogenic Pulmonary Edema. Although neurogenic pulmonary edema (NPE) represents a serious pulmonary complication, it is mediated by cardiovascular responses and is therefore included in this discussion. The mechanisms of NPE are not completely understood, but it is believed that the probable sequence of events is as follows: impaired cerebral oxidative metabolism and altered hypothalamic function results in an outpouring of neural impulses from the brain. Intense sympathetic stimulation results in a shift of blood volume from the systemic to the pulmonary circulation causing vascular congestion and pulmonary capillary damage. Protein and fluid leak out of the damaged capillaries. There is a breakdown of surfactant in the alveoli as this fluid transudates across the alveolar-capillary membrane. Atelectasis follows. These changes can occur within minutes after the CNS insult.[11] This sequence of events may be followed by respiratory distress syndrome.

The hemodynamic consequences of NPE include increased aortic, systemic arterial, pulmonary arterial, pulmonary venous, and superior vena cava pressures, and increased peripheral vascular resistance. These hemodynamic effects may last only 5–15 minutes, but the altered pulmonary capillary permeability accounts for the continued pulmonary edema seen.[11]

Clinical features. Clinical signs of NPE include tachypnea, frothy blood tinged sputum, and wet rales and rhonchi on auscultation of the lungs. Arterial blood gas analysis may reveal significant hypoxemia and hypocapnea. As the patient tires from the work of breathing, the $Paco_2$ rises and the Pao_2 falls even further leading to progressive acidosis. Chest x-ray may show diffuse haziness of the lung fields.[11]

Medical and nursing management. Treatment consists of controlling the primary problem which is intracranial hypertension. Elevation of the patient's head decreases intracranial pressure and allows for better pulmonary ventilation. Careful dehydration therapy while maintaining good tissue perfusion is undertaken. Mechanical ventilation is used to reverse oxygenation impairment and correct atelectasis. The application of positive end expiratory pressure (PEEP) may be necessary to effect adequate oxygenation. The deleterious effects of PEEP on intracranial pressure must be closely monitored.[11]

The nurse maintains the patient's head in an elevated position, but also turns the patient frequently to prevent worsening of atelectasis, and monitors the patient's neurological status, vital signs, urinary output, and arterial blood gases (ABGs). Frequent assessment of breath sounds and respiratory patterns is essential. Careful suctioning is preceded and followed by hyperoxygenation with several breaths of 100 percent oxygen from a bag-valve device (ambu). It may be necessary to administer paralyzing agents such as pancuronium bromide to prevent coughing and bucking, which could further increase intracranial pressure.[11]

Electrocardiographic Changes

ECG abnormalities consist of alterations in cardiac rhythm, conduction, and repolarization. These alterations lead to cardiac dysrhythmias, ST and T wave changes. Most of the ECG changes in patients with intracranial disorders are thought to be mediated by stimulation of the autonomic nervous system directly or by increased levels of circulating catecholamines, although increased parasympathetic activity may also contribute to some of the ECG changes seen.[12]

Alterations in Cardiac Rhythm. Alterations in cardiac rhythm may result from an imbalance between sympathetic and parasympathetic control over cardiac pacemaker function. Sinus arrhythmia and extremes of sinus tachycardia and sinus bradycardia may be observed in the same patient. Often these chances are not associated with patient activity at the time.

Other cardiac dysrhythmias associated with intracranial disorders include ventricular premature beats, atrial premature beats, wandering atrial pacemaker, atrial tachycardia, ventricular tachycardia, ventricular fibrillation, ideoventricular rhythm, and junctional rhythms.[9]

It is thought that disruption of the uniformity of myocardial cell recovery may encourage the appearance of reentrant-type dysrhythmias.[12] Premature ventricular beats are often precursors of more serious ventricular dysrhythmias. Overactivity of the sympathetic nervous system transiently lowers the vulnerable threshold period of the myocardium and predisposes it to ventricular fibrillation. Patients with subarachnoid hemorrhage seem particularly prone to develop dysrhythmias related to excessive sympathetic discharge.[9]

Alterations in Cardiac Conduction. Conduction disturbances that have been documented include atrioventricular block, bundle branch block, atrioventricular dissociation, and, in some cases, shortened P-R interval.[9,12]

Alterations in Myocardial Repolarization. Disorders of myocardial repolarization are reflected in the ST segment and T wave of the ECG. Tall, peaked, notched, flat, or deeply inverted T waves have all been reported. In addition, ST elevation, ST depression, prominent U waves, and prolongation of the QT interval are associated with patients with cerebrovascular accident and/or increased intracranial pressure (ICP). In a study by Jachuck et al,[13] QT prolongation was found in patients with ICPs in excess of 65 mm Hg. The authors considered QT prolongation in patients with intracranial hypertension to be an ominous sign, possibly indicating rostral-caudal deterioration and brainstem involvement with stimulation of the vagus nerves.

Excessive sympathetic discharge is thought to produce myocardial damage with subendocardial hemorrhage and focal necrosis. These changes often occur in the inner one-third of the left ventricle and in the papillary muscles.[12] Injured myocardial cells predispose the patient to develop cardiac dysrhythmias.

Medical and Nursing Management

While there may be other reasons for cardiovascular instability in neurological patients such as underlying cardiovascular disease, the nurse needs to recognize the significant role that the autonomic nervous system plays in regulating cardiovascular performance. Serious intracranial pathology can cause an imbalance in this regulation, leading to many cardiovascular complications, the effects of which can further compromise circulation to the brain as well as to other organ systems. Careful attention directed toward assessment of the cardiovascular and pulmonary status of those neurological emergency patients at risk allows the nurse to detect and report complications early, and to institute appropriate antiarrhythmic and other therapy.

DISORDERS OF TEMPERATURE REGULATION

Temperature variation occurs for many reasons. Since the nervous system controls body temperature, various neurological disorders have the potential for causing disorders of temperature regulation.

Regulation of Body Temperature

Body heat is regulated by the CNS through complex feedback mechanisms involving heat receptors in the brain, spinal cord, skin, and abdomen. The hypothalamus contains the ''thermostat'' and stimulates or inhibits autonomic responses to changes in internal temperature.[14] These responses include sweating and shivering, as well as vasodilation and vasoconstriction. These mechanisms, under normal conditions, maintain the temperature of the body within very narrow parameters.

When body temperatures exceed 41° C (105.8° F) to 42.2° C (108° F) the control mechanism in the hypothalamus is depressed and sweating is decreased. Thus, temperature continues in an upward spiral. Temperatures above 41° C for more than s short time may cause irreparable cell damage, particularly in the brain.[15]

It is also known that elevated temperatures increase cerebral metabolism and intracranial pressure, so that control of temperature is an important element in the management of any patient with actual or potential brain injury or disease.

Disorders of Temperature Regulation

Abnormal conditions which cause the temperature to shift above or below the normal parameters include toxic conditions affecting the temperature regulating centers, damage to the hypothalamus from injury or disease, failure of autonomic responses in disorders of the spinal cord, peripheral nerves, or skin, and extremes in external conditions that overwhelm the normal protective mechanisms.

Pyrogenic Fever

Pyrogens are the activating substances that produce fever.[14] Pyrogens are released from damaged body tissues, destruction of leukocytes, or from the activity of the invading organism itself. The pyrogenic substances, circulating in the bloodstream, directly affect the hypothalamic thermostat, causing the "set point" to rise. With the thermostat fixed at a higher than normal temperature, the rate of energy heat production is increased until the body temperature reaches the point at which the thermostat is fixed.[14,16]

When the body's normal heat conservation measures are exaggerated, the vasoconstriction of peripheral blood vessels may result in a chill, accompanied by shivering. As the body temperature reaches the thermostat "set," chilling and shivering cease. When the set is exceeded there is vasodilation and diaphoresis as the body attempts to maintain the temperature at the set point.[16]

Whether or not fever is an adaptive mechanism that assists the body in fighting the infection, or whether it is, in fact, a harmful by-product of infection remains controversial.[14]

Clinical Features. Patients with febrile illnesses often complain of generalized malaise, headache, and photophobia. They may be restless, with increased pulse and respirations, and dry, warm, flushed skin. There may be initial chilling even though the temperature is rising.

For debilitated patients and those with suppressed immune systems, severe infectious processes may occur without fever. In fact, such patients may actually have lower than normal temperatures.

High fever in young children and susceptible adults may result in seizures. Febrile seizures in children are most common from six months of age to about six years. Such children frequently have recurrent seizures with each febrile episode, and are seizure-free at other times.

Because fever greatly increases the metabolic rate, calories are utilized more rapidly than normal, and protein catabolism increases. Salt and water are lost through sweating. Thus, dehydration and malnutrition with weight loss can develop rapidly. Weakness and lethargy may persist for some time after the fever has abated.

Medical and Nursing Management. Treatment for the patient with fever will be directed toward the diagnosis and treatment of the underlying infection and management of the fever. Specific neurological infections resulting in fever were discussed in Chapter 7. This discussion focuses on the management of pyrogenic fever.

The goal of management of pyrogenic fever is to maintain the temperature within a safe range, and prevent dehydration and excessive protein catabolism. Promoting the patient's comfort and providing a quiet, restful environment minimizes the metabolic demands of the body.

Attainment of a normal temperature while the pyrogenic factors remain may be an unrealistic goal. If, in fact, fever is an adaptive mechanism which helps to fight the infection, a normal temperature may not even be a desirable goal. However, temperatures higher than 40° C (104° F) or widely fluctuating are to be avoided. Judicious use of antipyretic medications and external cooling devices can be used to maintain a stable, if somewhat elevated, temperature.

Aspirin and acetaminophen have been shown to be effective in reducing fever.[14] Caution should be used, however, in administering aspirin to children (see Reye's syndrome, Chapter 7). To be most effective in controlling the temperature, antipyretic drugs should be administered as the temperature is rising, not at it's peak, when the hypothalamic "set" will automatically serve to reduce fever. Since drug actions begin some 30 minutes after administration and remain active for several hours, the temperature flow record should indicate the times when medication was given, so that a pattern can be identified and used as a guide to further treatment.

When antipyretic drugs alone do not maintain the temperature below 39° C (102° F), other measures may need to be instituted. For short-term treatment, tepid sponge baths, perhaps using a mixture of alcohol and water, are often effective in reducing temperature by evaporation. Ice applied to the skin may be counterproductive since it may cause vasoconstriction and heat retention. Coverings should be light and loose, allowing free circulation of air around the body. Room temperatures should be cool. The body should be cooled slowly in order to avoid shivering, which raises the temperature.

For more prolonged management, a cooling blanket may be used. Care must be taken to protect the patient's skin from overexposure to the cooling apparatus. The blanket should be turned off before the temperature reaches the predetermined level, since the body temperature will continue to fall one or two degrees. The machine should be turned on again when the body temperature begins to climb. Operation of the machine in an automatic mode utilizing an indwelling rectal thermistor may accomplish temperature control more easily.

During periods of fever, special attention must be given to maintaining hydration and nutrition. The patient may lose as much as 3000 cc of fluid a day through perspiration. For patients to be able to drink, nourishing liquids may be provided that increase caloric intake as well as fluids and electrolytes. When intravenous fluids are given, volumes should be increased to compensate for fluid losses.

Central Nervous System Hyperpyrexia

When disease or injury directly affects the hypothalamic thermostat, the ability of the body to regulate its own temperature is lost. The temperature rises precipitously until death occurs. Sometimes the patient's temperature fluctuates widely in an apparently erratic fashion.

Since elevations of temperature further compromise an already damaged brain and increase ICP, aggressive management is critical. Because antipyretic drugs act on the hypothalamus to reduce temperature, they tend to be ineffective in the management of CNS system hyperpyrexia in which the hypothalamic thermostat is affected. External cooling devices are most effective and should be used as described earlier.

Heat Stroke

Heat stroke results from failure of the hypothalamic regulation of heat production and heat storage. Temperatures of 42°–43° C are usually required to produce coma, but delirium may be persent at lower temperatures.[17] Onset of delirium or coma may be sudden or may be preceded by headache, numbness, tingling, or mental confusion. Untreated, there is a high mortality rate, and residual neurological signs in survivors may include ataxia, hemiparesis, or dementia. Early, aggressive treatment usually results in good recovery, although the elderly and those with underlying hypertension or heart disease are at risk for pulmonary edema or circulatory collapse.

Clinical Features. The clinical features of heat stroke may be striking. The patient is delirious or comatose, with high fever (42° C or higher), and absence of sweating. The skin is hot and dry, and the pulse and respirations are increased. There may be involuntary limb movements, tremors, or even convulsions. Serum pH may be acidotic. Pupils are usually small and reactive and skeletal muscles hypertonic.[17]

Heat stroke is most common in elderly persons whose adaptive mechanisms are less efficient, and in others who engage in strenuous exercise in hot climates to which they are not acclimatized. Acclimatization is achieved by gradually increasing exercise in the hot environment over a period of several days to several weeks.

Medical and Nursing Management. The goals of management are to reduce the body temperature, reestablish sweating, and replace body fluids and electrolytes. When temperatures are extremely high, the temperature must be reduced quickly to avoid permanent cell damage. Since the autoregulatory mechanisms are not working, antipyretic agents may not be effective initially, but may help reestablish diaphoresis later. Immediate sponging with tepid alcohol and water, a cool environment, and increased air circulation along with the use of a cooling blanket will usually be successful in lowering the temperature to a safe level. Continued cooling can then proceed more gradually.

Careful monitoring during cooling is essential, since the sudden lowering of temperature may precipitate cardiac dysrhythmias or circulatory collapse. The patient should also be kept under close surveillance for several days, until the autoregulatory mechanisms are reestablished.

Administration of intravenous fluids with appropriate electrolytes is critical. When sweating is reestablished the patient may lose up to several liters of fluid in a matter of an hour or two, leading to another rise in temperature and circulatory collapse.

Heat Exhaustion

Heat exhaustion (heat shock) results from excessive loss of fluids and salt, with a decrease in blood volume. It usually develops slowly over a period of several days, with headache, fatigue, anorexia, vomiting, visual disturbances, and confusion or lethargy. If untreated, circulatory collapse will follow. The patient then appears pale, with a rapid pulse, decreased blood pressure, profuse sweating, and little or no rise in temperature.

Treatment includes bed rest in a moderate environment and replacement of fluids and electrolytes. With early treatment, recovery is usually complete and rapid. As with heat stroke, heat exhaustion is most common in the elderly and those exercising in hot weather without adequate fluid and salt intake.

Hypothermia

Hypothermia may be seen in a variety of clinical conditions, including disorders of the hypothalamus, myxedema, metabolic coma, and drug overdose. Temperatures below 35° C result in physiological changes including decreased cerebral blood flow, decreased cerebral metabolism, and decreased cerebral oxygen consumption. Thus, lowered temperatures may offer some protection to the brain and hypothermia is sometimes artificially induced during surgical procedures or as part of the management of intracranial hypertension (see Chapter 4). For this discussion, only accidental hypothermia is covered.

Clinical Features. Clinical features may vary with depth of hypothermia. In the absence of other pathology, a body temperature below 32° C is usually required to produce a change in the level of consciousness. Shivering ceases at temperatures below 30° C. Such patients are very pale and feel cold to the touch even in protected parts of the body. Respirations are slow and shallow, often with carbon dioxide retention. The pulse is slow, and blood pressure is often unmeasurable. Subcutaneous tissues are nonpliable, muscles are hypertonic, and reflexes may or may not be present. Pupils may be constricted or dilated and may not respond to light. Some patients will have initially been thought to be dead.[17] Atrial fibrillation is the most common cold-related dysrhythmia, although at body temperatures below 28° C ventricular fibrillation and cardiac standstill are likely.

Medical and Nursing Management. Treatment consists of rewarming the body until normal function returns. This must be undertaken cautiously, because as the body is rewarmed, its initial demand for oxygen is quite high, and cardiac output may not be adequate to meet this demand. The use of a thermal blanket at 36.6°–37.7° C can increase the body temperature by 1°–2° per hour. Intubation and mechanical ventilation may be needed. Electrical defibrillation is usually successful in terminating ventricular fibrillation if the temperature is greater than 28°C. Cardiac resuscitation medications should be given sparingly because as the body warms, peripheral vasodilation occurs. Drugs that have been sequestered are released leading to a "bolus effect" that may cause fatal dysrhythmias.

Intravenous fluids should be given cautiously, since decreased urinary output may lead to pulmonary edema. Warming intravenous (IV) fluids to 37° C may assist in the rewarming process. Nasogastric or rectal lavage with warm normal saline may be done to rewarm the gastrointestinal tract. Warmed peritoneal lavage with normal saline is also sometimes used. Peripheral circulation must be monitored since gangrene of the fingers and toes is a common complication of accidental hypothermia.

Patients who survive rarely suffer permanent neurological deficits unless body temperatures fall below 28° C. When brain damage does occur, it usually is characterized by disturbances of memory, brainstem dysfunctions, and muscle hypotonia.

It should be kept in mind that most clinical thermometers do not register very low temperatures. When hypothermia is suspected, a special thermometer should be obtained to ensure accurate monitoring during the recovery period.

REFERENCES

1. Bogrand BA: Impairment of respiratory function, in Snyder M (ed): *A Guide to Neurological and Neurosurgical Nursing*. New York, Wiley, 1983.

2. Taylor JW, Ballenger S: *Neurological Dysfunctions and Nursing Intervention*. New York, McGraw-Hill, 1980.

3. Kess R: Suddenly in crisis: Unpredictable myasthenia. *Am J Nurs*, August 1984.

4. Hickey J: *The Clinical Practice of Neurological and Neurosurgical Nursing*. Philadelphia, Lippincott, 1981.

5. Drachman D: Myasthenia gravis, Part II. *New Engl J Med*, Jan 19, 1978.

6. Adams RD, Victor M: *Principles of Neurology*, ed 3. New York, McGraw-Hill, 1985.

7. Kennedy R, Danielson MA, Mulder DT, et al: Guillain-Barré syndrome: A 42 year epidemiologic and clinical study. *Mayo Clin Proc* 1978;53:93–99.

8. Berne RM, Levy MN: *Cardiovascular Physiology* ed 4. St Louis, Mosby, 1981.

9. Zegeer LJ: Systemic cardiovascular effects of intracranial disorders: Implications for nursing care. *J Neurosurg Nurs* 1984;16:161–167.

10. Price SA, Wilson LM: *Pathophysiology: Clinical Concepts of Disease Processes*. New York, McGraw-Hill, 1978.

11. Neumann D, Bailey L: An overview of neurogenic pulmonary edema. *J Neurosurg Nurs* 1980;12:206–209.

12. Nikas DL (ed): *The Critically Ill Neurosurgical Patient*. New York, Churchill-Livingstone, 1982.

13. Jachuck SJ, Ramani PS, Clark T, et al: Electrocardiographic abnormalities associated with raised intracranial pressure. *Brit Med J*, February 1975, pp 242–244.

14. Heideman CA: Alterations in temperature, in Snyder M (ed): *A Guide to Neurological and Neurosurgical Nursing*. New York, Wiley, 1983.

15. Levine ME: *Introduction to Clinical Nursing*. Philadelphia, FA Davis Co., 1971.

16. Guyton A: *Textbook of Medical Physiology*, ed 5. Philadelphia, WB Saunders, 1976.

17. Plum F, Posner JB: *The Diagnosis of Stupor and Coma*, ed 3. Philadelphia, FA Davis Co, 1980.

Chapter 12

Pain

INTRODUCTION

Pain is a phenomenon about which much remains unknown. It has been variously described as a subjective response to a noxious stimuli; a private, personal sensation of hurt; and a neurophysiological mechanism including both a peripheral and a central component.[1,2] It is generally agreed that pain is more than a sensation. While it is clear that noxious stimuli are received by free nerve endings in skin, muscle, and other organs, the exact mechanisms by which such stimuli are perceived as painful is problematical.[3]

Furthermore, it is well recognized that pain can exist in the absence or after the disappearance of noxious stimuli, as typified by phantom limb pain. Thus, the surgical interruption of pain pathways in the periphery, spinal cord, or brain does not always relieve pain. Pain may also recur after the cause has apparently been successfully treated.[4]

The discovery of neurosecretory substances known as endorphins has stimulated renewed research into the nature and control of pain.[5,6] Endorphins are opiatelike substances produced in the brain, and are capable of occupying the same receptor sites as morphine. It is believed that endorphins relieve pain by affecting the perception of pain, just as occurs with morphine and other opiates. Research studies have demonstrated that individuals with less pain than might be expected have high endorphin levels, while those with chronic pain syndromes have depleted endorphins.[5,6] It has also been demonstrated that electrical stimulation, stress, and perhaps other external influences may increase the level of endorphins.[5,7,8] Thus, understanding the behavior of endorphins may help to explain the delayed pain response in individuals who have suffered severe injuries; the euphoria and altered pain perception in long-distance runners; and the effectiveness of some nontraditional pain management techniques such as acupuncture and biofeedback.

It has also been speculated that endorphin receptors play a role in narcotic tolerance and withdrawal. The exogenous opiates bind the receptors, and after prolonged use of exogenous narcotics, a signal is relayed that inhibits the release of endorphins.[8] This increases the dependency on external sources of narcotics, leading to withdrawal symptoms when the source is removed. Several theories, although not entirely proved, help in understanding some of the pain phenomena and provide a rationale for treatment.

Pattern Theory

The pattern theory suggests that the pain impulses must be of a certain intensity and are summated with other incoming nerve fibers in the dorsal horns of the spinal cord. This "summation" provides a pattern that is perceived at the cortical level as pain.[3] A variation of this theory postulates that stimuli of various intensities travel through different pathways, one fast (large fibers) and one slow (small fibers). Normally there is a system for limiting incoming impulses and preventing the summation. When the system breaks down, chronic pain results. The pain message is stored in the gray matter of the dorsal horns and any stimuli moving through the pathway elicits the sensation of pain, thus setting up reverberating circuits in which pain begets pain, even when the originating stimulus has been removed.[1,8]

Gate Control Theory

The gate control theory suggests that there is a gate mechanism in the dorsal horns that edit or modify the impulses moving upward through the spinal cord.[3,9] This theory proposes that stimulation of the large (fast) fibers decreases the effectiveness of the small (slow) fibers to transmit messages. The fast fibers receive messages from the periphery as well as from the cortex, brainstem, and limbic area, thus modifying the emotional response. The theory postulates that when the large fibers are stimulated by nonpainful stimuli (heat, touch, etc.), the painful impulses are blocked and thus the "gate" is closed and pain is relieved.[3,5] The pattern and gate control theories help explain the effectiveness of dorsal column stimulation, heat, massage, and counterirritants in reducing pain.[9]

CLINICAL FEATURES

Pain is often classified according to its expected duration, since both patient response and methods of treatment are affected almost as much by the duration of the pain as by its severity.[10] Furthermore, pain management is tempered by knowing the reason for the pain, or conversely, by the need to establish a cause.

Acute Pain

Acute pain is the term usually used to describe pain that is of relatively sudden onset and of limited duration due to a specific and readily identifiable injury or disease state. Typical examples of acute pain include postoperative incisional pain, pain from kidney or gall stones, burns, bites, needle pricks, fractured bones, or myocardial infarction. Acute pain can vary from mild to severe, with a duration of seconds to days or even weeks.

Acute pain is usually accompanied by autonomic responses such as increased pulse rate, diaphoresis, pupil dilation, increased blood pressure, decreased urinary output, and decreased peristalsis. The patient's behavior is characterized by splinting or protecting the painful part, making efforts to relieve the pain by rubbing or holding the painful part, and grimacing, crying, or moaning.

Acute pain acts as a warning of injury or illness and helps in identifying the location or underlying cause of the problem. The intensity of the pain is an indication of the severity of the illness or injury.

Intractable Pain

Intractable pain is a term often used interchangeably with chronic pain, but in this chapter it will be used to distinguish the constant, unvarying pain that persists because of a clearly identifiable but untreatable or incurable pain source. Intractable pain progresses rather than recedes. The best known example is the pain of terminal cancer, particularly that caused by infiltrating or metastatic lesions. The autonomic responses described earlier may or may not be present. The patient's behavior is characterized by focusing on the pain to the exclusion of all else, the appearance of a dull, glassy expression, reduced activity, feelings of isolation and loneliness, and the persistent fear that the pain will become unendurable and uncontrollable. The physical pain and discomfort experienced by such patients is intensified by the mental anguish associated with the fear of impending death or mutilation. The patient becomes exhausted, feels hopeless, and may be severely depressed.

Chronic Pain

Chronic pain, as differentiated from intractable pain, refers to relatively benign pain that is without predictable time limit and is not associated with a progressive or terminal condition. The pain may be continuous or intermittent, of acute or insidious onset, and mild or severe. It may have a demonstrable but untreatable source, or the source may not be identifiable or may have been removed. It is pain that the patient must ''learn to live with.'' Typical examples of chronic pain are arthritis pain, low back pain, neuropathic pain (neuralgia, peripheral neuritis), and phantom limb pain. Characteristically, patients with chronic pain have no autonomic signs, do not adapt to the pain, but seem to suffer increasingly the longer the pain persists, appear tired, depressed, and hopeless, focus on the pain to the exclusion of all else, react to stress or additional discomforts with increased pain, and become angry, hostile, or manipulative when care givers are unsuccessful in relieving the pain.

It has been stated that the benign chronic pain states described assume a disease status, to be treated as an entity separate from the pain source.[8]

Headache

Headache is one of the most common ills and a frequent symptom in neurological conditions. Most intracranial structures are without sensation, so that headache is related to distention or traction involving the veins or arteries; compression, traction, or inflammation of sensory or cranial nerves; or spasm of cranial or cervical muscles. A complete discussion of the various categories of headache is beyond the scope of this book. Emphasis is placed on the characteristics that distinguish ordinary headaches from those that may be symptomatic of serious neurological disease.

Headaches from Structural Lesions

Headaches can occur from structural lesions such as brain tumors, subarachnoid hemorrhage, arteritis, and meningitis. These headaches vary in frequency, intensity, and location, so that differentiation depends on the history of onset, course, and the presence of persistent neurological signs.

Vascular Headaches

Vascular headaches include classic migraine, common migraine, and cluster headaches.

Classic Migraine. Classic migraine, or the so-called ''sick headache,'' tends to run in families and often begins in late childhood or early adolescence. This recurrent headache is often preceded by an aura, which may consist of flickering lights, usually unilateral, transient blindness, or other sensory disturbances. The headache is unilateral, throbbing, and frontal, and is often accompanied by nausea and vomiting. The patient is usually incapacitated for one or two days. The attack ends with a period of sleep.

Common Migraine. The common migraine headache is similar to the classic migraine, but there is no aura. There is less likely to be a family history, and the attacks rarely begin before early adulthood.

Cluster Headache. Cluster headache, as its name implies, occurs in clusters, with a daily attack for several days or even a week or two, followed by weeks or months without an attack. The pain is intense, often occurring at night, and lasts for an hour or two. The pain is in the area of the orbit and is often accompanied by tearing, rhinorrhea, and flushing or swelling of the affected side of the face.

Nonmigrainous vascular headaches may occur episodically as a result of fever, hunger, fatigue, or the use of certain drugs such as nitroglycerin or histamine.

Nonvascular Headaches

Nonvascular headaches are generally of the tension or muscle contraction type. They tend to be bilateral, originating in the occipital area. They are described as constant, and are often associated with a period of stress or a chronically stressful lifestyle. There is often a sensation of neck stiffness, and the muscles of the neck and shoulders may be tender.

MEDICAL AND NURSING MANAGEMENT

To appropriately intervene with the various pain syndromes, an understanding of certain principles is essential. Treatment of pain must be holistic, that is, it must address both the physiological mechanisms and the interacting influences that affect the individual's perception of and response to pain.

Pain Tolerance

The intensity of sensation required to elicit the sensation of pain (threshold) is measurable and is relatively stable from one person to another and from one time to another. Pain tolerance (the intensity of pain that will be accepted by the individual without seeking relief) varies considerably among individuals, and at different times for the same individual.[10,11] Tolerance to pain is affected by the following:[11]

- older individuals seem to tolerate pain less well than younger people
- women appear to tolerate pain less well than men
- high anxiety and denial correlate with lowered pain tolerance
- predictability (reason for the pain and its probable course) increases pain tolerance
- the amount of control the individual has over pain affects tolerance. Self-regulated medications, relaxation techniques, self-administered stimulation techniques, and similar modalities are helpful in increasing pain tolerance.

Attitudes of Health Care Professionals

It has been demonstrated that the attitudes of health care professionals strongly influence the degree to which pain is effectively managed. Some of the attitudes and beliefs of physicians and nurses about pain that negatively influence pain control include:[12-16]

- pain tolerance is a reflection of character
- the patient's report of pain is unreliable
- if no cause can be found for the pain, the patient is either neurotic or a malingerer
- if the ordered dose of medication does not relieve the pain, the patient is probably malingering or is exaggerating the pain
- patients who respond well to a placebo do not have real pain. Conversely, the patient who has real pain will not respond to a placebo
- if the patient asks for pain medicine before the time a dose is due, the patient is probably becoming addicted, and the medication should be reduced
- the patient who falls asleep after asking for pain relief (or is asleep at the time an ordered dose is due) is probably not having very much pain
- only narcotics are effective in relieving pain
- it is best to begin treating pain with smallest possible doses of medication and gradually increase the dose if relief is not obtained.

Placebo Effect

A placebo is any form of treatment that produces an effect in a patient because of its implicit or explicit intent, not because of its specific physical or chemical properties.[14] There is strong evidence that at least 30–40 percent of subjects in an experimental situation showed some benefits from a placebo.[14,17] Efforts to determine the personality type of placebo responders has been ineffective because many individuals will respond at one time and not at another. Furthermore, research has demonstrated that the benefits a patient receives from pharmacologically potent treatments is augmented when the ordering physician has confidence in the treatment and the physician is viewed by the patient as being supportive. Several studies have indicated that even when patients have been told that the treatment being administered is inert, many report improvement.[17] Thus, the placebo effect can be defined as the change in the patient's condition that is attributable to the symbolic import of the healing intervention rather than to the specific treatment modality.[17]

The placebo effect can be used to augment the effects of potent pain relieving medications and treatments. McCaffery[14] recommends that all pain medications be augmented in the following ways.

Use Convincing Stimuli

The pain regimen must make sense to the patient. This may explain why injections may be more effective than oral medication. The use of complex equipment, detailed explanations, change of position, comfort measures such as back rubs and clean linen, a change in room temperature, and reduction of stimuli such as light and noise may all facilitate the placebo effect. The patient may be taught breathing and relaxation techniques, with careful explanations as to their relevance to pain relief.

Be the Trusted Expert

Pain medication should be administered by a trusted expert. The patient must have faith in the care giver as well as the prescribed regimen. It is important that the patient have confidence in the physician, and is secure in the concern and competence of the nurse.

Focus Attention on Symptoms

Attention should be focused on the symptoms which the medicine is designed to ameliorate. A thorough assessment should be made before each administration, with consideration of both subjective and objective signs.

Explain the Intent

Explain the intent of the medicine or treatment. Such statements as "This medicine is especially effective for the kind of pain you have," or "We have found this regimen to be very effective in breaking the pain cycle," add to the effectiveness of the treatment.

Assessment of Pain

Johnson[10] suggests that the assessment of pain includes determining if pain exists and evaluating the descriptive characteristics of pain, the physiological and behavioral responses that occur with pain, the individual's perception of pain, and the adaptive mechanisms being used to cope with the pain.

Determine that Pain Exists

The most reliable guide to determining whether or not the patient is in pain is the patient's verbal report of pain or discomfort. Every complaint of pain should be followed up by a thorough investigation. While acute pain is usually accompanied by physiological signs such as increased pulse, elevated blood pressure, diaphoresis, or pupil dilation, such signs are often not present with chronic or intractable pain. Even such signs as splinting, grimacing, or moaning are frequently absent in patients with chronic pain.

Patients whose level of consciousness is depressed due to drugs or disease may indicate pain only by increased restlessness. Patients with intractable or chronic pain sometimes are hesitant to complain, but may reveal that they are uncomfortable when asked about how they feel or how well they sleep.

The history of the pain is important because it may reveal the cause of the pain, as well as help to identify the kinds of management problems that may be anticipated. For example, pain tolerance decreases as the pain persists over time. Patients with chronic or intractable pain respond differently to pain than do those in acute pain.

Evaluate Descriptive Characteristics of Pain

The patient may be asked to describe the pain in relation to its location, type, and intensity.

Location. The patient may be asked to point to the place that hurts. The pain may be localized, that is, occurring at only one site; may be radicular, that is, occurring along the pathway of a nerve root within a dermatome; may radiate or spread from the site of origin to other areas; or be referred or felt in an area other than the site of origin.

Type of Pain. Pain may be described as sharp, dull, aching or lancinating, etc. Patients may describe abnormal sensations such as dyesthesia, an unpleasant or painful sensation caused by a stimulus that is not normally painful; hyperalgesia, an excessive sensitivity to painful stimuli; or paresthesia, abnormal sensations such as burning, itching, or prickling without obvious stimuli. The patient may also describe feelings of tightness, pressure, distention, or throbbing.

Intensity. There are no objective measures of pain intensity. The patient's report is the only useful guide. Sometimes the patient may be assisted in providing a more accurate description of pain intensity by comparing the present pain to one previously experienced, e.g., like a toothache; better than yesterday; the worst pain I have ever had; or worse than when I had surgery. Of course, pain intensity is influenced not only by the stimulus, but by the patient's emotional state, fatigue, and other subjective factors.

Evaluate Responses to Pain

Patients' responses to pain vary from individual to individual and from one time or set of circumstances to another even for the same patient. Responses to acute pain are different from those of patients with pain of longer duration. Acute pain may be accompanied by automatic and reflexive efforts to protect the part from further injury. The voluntary response is directed toward obtaining relief.

The response to chronic or intractable pain is often to turn inward, focusing on the pain, with regression and dependent behaviors. Regardless of the patient's particular mode of responding to the pain, a careful assessment will assist in planning appropriate interventions and in identifying progress toward recovery.

Evaluate Perception of Pain

How the pain is viewed by the patient is important in planning interventions. For example, the patient who believes the pain is a punishment for past misdeeds will respond differently to treatment than the patient who views pain as a challenge to be overcome. The meaning pain has for any individual is a product of past life, philosophy, religious orientation, and the effects that the pain (and disease) has had on the patient's life and relationships. Assisting patients to clarify their feelings and attitudes about the pain is particularly important for those with long-term pain.

Evaluate Adaptive Mechanisms

Knowing how the patient copes with pain will provide a guide for treatment. Does the patient try to ignore or minimize the pain? Do the coping strategies used increase or decrease the pain? What measures does the patient take to decrease the pain? Are these coping mechanisms successful or unsuccessful in assisting the patient to maintain a normal lifestyle and healthful activity?

Principles of Management

Pain experts agree that physicians and nurses are more likely to undertreat than overtreat pain.[12,13,16] As discussed earlier, pain begets pain, the noxious stimuli setting up memory pathways and reverberating circuits that continue to produce pain even when the original pain source has been removed.[1,8] Thus, the goal of pain therapy is to break the pain cycle, treat the source, and modify the pain behaviors in a positive way.

To break the pain cycle it is necessary to initiate therapy with large enough doses of pain medication, augmented by the use of the placebo effect and other nonpharmacological modalities to produce comfort. When pain has been relieved, treatment can be modified as indicated to maintain an acceptable level of comfort. It has been suggested that analgesic drugs are most effective when used to prevent the recurrence of pain.[5,8,16] Doses of medication ordered to be given "as needed" often places patients in the position of having to watch the clock, assess their own pain, and convince the nurse that a dose of medication is justified. Most authorities agree that regularly scheduled medications based on the drug's known potency and duration of action are more likely to maintain comfort and prevent the patient from focusing exclusively on the pain and the behaviors associated with pain.[5,8,12,13,16]

Whether narcotic or non-narcotic drugs are the best choice for a particular patient depends on the nature and severity of the pain and its expected duration. The narcotic analgesics, administered parenterally, are the most rapidly effective drugs and therefore are used most often for acute pain. For such patients, the problems of tolerance (decreased responsiveness due to prior administration), physical dependency (abnormal physiological state produced by repeated administration of the drug which will result in withdrawal symptoms when the drug is discontinued), and addiction (psychological dependence on drugs resulting in compulsive drug use) do not arise.

For patients with intractable pain resulting from a progressing and terminal condition, tolerance and physical dependency will develop with continued narcotic use, but this should not be confused with addiction, which is a rare occurrence when drugs are used in a medical setting. In any case, such patients should not be denied pain relief because of the fear of dependence or addiction.[12,16,18]

Patients with chronic pain (benign condition of undetermined duration) present a more complicated problem in management. In general, non-narcotic drugs used in conjunction with nonpharmacological treatment modalities offer the best hope for long-term pain relief. Many such patients will benefit from referral to a pain management clinic where a total treatment plan may be developed and implemented. When the patient with chronic pain has been using narcotic analgesics, sudden discontinuance should be avoided since physical dependence may have developed.

REFERENCES

1. Livingstone RB: Neural integration, in Frohlich, ED (ed): *Pathophysiology, Altered Regulatory Mechanism in Disease.* Philadelphia, Lippincott, 1976.

2. Sternbach RA: *Pain: A Psychophysiological Analysis*, New York, Academic Press, 1968.

3. Melzach R, Wall PD: Psychophysiology of pain, in Jacox AK (ed): *Pain: A Sourcebook for Nurses and Other Health Professionals,* Boston, Little, Brown, 1977.

4. Adams RD, Victor M: *Principles of Neurology*, ed. 3. New York, McGraw-Hill, 1985.

5. Brand KP: Alterations in comfort, in Snyder M (ed): *A Guide to Neurological and Neurosurgical Nursing.* New York, Wiley, 1983.

6. Wilson RW, Elmassian BJ: Endorphins. *Am J Nurs*, April 1981, pp 722–725.

7. Akil H: Enkephalin-like material elevated in ventricular cerebrospinal fluid of pain patients after analgetic focal stimulation. *Science* 1978;201:463–465.

8. Luce JM, Thompson TL, Getto CJ, et al: New Concepts of chronic pain and their implications. *Hosp Pract,* April 1979, pp 113–123.

9. Whidden A, Fidler MR: Pathophysiology of pain, in Jacox AK (ed): *Pain: A Sourcebook for Nurses and Other Health Professionals.* Boston, Little Brown, 1977.

10. Johnson M: Assessment of clinical pain, in Jacox AK (ed): *Pain: A Sourcebook for Nurses and Other Health Professionals.* Boston, Little Brown, 1977.

11. Jacox AK (ed): Sociocultural and psychological aspects of pain, in *Pain: A Sourcebook for Nurses and Other Health Professionals.* Boston, Little Brown, 1977.

12. Marks RM, Sacher EJ: Undertreatment of medical inpatients with narcotic analgesics. *Ann Intern Med* 1973;78:173.

13. Charap AD: The knowledge, attitudes and experience of medical personnel treating pain in the terminally ill. *Mt Sinai J Med* 1978;45:561–580.

14. McCaffery M: Would you administer placebos for pain? *Nursing 82*, February 1982, pp 80–85.

15. Goodwin JS, Goodwin JM, Vogel A: Placebo misuse. *Nursing 82*, February 1982, pp 82–83.

16. Dexter DM: The narcotic analgesics. *Am J Nurs*, July 1981, p 1364.

17. Brody H: The lie that heals: The ethics of giving placebos. *Ann Intern Med* 1982;97:112–118.

18. Gebbart G: Narcotic and non-narcotic analgesics for relief of pain, in Jacox AK (ed): *Pain: A Sourcebook for Nurses and Other Health Professionals.* Boston, Little Brown, 1977.

Chapter 13

Neurobehavioral Emergencies

There is an almost infinite number of acute and subacute conditions that bring patients to the emergency department because of an inexplicable change in the patient's behavior, with or without other signs or symptoms. A definitive review of all of these disorders is outside the scope of this book. However, a general understanding of the various behavioral abnormalities may assist the nurse in providing appropriate care and referral for the individual patient and at the same time cope with the disruption that often ensues when a patient with grossly abnormal behavior arrives in a busy emergency department.

Research indicates that behavioral changes may result from disturbances in the synthesis, release, storage, or inactivation of transmitter substances and changes in the dendritic receptor sites[1] as well as from structural changes in the brain substance. Even conditions classically labeled "affective" or "functional" are now believed by some authorities to be influenced by genetic or other organic abnormalities.[1,2] Thus, the border zones between neurology and psychiatry are becoming blurred,[1] and the patient who comes to the emergency department as a result of a sudden episode of "psychotic" or bizarre behavior presents both a diagnostic and management challenge.

Since organically mediated disturbances tend to respond poorly to, and may even be worsened by, the usual psychiatric interventions, early recognition of the organic nature of the behavioral disturbance allows more appropriate interventions and referrals to be made. Thus, the purpose of this chapter is to alert emergency department personnel to the diagnostic possibilities and to offer some suggestions in the management of patients who do not fit into the usual categories of psychiatric disease.

DISTURBANCES OF CONSCIOUSNESS (HYPERVIGILANCE)

Disturbed consciousness as it relates to coma is discussed in Chapter 14. Consciousness has two components, arousal and content. Stupor, coma, and obtundation are essentially disturbances of arousal (hypovigilance), while delirium and the acute confusional state represent disturbances of content and are often accompanied by heightened awareness (hypervigilance). When delirium or the confusional state appear during the evolution or devolution of stupor or coma, they can be appropriately discussed as a disturbance of consciousness as they are in Chapter 14. When they occur as isolated phenomena, they can be considered behavioral abnormalities and are therefore reviewed in this chapter.

Acute Confusional State

The acute confusional state is a condition of hyperexcitability and irritability (see Chapter 14). An individual, previously well, suddenly becomes restless, agitated, fearful, and emotionally unstable.[2,3] Such a patient appears inattentive and is easily distracted. He or she may have both auditory and visual hallucinations; may be paranoid and suspicious; is usually sleepless, unable or unwilling to follow commands; and may refuse to eat or drink. The patient is disoriented and confused and may be resistive and uncooperative either through inability to remain still or as an inappropriate response to misinterpreted environmental stimuli.

There are many possible causes of an acute confusional state. Some of these are discussed as separate syndromes later in this chapter. Elderly, brain-damaged, or demented individuals appear to be most prone to develop such a problem, perhaps because there is less reserve to draw upon. A relatively mild infection with fever, dehydration, hypoglycemia, electrolyte imbalance or anoxia may trigger symptoms. A mild head injury (sometimes forgotten or not reported), subarachnoid hemorrhage, heart disease, or other medical condition may precipitate the onset, as can idiosyncratic reactions to otherwise benign medications (see later in this chapter).

Delirium

Delirium has features in common with the acute confusional state, but in addition the patient usually has associated autonomic signs such as hypertension, tachycardia, diaphoresis, pupil dilatation, and sometimes fever. There may also be psychomotor signs such as tremors, asterixis, or myoclonus. The patients are extremely restless, with severe agitation and loss of contact with reality. Some authors do not distinguish between acute confusional state and delirium, believing one to be a mild form of the syndrome. Other authors believe there are two separate mechanisms.[2] The exact mechanism for either of these conditions remains uncertain, but it is generally accepted to be a matter of diffuse brain dysfunction, rather than localized disease.

DEMENTIA (ORGANIC BRAIN SYNDROME)

Dementia is the loss of intellectual capacity arising from organic changes within the brain. Organic brain syndrome is a catch-all phrase that includes a wide variety of dementing diseases. Senile dementia or senility is a term frequently used to designate the changes in mental status seen in some aged individuals. It is probably a misnomer since it is obvious that old age alone does not result in dementia,[4] although it is possible that the aging brain is more vulnerable to the diseases that cause dementia.[2]

Many of the same diseases that may cause dementia in elderly patients are sometimes seen in younger individuals and are then termed presenile dementia. Like acute confusional states and delirium, dementia has many causes (or rather is many diseases). Adams and Victor[2] classify the dementing diseases as follows:

1. those that are associated with other medical conditions such as hypothyroidism or Cushing's syndrome
2. those associated with other neurological signs as in Huntington's chorea or Jacob-Creutzfeldt disease
3. those in which dementia is the primary symptom such as in Alzheimer's or Pick's disease

Characteristic of all of these diseases is the gradual onset (as contrasted to the rapid onset) of acute confusional state and delirium. In general, most patients will first demonstrate a mild change in personality, becoming less spontaneous and mentally slower. Memory problems follow with gradual deterioration of all mental functions, but without change in the level of consciousness. Since the changes described all occur over time, such patients are less likely to appear in the emergency department than are patients with behavioral disorders of rapid or sudden onset. An intercurrent illness or a family crisis may, however, precipitate the recognition of impending problems and thus result in seeking medical care.

All such patients deserve a thorough work-up, regardless of age, since many of the diseases can be treated. Those that are progressive and untreatable require that family members begin as soon as possible to plan for the future care of the demented individual.

AMNESIA

Amnesia is the loss of the ability to form memories despite an alert mind.[2] Loss of memory forms a prominent part of dementia (see earlier), but in dementia all mental functions are affected, whereas in amnesia the memory disturbance appears in an individual whose other mental functions are relatively normal. The most common conditions causing amnesia are Korsakoff's syndrome, post-traumatic amnesia, transient global amnesia, and affective amnesia.

Korsakoff's Syndrome

Sometimes referred to as amnestic-confabulatory psychoses, Korsakoff's syndrome is characterized by severe memory loss, with or without confabulation and with relatively intact mental functions that do not depend on recall or the acquisition of new information.[2] The patient has good social skills and intact language but has both retrograde (covering the period prior to onset of amnesia) and anterograde (covering the period since onset of amnesia) memory loss. Such patients respond in appropriate ways to immediate events but become easily confused in new situations or places. For example, the patient will eat normally when presented with a tray of food, but become lost in the corridor if sent to the bathroom. The physician or nurse who leaves the room for a moment may be greeted as a stranger on return. When asked questions the patient may ''make up'' an answer that sounds logical but is unrelated to the truth (confabulation). The patient is indifferent to the memory loss and shows no embarrassment when the truthfulness of the statements are challenged. When accompanied by ataxia, nystagmus, and gaze palsies, the condition is referred to as Wernicke-Korsakoff's syndrome.[2]

The cause of Wernicke-Korsakoff's syndrome is a deficiency in thiamine. It is most commonly seen in the malnutrition of alcoholism but may also be found in other conditions that affect the absorption of thiamine. Treatment is administration of thiamine and institution of a well-balanced diet. When thiamine is administered promptly to patients exhibiting only the ataxia, nystagmus, and gaze palsy, the amnestic psychoses may be prevented and the other symptoms usually clear up within a few days. The amnestic syndrome, once it has developed, responds more slowly to thiamine and may never completely clear.

It is believed that in a severely malnourished individual, infusion of glucose may speed metabolism and use up the last vestiges of thiamine, thus precipitating the Wernicke-Korsakoff syndrome. In alcoholic and other malnourished persons every glucose infusion should include a vitamin supplement and additional thiamine.

Post-traumatic Amnesia

Following head injury (either mild or severe) there may be both retrograde and anterograde amnesia, in which the patient remembers nothing of the events prior to the injury, the injury itself, or the events following the injury. During recovery, the time period that is blacked out gradually shrinks so that the patient may eventually remember all or most of the events up to the time of the injury and events shortly after the injury.[2] Unlike Korsakoff's psychoses, these patients generally are able to learn new material and rarely confabulate. Similar forms of amnesia may be seen in patients following encephalitis, strokes, tumors, head surgery, or anoxic episodes.

Transient Global Amnesia

Transient global amnesia is the sudden onset of retrograde amnesia in an apparently healthy normal individual.[2] It is seen most commonly in late middle or older age groups. Typically, the patient is found by family members to be confused about the immediate past, but to have good recall of distant events. For example, the patient will express surprise at the presence in the house of a guest who has been there several days, or will think it is time for lunch when lunch has already been eaten. The patient will often seem anxious and worried but otherwise responds appropriately to immediate events and is able to retain new information. The amnesia persists for several hours and then begins to clear. Within a day or two (and sometimes by the time the patient arrives at the hospital) the patient appears to be perfectly normal, with only a brief period for which there are no memories.

There is rarely a recurrence of the amnesia. The cause of transient global amnesia is unknown, but may represent a very localized stroke or ischemic event.

Affective Amnesia (Fugue States)

There are instances of amnesia without identifiable organicity, believed to result from situational stress. Such episodes may be of short duration or, rarely, may have persisted for a fairly extensive time. Persons with affective amnesia may appear at a medical facility or police station asking for assistance, or may be found wandering dazedly in a location far from home. Even more rare are the individuals who suddenly reappear in familiar haunts, after being missing for some time; or those who ''wake up'' in a strange town wondering how they arrived there with no memory of having left home.

These patients appear to have no cognitive deficits other than the retrograde amnesia. Since an accurate history is unobtainable, and objective signs may be absent, diagnosis can present a problem. Affective amnesia has certain qualities that may help to differentiate it from the organic amnesias described earlier[1]:

1. Overlearned information such as personal identity may be forgotten in affective amnesia but is usually remembered with other forms of amnesia.
2. Memory defects may be selective: some information is remembered and some forgotten for the same time period.
3. The forgotten material or forgotten time period may be clearly identified with a stressful life event.
4. Recovery of memory may be sudden rather than gradual.

It must be stressed that while all of these clues are helpful in establishing a diagnosis, none is definitive. Mild head injury could have been sustained and forgotten; psychomotor seizures may end with a fugue state; all of the characteristics described can apply to patients with transient global amnesia. Some authorities suggest that a diagnosis of "hysterical" or affective amnesia should never be made unless there is a previous history of psychosomatic illness.[1] Sometimes under hypnosis or in an amytal interview, amnesic patients will reveal their true identity, remember events of the immediate past, or reveal details of the stressful precipitating situation. However, this usually will not effect a "cure" although most such patients will regain memory if cared for in a calm, non-threatening, supportive milieu.

ALCOHOL-RELATED SYNDROMES

Perhaps one of the most common causes of behavioral abnormalities seen in the emergency department are those related to the ingestion of or withdrawal from alcohol.

Intoxication

Intoxication alone rarely requires medical attention. However, excessive alcohol use frequently results in injury or other conditions that bring the patient into the emergency department. Furthermore, other medical problems have, on occasion, been mistaken for drunkenness, so the patient is entitled to a careful examination. In general, if no injury or illness is found, patients who are easily arousable and who have normal vital signs and no focal neurological deficits probably will "sleep it off" in a few hours. They should, however, be observed closely until it is certain that they are recovering normally.[3]

Alcoholic Coma

Usually excessive use of alcohol causes nausea and vomiting before the amount of alcohol consumed is enough to result in coma. However, when coma does occur, it is a medical emergency, since such patients may suffer respiratory depression or may aspirate while unconscious. In addition, alcohol ingestion does not lend immunity to other diseases that might result in coma. Before the diagnosis is made, head injury, diabetes, stroke, seizures, and other causes of coma must be ruled out. The patient should be admitted to the hospital and treated as any other comatose patient. If methanol or isopropyl alcohol or other drugs are suspected, dialysis may be indicated.

Pathological Intoxication (Acute Alcoholic Paranoid State)

It is frequently reported that some individuals will engage in a violent act after ingestion of a small amount of alcohol. These individuals usually do not demonstrate the slurred speech and incoordination generally associated with intoxication; have no history of criminal or violent behavior (except after alcohol use); are not chronic alcoholics; and have no memory afterward of the period in which the violence occurred. The violent act is usually unprovoked or out of proportion to the provocation, and the episode ends as abruptly as it began.[1]

It has been suggested, but with very inconclusive evidence, that there may be a relationship to seizure activity. The electroencephalograms (EEGs) of these patients are usually normal between episodes but are often abnormal during an attack.[1] It is well known that alcohol use may precipitate a seizure in susceptible persons. The patient should be strongly advised to abstain from alcohol use in the future. (See also "Dyscontrol Syndrome" later in the chapter.)

Abstinence and Withdrawal Syndromes

Chronic alcoholics and periodic drinkers (binge drinkers) often develop withdrawal symptoms when they stop drinking. Each of the syndromes described may occur in isolation, in combination, or in sequence.

Tremulousness

Tremulousness is referred to by the drinker as the "shakes" or the "jitters." Following heavy drinking the individual falls asleep and awakens after a period of abstinence feeling jittery; may have tremors; is often nauseated and vomits; has headache; and is nervous and irritable. The symptoms are relieved by alcohol, so the binge may continue until funds run out, an injury occurs, or for some other reason the supply of alcohol is unavailable. The symptoms peak in about 24–36 hours, then gradually subside, leaving the individual severely depressed. At its peak, the patient is severely tremulous (may be unable to walk or engage in self-care); is flushed, tachycardic and anorexic; startles easily, and is over-alert and unable to sleep.[2]

In addition, some patients will have hallucinations, which are often of a frightening nature. These represent misperceptions or misinterpretations of environmental stimuli. The patient may complain of seeing things or hearing things, of having bad dreams, and has difficulty separating the real from the unreal.[2]

If released from the hospital while recovering, the patient is likely to resume drinking in order to escape the troublesome symptoms or the feeling of depression that follows.

Withdrawal Seizures

Withdrawal seizures (see Chapter 10) may be referred to by patients as "rum fits."[2] They are most likely to occur within the first 24–48 hours after the cessation of drinking. The seizure activity may consist of a single grand mal seizure or a burst of several seizures. An occasional patient will develop status epilepticus. These seizures must be differentiated from other causes of seizures. Even small amounts of alcohol may trigger seizures in idiopathic epilepsy. Intoxicated patients may sustain injuries and suffer from post-traumatic seizures. Focal seizures can never be attributed to alcohol.

Since "rum fits" occur only in conjunction with alcohol use, long-term treatment with anticonvulsant drugs is usually not indicated.

Delirium Tremens

Delirium tremens may follow one or more of the syndromes described previously or may be the first evidence of withdrawal. Heavy drinkers who come to the hospital for treatment of other conditions are likely candidates. Symptoms are likely to develop 48–72 hours after abstinence begins.[2] Delirium tremens is characterized by severe confusion, delusions, hallucinations, tremor, agitation, and sleeplessness. There are also autonomic signs such as pupillary dilatation, diaphoresis, tachycardia and fever.[2] The mortality rate varies from 5 to 15 percent, so it is essential that aggressive management be instituted promptly. Close observation, frequent vital signs, correction of fluid and electrolyte abnormalities, maintenance of hydration and fluid volume, and sedation to prevent exhaustion and cardiovascular collapse are the basis of therapy. Obviously, attention must be given to ruling out related medical problems, such as head injury, liver, or gastrointestinal disease. The condition usually lasts about three days and then gradually improves.

Alcohol Addiction

Both the individual and society pay a heavy price for alcoholism. Patients who appear in a medical facility as the result of alcoholism require treatment both for the immediate problem and for the addiction itself. Sometimes waking up in the hospital after a life-threatening illness may motivate the problem drinker to seek long-term care. In any case, health care professionals have an obligation to offer such help in a nonjudgmental, nonpunitive way and to make appropriate referrals for follow-up care.[2]

DRUG-RELATED BEHAVIORAL EMERGENCIES

Most drug-related conditions seen in the emergency department result from overdoses caused by attempts at suicide or from illicit drug use. The diagnosis is usually fairly obvious, and the treatment directed toward the specific drug involved. Sometimes, however, the patient is brought to the attention of family or police because of a sudden change in behavior.

Delirium Associated with Common Medications

Almost any medication can result in a "paradoxical" or "idiosyncratic" reaction in some individuals. Elderly, debilitated, brain-damaged persons and those with incipient renal or kidney failure are particularly susceptible to such reactions. Certain drugs are more likely to result in untoward effects than others. Diet pills with amphetamines, sleeping pills with atropine or scopolamine, corticosteroids, and the tricyclic antidepressants are all common offenders. However, even diuretics or cardiac drugs may cause problems for certain individuals. Elderly and brain-damaged patients tend to tolerate neuroleptic drugs poorly and may become increasingly agitated and confused, for which they may be given larger doses, thereby complicating the problem.

The patient may become unaccountably confused, disoriented, restless and insomniac. They may have delusions, paranoid ideation or hallucinations. There may also be autonomic signs (see "Delirium" earlier in this chapter).

Any patient with the sudden onset of confusion or delirium should have a complete drug history recorded (including both prescription and over-the-counter drugs). All but essential medications should be discontinued and necessary medications should be reduced to the lowest possible dosage. Work-up for other causes of delirium should, of course, be undertaken.

Delirium Associated with Illicit Drug Use

Certain drugs that are subject to abuse because of their psychotropic effects often cause behavioral abnormalities.[1-3] Psychedelic drugs such as phencyclidine (PCP) and mescaline, sometimes at first use and in small amounts, may result in severe confusion, agitation, disorientation, perceptual distortions, and distractibility. Occasionally, an individual will exhibit extremes in behavior such as running, fighting, and hiding while appearing to be completely out of contact with the environment.

Methaqualone (Quaalude) produces hallucinations and agitation, which then progresses to coma.

LIMBIC SYSTEM PHENOMENA

The limbic system (limbic lobe, circle of Papez; see Chapter 2) is involved in both the experience and the expression of emotion.[1,2] Many acute and chronic neurological diseases may be accompanied by gross behavioral changes. In addition there are several well-defined syndromes that some authorities believe may be mediated in some poorly understood way by the limbic lobes.

Rage Reactions

Stimulation and oblation experiments in animals have produced aggressive behavior in normally placid animals, and placid behavior in normally aggressive animals. Similar unexplained behavior has been seen in humans following surgical procedures, head injuries, and encephalitis. The patient may lash out at any stimulus, and will kick, bite, spit, smash things, shout, and curse. The same response is elicited by every stimulus, however benign. The patient appears to be terrified or extremely angry and is totally beyond reason or logic.[1,2] When the behavior occurs without the accompanying emotion (that is, the patient fights or throws but seems calm), it is called ''sham rage.''[2] Such patients often respond ''paradoxically'' to sedating drugs, becoming even more aggressive or violent. Similarly, such techniques as behavior modification or psychiatric interventions are usually totally ineffective. The behavior may end as suddenly as it began or may gradually improve as the patient's disease improves.

Dyscontrol Syndrome

Dyscontrol syndrome or episodic violence is usually seen in young men (teens or early twenties) and generally disappears as the individual reaches the forties or fifties. A person who is described as usually good natured and peaceful suddenly becomes violent, breaking things or even inflicting bodily injury to himself or others. The episode is usually brief and ends as suddenly as it began. There is usually little or no provocation, or the provocation is out of proportion to the response. The individual may have used drugs or alcohol prior to the episode (see ''Pathological Intoxication'' earlier in this chapter), but this is not always the case. Some authorities dispute the organic cause of the syndrome, and others believe it may be a manifestation of complex partial seizures (see later).[1,2] However, there does appear to be a high incidence of EEG changes in these individuals. There is no known effective therapy, and the affected individuals often join the prison population.[1]

Complex Partial Seizures

Complex partial seizures, often referred to as psychomotor seizures (see Chapters 10 and 16), may result in aggressive or combative behavior as part of an automatism. In general, the aggression of seizures is nondirected, that is, there appears to be no real intent to do harm to any particular individual or object. It is most likely to occur when someone attempts to stop or interfere with the patient's automatic behavior. For example, the nurse attempts to restrain a patient who is running down the hall or attempting to get out of bed. The patient will usually appear to be out of contact and does not respond to verbal commands. Such patients rarely direct an attack except when they themselves are disturbed.

Whether or not a sustained violent act can be part of a seizure is controversial. Most authorities reject seizures as a defense for "criminal" behavior.[1]

NURSING MANAGEMENT

In the preceding sections, various conditions that may cause a change in behavior have been discussed in terms of signs and symptoms, etiology and medical management. Priorities of nursing management are based on the goals of maintaining the safety of the patient, other patients, and the staff; initiating diagnostic procedures; and making appropriate referrals for follow-up care. Specific nursing interventions for patients with behavioral emergencies are presented in Chapter 18.

REFERENCES

1. Pincus IH, Tucker GJ: *Behavioral Neurology,* ed 2. New York, Oxford University Press, 1978.
2. Adams, RD, Victor M: *Principles of Neurology,* ed 3. New York, McGraw-Hill, 1985.
3. Plum F, Posner JB: *The Diagnosis of Stupor and Coma,* ed 3. Philadelphia, FA Davis Co, 1980.
4. Taylor JW: Mental status and dependency in the elderly, in Hall BA (ed): *Mental Health and the Elderly,* Orlando, Grune & Stratton, 1984.

BIBLIOGRAPHY

Brigman C, Dickey C, Zegeer J: The agitated aggressive patient. *Am J Nurs,* Oct 1983, pp 1409–1411.

Misik I: About using restraints. *Nursing '81,* August 1981, pp 50–55.

Taylor JW, Ballenger S: *Neurological Dysfunctions and Nursing Interventions.* New York, McGraw-Hill, 1980, Chaps 7 and 12.

Part III

Quick Guide to Immediate Care of Patients with Neurological Emergencies

Chapter 14

Immediate Care of the Patient with Coma or Other Disturbances of Consciousness

DEFINITIONS

Consciousness	The state of awareness of self and environment. Components of consciousness include *arousal* and *content*
Coma	Unresponsiveness from which the individual cannot be aroused; total absence of awareness of self and environment even with stimulation
Stupor	Unresponsiveness from which the individual can be aroused by strong stimuli. When aroused, is usually confused and unable to cooperate or answer questions appropriately
Obtundation	Reduction in alertness, with inattention and indifference to the environment. Responds slowly and appears drowsy even when awake
Confusional state	Reduced wakefulness with hyperexcitability and irritability. Stimuli are often misinterpreted, resulting in difficulty in following commands. Appears bewildered and frightened. May resist or fight efforts to provide care and treatment
Delirium	Characterized by severe disorientation, fear, suspiciousness, irritability with misperception of stimuli and visual hallucinations. May be loud, talkative, and agitated. Often resistive and uncooperative. Delirium may occur with high fever and is seen in alcoholic withdrawal as well as other conditions

Akinetic mutism, coma vigil, vegetative state, cerebral death (not brain death)	All of these terms refer to a state in which sleep-wake cycles are present but without evidence of cognition. The various terms connote variations in appearance and motor function, but tend to be used interchangeably
Locked-in syndrome	Evidence of mental functioning persists even though there is no verbal or motor response because of selective de-afferentation that produces paralysis of all four extremities and the lower cranial nerves, but without loss of consciousness. Awareness may be demonstrated by eye blinking on command. Must be differentiated from akinetic mutism or coma vigil, described previously
Brain death	All brain functions, including those of the brainstem controlling respirations, blood pressure, and the cranial nerves are absent. Even with life-support systems, survival rarely exceeds a few days. Must be distinguished from irreversible coma in which the brainstem maintains internal homeostasis but without apparent awareness, as described under akinetic mutism

ETIOLOGY

Coma, as well as other disturbances of consciousness, results from conditions that depress or destroy the reticular activating system (RAS) in the brainstem, or by diffuse conditions that affect both cerebral hemispheres. These conditions can be categorized as follows:

1. *supratentorial mass lesions* that encroach on deep brainstem structures, such as subdural hematoma, massive stroke, tumor, or abscess
2. *subtentorial lesions* that damage the brainstem or surrounding areas, such as cerebellar or brainstem stroke, abscess, or tumor
3. *metabolic disorders* that affect all areas of the brain. These disorders may include electrolyte disturbances, drug-alcohol overdose, anoxia, encephalitis, encephalopathy, diabetic coma, and seizures
4. *psychogenic states* that resemble coma but have no apparent physiological cause such as depression, catatonia, and conversion reaction

There is a frequently used mnemonic that is helpful in remembering the various conditions that must be considered when evaluating the patient in coma:

A   alcohol
E   epilepsy, encephalopathy
I   insulin
O   overdose (drugs, medications)
U   uremia
T   trauma
I   infection
P   psychogenic condition
S   stroke, cerebrovascular accident (CVA), syncope

NURSING MANAGEMENT

Goals

- Protect the brain from further injury
- Stabilize the vital signs
- Preserve the evidence and assist with medical diagnosis
- Document critical information
- Support the family

Process

- Initial assessment
- Diagnoses (medical/nursing)
- Rapid response
- Documentation/planned continuity

Table 14–1 Nursing Management of Patients with Coma or Other Disturbances of Consciousness

Assessment	Diagnoses (Medical/Nursing)	Rapid Response	Documentation, Planned Continuity
Initial Rapid Assessment			
1. Airway for: • occlusion • aspiration • presence of foreign material	1. Ineffective airway clearance related to: • pharyngeal/glossal hypotonia • vomitus • secretions • inability to swallow	1. Open airway by: • reposition • suction • insert oral/nasal airway • prepare for intubation • c-spine precautions if trauma suspected	1. Documentation: • begin flow chart • establish baseline
2. Respiratory status for: • rate • volume • rhythm • breath sounds • arterial blood gas	2. Ineffective breathing pattern; impaired gas exchange related to: • failure of central controls • failure of mechanics of breathing • alveolar membrane changes (aspiration, atelectasis) • metabolic abnormalities • unknown causes	2. Institute respiratory rescue procedures: • mouth-to-mouth or mask-to-mouth resuscitation • assist with intubation • initiate mechanical ventilation • administer oxygen	2. Record: • time • sequence • dosages • tests • interventions • responses
3. Cardiovascular status for: • apical pulse rate • blood pressure • dysrhythmias (ECG/ cardiac monitor)	3. Cardiovascular instability related to: • failure of central controls • autonomic dysfunctions • vagal dysfunction	3. Maintain circulation by: • insert intravenous line(s) • infuse glucose solution (after drawing blood sample)	3. Record: • intake and output • see number 2, above

- skin color, moisture,
  temperature

4. Temperature for:
   - hyperthermia
   - associated signs:
     sweating
     chilling, shivering
     headache,
     photophobia
     rash, petechia
     meningeal signs
   - hypothermia (obtain
     special thermometer for
     temperatures below
     35° C)
   - associated signs:
     slow pulse
     shallow respirations
     low to nonpalpable
       blood pressure
     hypertonic muscles

4. Alteration in temperature
   related to:
   - failure of central controls
   - presence of pyrogens
   - external conditions:
     heat stroke
     heat exhaustion

- acd thiamine if alcoholic or
  malnourished
- replace fluid/blood loss
- MAST suit if indicated
- prepare vasoactive drugs
  (dopamine may be
  preferred in presence of
  brain damage)
- prepare to treat
  dysrhythmias
- irsert indwelling catheter

4. Control temperature (fever)
   by:
   - light covering
   - cool environment
   - antipyretic medications (no
     aspirin for children)
   - alcohol/tepid water sponge
     bath
   - cooling mattress, blanket
   - replace fluids, electrolytes
   - gradual cooling to prevent
     shivering
   - promote air circulation
   - promote comfort, reduce
     stimulation; quiet, dark
     room, gentle handling
   - culture nose, throat, blood,
     wounds

4. Maintain flow record:
   - temperature
   - medications
   - other interventions
     time
     sequence
   - patient response

Table 14–1 continued

Assessment	Diagnoses (Medical/Nursing)	Rapid Response	Documentation, Planned Continuity
pupils constricted or dilated/nonreactive ventricular fibrillation		• isolate from others *Hypothermia* (not due to exposure) • warm environment • warm covering *Hypothermia* (due to exposure) • restore respirations • monitor for and treat dysrhythmias • rewarm	

5. Metabolic status for:
• blood glucose
• alcohol level
• drug screen
• serum electrolytes
• BUN, creatinine
• serum ammonia (if Reye's syndrome suspected)
• CBC
	5. Altered metabolic status related to:
	• metabolic disease
	• alcohol/drug overdose
		5. Restore metabolic balance by:
		• adjust infusions
		• administer insulin if indicated
		• administer antidotes if indicated (naloxone, etc.)
		• control respirations
			5. Record:
			• specimens obtained
			  time
			  sequence
			• laboratory data
			  time
			  sequence
			• interventions
			  time
			  sequence
			  response

6. Neurological status for:
   - level of consciousness
   - pupils
     size
     reactivity
   - papilledema
   - eye opening
   - verbal response
   - motor response
   - increasing systolic
     blood pressure
   - slowing pulse rate
   - change in respiratory
     pattern
   - bulging fontanels
     (infants)
   - decortication
   - decerebration

6. Altered tissue perfusion
   (cerebral) related to:
   - intracranial hypertension
   - increased brain mass
     mass lesion
     edema
   - increased cerebral blood
     volume (vasodilation)
   - increased cerebrospinal
     fluid volume

6. Control/reduce intracranial
   pressure by:
   - controlled ventilation
     $Paco_2$ at 25–30 mm Hg
     Pao_2 at 100 mm Hg
   - osmotic diuretics
     mannitol 20% (IV bolus
     or drip); *use filter*
   - steroids: dexamethasone,
     4–100 mg IV bolus
   - control seizures (see
     Chapters 10, 16)
   - control agitation (see
     Chapters 13, 19)
   - elevate head to 30–45
     degrees
   - avoid Valsalva maneuver
   - maintain blood pressure
     (see number 3 above)
   - control temperature (see
     number 4 above)
   - prepare for CT scan of
     head
   - prepare for intracranial
     pressure monitoring if
     indicated
   - lumbar puncture if
     indicated only after CT
     scan

6. Initiate neuro flow record:
   - LOC
   - pupils
   - Glascow Coma Scale
   - vital signs
   - arterial blood gas
   - respirator settings
   - medications
     time
     sequence
   - other interventions

Table 14–1 continued

Assessment	Diagnoses (Medical/Nursing)	Rapid Response	Documentation, Planned Continuity

7. Other critical data
• clothing and effects for:
  dirt, tears, excreta, vomitus, blood
  drug, medication containers
  Medi-alert tags
  other medical information
  living wills, donor consents
• Head-to-toe examination for:
  cuts, bruises, fractures
  skin: ecchymosis
  lividity
  rash, petechiae
  ears, nose, throat:
  redness
  exudate
  urinary output
  trismus, opisthotonus
  focal neurological signs:
  paresis
  cranial nerve signs
  abnormal reflexes
  abnormal muscle tone
  other
	7. Unknown medical diagnoses	7. Assist in establishing medical diagnosis:
		• remove and preserve clothing intact
		• avoid obliterating evidence
		• obtain specimens of all excreta/vomitus
		• label all clothing and effects
		• inform physician of all findings
		• obtain specimens (cultures) from nose, throat, ears, if indicated
		• urine for specific gravity, osmolality
		• question ambulance personnel, family
		• hold witnesses for physician
		• question patient if possible
		• call previous physician if known
			7. Record:
			• condition of clothing
			• list and describe all effects
			• description of all cuts, bruises, wounds, fractures
			• results of physical examination
			• specimens collected; time sequence
			• document all changes in signs as they occur; time sequence
			• document all responses
			• document history and all preceding events

- history for

  A allergy
  M medications
  P past medical history
  - recent illnesses
  - recent accidents
  - drug, alcohol
    - use
  - seizures
  L last meal
  E events surrounding
  - incident
  - onset
  - course:
    - improving
    - deteriorating
  - early signs
  - precipitating
    - events

- Diagnostic studies
  - CT scan for:
    - mass
    - edema
    - herniation
  - lumbar puncture for:
    - pressure
    - WBC
    - protein
    - glucose
    - chlorides
    - gram stain
    - cultures

Table 14–1 continued

Assessment	Diagnoses (Medical/Nursing)	Rapid Response	Documentation, Planned Continuity
8. Family or significant other for: • understanding of illness and emergency department routines • family coping patterns: crying anger fainting visceral reactions complaints failure to cooperate inability to make decisions • understanding of prognosis: anger denial bargaining • expressions of: guilt despair "Why?," "Why me?" anger at God conflict with value system	8. Alteration in family process related to: • knowledge deficit new illness limited experience • ineffective coping sudden onset catastrophic event unfamiliar surroundings distrust of health care providers • grief (anticipatory), potential or impending death of loved one • spiritual distress catastrophic event impending loss • recommended treatment conflicts with belief system, perceived wishes of patient	8. Provide information and support for family: • provide information at frequent intervals • explain procedures, policies, routines • maintain regular contact • calm, gentle approach in response to anger, complaints • provide privacy, coffee, tissues, place to sit or lie down • provide counselor pastor, chaplain nurse medical social worker • encourage verbalization • offer hope but discourage unrealistic expectations • assist family to identify feelings and their cause • demonstrate respect for family's belief system • support family's decisions within legal, ethical boundaries	8. Record: • family behavior • interventions • family response

Re-assessment (prior to transfer)

9. Review critical data
   - airway
   - respiratory status
   - ventilator settings
   - cardiovascular status
   - metabolic status
   - neurological status
   - outstanding lab tests
   - intake and output
   - appearance and present signs, symptoms
   - ongoing therapy:
     intravenous infusions
     medications
     oxygen
   - family response

9. Physiological stability related to:
   - safety for transfer

9. Prepare to transfer patient:
   - replenish all infusions
   - suction to clear airway
   - attach to portable monitor (if indicated)
   - remove excess equipment
   - clean patient, bed
   - store effects safely
   - inform family
   - review data with receiving nurse
   - transfer patient
   - check neuro status with receiving nurse
   - introduce family to receiving nurse

9. Record:
   - update all flow records
   - review all documents for:
     completeness
     medications
     treatments
     infusions
     laboratory data
     total intake and output
   - patient response
   - transfer all documents with patient

BIBLIOGRAPHY

Alcorn MH: Altered levels of responsiveness: Decreased response, in Snyder M (ed): *A Guide to Neurological and Neurosurgical Nursing.* New York, Wiley, 1983.

Plum F, Posner JB: *The Diagnosis of Stupor and Coma,* ed 3. Philadelphia, FA Davis Co, 1980.

Taylor JW, Ballenger S: *Neurological Dysfunctions and Nursing Interventions.* New York, McGraw-Hill, 1980.

Rainer JK, Hollis J: Evaluation of the comatose patient. *J Neurosurg Nurs* 1983;15:283–286.

Ropper AH: Coma in the emergency room, in Michael P (ed): *Neurological Emergencies.* New York, Churchill-Livingstone, 1983.

Chapter 15

Immediate Care of the Patient with Motor and Sensory Dysfunction

DEFINITIONS

Hemiplegia	Paralysis of one side of the body, usually resulting from disease or injury involving the contralateral cerebral cortex or the cerebrospinal (pyramidal) tracts
Monoplegia	Paralysis of one extremity, usually indicating injury or disease of the nerve root or peripheral nerve leading from the spinal cord to the extremity
Quadriplegia	Paralysis of all four extremities, resulting from injury or disease of the upper thoracic or cervical spinal cord with loss of all motor and sensory function below the level of the lesion; the nerve roots or peripheral nerves affecting all levels of the spinal cord; the brainstem where the motor, sensory pathways decussate; or bilateral involvement of the motor cortex, and/or the cerebrospinal pathways. Usually in the latter conditions the cranial nerves are also affected, resulting in bulbar weakness and other cranial nerve abnormalities
Paraplegia	Symmetric weakness of both lower extremities resulting from injury or disease of the lower spinal cord with loss of all motor and sensory function below the level of the lesion, the cauda equina, or the roots or peripheral nerves leading to the lower part of the body. Bladder, bowel, and sexual functions are often involved

Upper motor neuron lesion	Impaired motor function resulting from injury or disease of the motor cortex or the corticospinal (pyramidal) tracts. Signs include spasticity (spastic paralysis), hyperreflexia, and abnormal reflexes such as the Babinski or Hoffman's. Examples include stroke, spinal cord injury, multiple sclerosis
Lower motor neuron lesion	Impaired motor function resulting from injury or disease of the anterior horn cells in the spinal cord, the cranial nerve nuclei, the spinal nerve roots, or peripheral nerves. Signs include flaccidity (flaccid paralyses), decreased or absent reflexes, atrophy, and sometimes fasciculations. Examples include Guillain-Barré syndrome, poliomyelitis
Extrapyramidal lesion	Impaired motor function resulting from injury or disease of the basal ganglia or cerebellum. Signs include rigidity, bradykinesia, abnormal movements, ataxia. Examples include Parkinson's disease and Wernicke's disease
Motor system disease	Impaired motor function that involves both the upper and lower motor systems. The most common example is amyotrophic lateral sclerosis
Neuromuscular disease	Impaired motor function resulting from abnormalities at the neuromuscular junction. Signs include fluctuating weakness of affected muscles. The most common example is myasthenia gravis. Curare-like drugs also cause motor dysfunction at the neuromuscular junction
Exteroceptors	Sensory receptors in the skin that convey sensations of heat, cold, touch and pain
Proprioceptors	Sensory receptors in deep structures that convey information about the position of the body in space, the force and direction of movement and of pressure
Dermatomes	The body segment (somite) supplied by a single sensory nerve root
Anesthesia	Loss of all sensation in the areas affected
Paresthesia	Abnormal sensations such as crawling, tingling, itching or burning
Hypesthesia	Decrease in sensation

Hyperesthesia	Abnormal sensitivity to all forms of sensation
Glove and stocking distribution	Loss of sensation in the distal areas of both upper and lower extremities. Usually seen in peripheral nerve disease
Segmental sensory loss	Loss of sensation in the area of one or more discrete dermatomes
Brown-Séquard syndrome	Loss of pain and temperature sensation on the side contralateral to the lesion with loss of proprioception on the ipsilateral side. Results from a localized lesion involving only one-half of the spinal cord
Dejerine-Roussy syndrome	Loss of all sensation on the side of the lesion, usually due to injury or disease involving the thalamus. Sometimes accompanied by spontaneous pain or discomfort (thalamic or central pain). May be seen following stroke
Astereognosis	Inability to recognize objects by touch. Results from lesions of the contralateral parietal lobe
Extinction	Patient acknowledges only sensation on the intact side when both sides are stimulated, even though he or she is able to appreciate the sensation when applied only to the affected side
Respiratory failure	Life-threatening condition in which the amount of oxygen available to the body is inadequate
Muscles of respiration	Include diaphragm and intercostal muscles. Accessory muscles include the sternocleidomastoid, trapezius, and muscles of the face, tongue, and pharynx
Vital capacity	Volume of gases expired after maximal inspiratory effort. It is decreased when inspiratory effort is compromised by neuromuscular disease. Normal vital capacity is about 3000–4000 cc. Below 1000 cc the respiratory reserves are compromised. A minimum of 500 cc is required to sustain life

ETIOLOGY

Motor and sensory abnormalities may result from a wide variety of neurological injuries and diseases. In many instances the motor or sensory dysfunction is of secondary or incidental importance in relation to a more critical problem such as coma following head trauma or subarachnoid hemorrhage (see Chapters 8, 9, 11, and 14). However, there are some situations that bring the patient to the emergency department when the major symptom is the acute onset of motor or sensory dysfunction. It is the immediate assessment and management of these patients that are considered in this chapter.

Neurological conditions that may result in respiratory failure due to impaired function of the muscles of breathing were discussed in Chapter 11. In addition to the diseases described there (myasthenia gravis, Guillain-Barré syndrome and amyotrophic lateral sclerosis), patients with injury or disease of the cervical spinal cord (see Chapter 8) may be admitted with actual or incipient respiratory failure. Patients with weakness of the bulbar muscles from stroke or other brainstem conditions may have difficulty breathing due to airway obstruction from secretions or vomitus.

A second group of patients with motor and sensory impairment who may require emergency intervention are those who, without appropriate and immediate treatment, may suffer from an extension of the functional loss. Proper immobilization of a patient with a vertebral injury is an example. Patients with compression from spinal cord tumors or other lesions may also develop permanent damage to the spinal cord if treatment is delayed.

In some instances the major significance of the onset of motor or sensory abnormalities may be that the symptoms assist in making a prompt diagnosis of a condition that requires treatment to reduce the probabilities of serious consequences. An example is that of the hemiplegic patient who is having transient ischemic attacks or a progressing stroke.

NURSING MANAGEMENT

Goals

- Anticipate and prevent (intercept) respiratory failure
- Prevent or minimize permanent disability

Process

- Initial rapid assessment:
  respiratory function
  level of impairment
- Diagnoses (medical and nursing)
- Rapid response
- Documentation
- Planned continuity

Table 15–1 Nursing Management of Patients with Motor and Sensory Dysfunction

Assessment	Diagnoses (Medical/Nursing)	Rapid Response	Documentation, Planned Continuity
1. Respirations for • rate, counted for full minute • volume: palpation auscultation over all segments vital capacity (spirometer) • use of accessory muscles • arterial blood gases: increase in P_{CO_2} (early) decrease in P_{O_2} (late)	1. Ineffective breathing pattern, impaired gas exchange related to neuromuscular impairment	1. Administer oxygen as indicated • reduce energy consumption relieve anxiety position for comfort and muscle support plan care to minimize fatigue • maintain clear airway: positioning suctioning oral, nasal airways • mouth-to-mouth or mask-to-mouth rescue • prepare for intubation • prepare for mechanical ventilation	1. Initiate flow chart • record all findings as baseline • document interventions and response
2. Bulbar functions for • gag reflex • ability to swallow • ability to vocalize • ability to chew	2. Ineffective airway clearance (actual or potential) related to: • pharyngeal/glossal hypotonia	2. Position to: open airway promote drainage of secretions/vomitus • suction as needed	2. Continue documentation

Table 15–1 continued

Assessment	Diagnoses (Medical/Nursing)	Rapid Response	Documentation, Planned Continuity
• ability to open and close mouth • cough/sneeze reflex	• excessive/pooled secretions • inability to clear airway independently	• insert oral/nasal airway • maintain NPO • prepare to intubate	
3. Vital signs for: • temperature • blood pressure lying/sitting/standing fluctuations • pulse: monitor for dysrythmias	3. See Chapter 14 • cardiovascular instability related to autonomic dysfunction	3. See Chapter 14 • maintain circulation by: insertion of intravenous line(s) infuse solutions as ordered (volume expanders may be indicated) • prepare to treat dysrhythmias	3. See Chapter 14 • vital sign flow chart • record all findings • document interventions and response
4. Bladder for: • incontinence • retention: with/ without overflow	4. Alterations in urinary elimination related to autonomic dysfunction	4. Insert indwelling catheter (temporary) or: • initiate intermittent catheterization • in presence of bladder distention (over 500 cc) drain bladder slowly • maintain residuals below 500 cc	4. Initiate intake and output records • document interventions • record residuals

5. Abdomen for:
   - bowel sounds
   - flatus
   - stool
   - abdominal distention
   - vomiting

6. Motor function of upper/lower extremities for:
   - muscle strength
   - muscle tone
     flaccidity
     spasticity
     rigidity
   - muscle mass:
     atrophy
     hypertrophy
   - reflexes:
     hyperreflexia
     hyporeflexia
     abnormal reflexes:
       Babinski
       Hoffman's
       others as indicated
   - abnormal movements:
     tremors

5. Alteration in bowel function related to
   - autonomic dysfunction
   - paralytic ileus

6. At risk for:
   - permanent disability
   - extension of disability

5. In absence of bowel sounds or if abdomen distended
   - give nothing by mouth
   - prepare to place nasogastric tube for suctioning
   - increase intravenous fluid rate to compensate for gastric drainage

6. Monitor for progression of symptoms
   - assist with medical diagnostics
   - minimize progression/extension:
     immobilize unstable vertebrae (Chapter 8)
     institute aneurysm precautions in subarachnoid hemorrhages:
       quiet, dark room
       avoid Valsalva
       avoid straining
       relieve anxiety
     assist with measures to prevent stroke in TIA:
       administer anticoagulants as ordered

5. Record all findings
   - document intervention and response
   - record gastric suction output on flow charts

6. Record baseline data
   - maintain flow chart
   - record all diagnostic tests and results
   - document interventions and response

Table 15–1 continued

Assessment	Diagnoses (Medical/Nursing)	Rapid Response	Documentation, Planned Continuity
chorea/athetosis others		assist with measures to relieve compression in spinal cord disease assist with other treatments as indicated by disease/injury	

7. Sensory function of:
upper extremities
lower extremities
trunk (level) for:
• ability to recognize touch
• ability to recognize temperature
• ability to feel pain
• ability to recognize position of body parts
	7. At risk for:
	• permanent disability
	• extension of disability
	• altered sensation
	  inability to feel touch
	  inability to feel pain
	  distorted pain sensation
	  inability to recognize
	    distended bladder
	    distended bowel
	• potential for injury related to inability to feel pain, temperature, position of body parts
		7. See earlier (Motor function)
		• observe for covert evidence of pain, i.e.:
		  sympathetic response
		  involuntary splinting
		  swelling, inflammation, injury
		• observe for unreported signs and symptoms, i.e.:
		  bladder distention
		  dribbling of urine
		  abdominal distention, rigidity
		  nausea, regurgitation, reflux
		• Protect from injury:
		  test temperature of
		    food, fluids, bath water
			7. See earlier (Motor function)
			• record and report all observations
			• document all intervention and patient response

8. History • onset • course • antecedent illness • injury	8. Exacerbation of known illness • unknown diagnoses	use siderails, padding, slings, other protective devices examine body surfaces regularly for evidence of cuts, bruises, blisters 8. Obtain history from patient, family, ambulance attendant • call family physician if indicated • determine type of injury, accident • examine for presence of other illnesses/injuries	8. Record all data
9. Laboratory data as indicated: • x-rays • CT scan • myelogram • lumbar puncture • other	9. See number 8	9. Assist/prepare patient for diagnostic tests	9. Record all data • time/sequence of tests
10. Reassessment (prior to transfer): • review critical data: respiratory status airway	10. Physiological stability related to: safety of transfer continuity of care	10. Prepare to transfer: • replenish all infusions • suction to clear airway • attach to portable monitor if indicated	10. Record/update all flow charts • review all documents for completeness: observations

Table 15–1 continued

Assessment	Diagnoses (Medical/Nursing)	Rapid Response	Documentation, Planned Continuity

cardiovascular status
bladder function
bowel function
motor/sensory function
outstanding laboratory
  tests
ongoing therapy:
  intravenous
    infusions
  medications
  oxygen
  respiratory support
  stabilization
    measures
ongoing nursing
  measures
		• obtain portable oxygen supply if indicated
		• obtain portable respiratory support equipment if indicated
		• remove excess equipment
		• assure cleanliness of patient, bed
		• inform/reassure patient/family
		• review data with receiving nurse
		• introduce patient/family to receiving nurse
			treatments
			medications
			infusions
			intake/output (including gastric secretions)
			laboratory data
			patient response and present condition
			• transfer all documents with patient

BIBLIOGRAPHY

Adams RD, Victor M: *Principles of Neurology,* ed 3. New York, McGraw-Hill, 1985.

Bograd BA: Impairment of respiratory function, in Snyder M (ed): *A Guide to Neurological and Neurosurgical Nursing.* New York, Wiley, 1983.

Kess, R: Suddenly in crisis: Unpredictable myasthenia. *Am J Nurs*, August 1984.

Buchanan, LE: Patient preparation and transfer to a regional spinal cord injury center. *J Neurosurg Nurs*, June 1982;14(3):137–139.

Chapter 16

Immediate Care of the Patient with Seizures

DEFINITIONS

Seizure	The sudden, recurrent, transient disturbance in mental functioning, body movement or both caused by excessive electrical discharges of groups of brain cells
Convulsion	A seizure with loss of consciousness and tonic-clonic muscle contractions
Epilepsy or ideopathic epilepsy	A seizure disorder of unknown etiology. The term, though somewhat outdated, is still sometimes used in a generic sense to refer to any chronic seizure disorder
Status epilepticus	Recurrent generalized convulsions following one another so rapidly that there is no return of consciousness between seizures
Epilepsia partialis continua	Persistently recurrent simple partial seizures with focal motor signs confined to a part of the body in which they originate. Usually takes the form of a clonic spasm with no change in consciousness
Aura	The portion of a seizure that occurs before consciousness is lost and for which memory is retained after the seizure. The aura is usually a ''feeling'' or sensation or a psychic experience (see Chapter 10) that heralds the onset of the ''event'' or ictus
Ictus	The ''event'' or the entire seizure, measured from the moment the patient's mental status changes or movement begins and ending when the patient has returned to normal

Postictal period	The period immediately following the seizure, and lasting until the patient's mental status and mental functioning has returned to normal
Todd's palsy	A residual neurological deficit such as weakness of an extremity that, along with other deficits such as aphasia, may last for a few minutes or a few hours after a seizure

ETIOLOGY

A seizure disorder is a symptom, not a disease. Neurons are intrinsically excitable and there is normally a balance between excitatory and inhibitory influences, allowing for orderly transmission of electrical impulses. When neurons or groups of neurons are damaged or diseased, from whatever cause, normal input is decreased, allowing abnormal synchronous discharges to persist and spread. The specific pathology that can cause seizures varies but includes:

- congenital and birth injuries
- metabolic disorders
- trauma
- infections
- alcohol or drugs/poisoning
- brain tumors
- vascular disorders

Since some of the conditions listed are treatable, every patient suffering a first seizure deserves a thorough work-up to ascertain the cause. In many instances no cause will be found, and the diagnosis of ''idiopathic epilepsy'' or seizure disorder will be made. This is most often the case when the first seizure occurs in childhood. In young adults and older individuals, brain tumor, trauma, vascular disorders, infections, or other conditions are more likely to account for the onset of seizures.

NURSING MANAGEMENT

It should be kept in mind that a single seizure in a patient known to have a seizure disorder is rarely a cause for alarm. The greatest danger to such a patient is from falling or other injury sustained during the episode.

For the patient who suffers a single seizure with no previous history, the immediate care is little different. The emphasis for such a patient is on immediate referral and diagnosis. The patient who has frequently recurring seizures (status epilepticus) represents a medical emergency and requires aggressive therapy.

Goals

- Prevent injury
- Prevent respiratory failure
- Prevent cardiovascular collapse
- End the seizure(s)
- Prevent complications
- Provide supportive care
- Document critical information
- Appropriate referral

Process

- Initial assessment
- Diagnoses (medical and nursing)
- Rapid response (intervention)
- Documentation
- Planned continuity

Table 16–1 Nursing Management of the Patient with Seizures

Assessment	Diagnoses (Medical/Nursing)	Rapid Response	Documentation, Planned Continuity
Seizure in Progress			

1. Motor activity
• tonic/clonic
• focal/generalized
• intermittent/continuous
• automatisms
 	
Level of consciousness
• responds to environmental stimuli
• unresponsive to environmental stimuli
	1. Potential for injury related to:
	• uncontrolled motor activity
	• automatic behavior
	• tongue biting
	• impaired consciousness
		1. Provide protection:
		• continuous presence
		• avoid restraint
		• pad siderails
		• prevent falling
		• insert oral airway when possible
			1. Documentation:
			• time
			  sequence
			  duration
			  description
			• interventions

2. Respiratory status for • chest excursions • color • breath sounds • secretions/vomitus	2. Impaired gas exchange, ineffective airway clearance (actual/potential) related to: • interrupted respiratory effort • aspiration • obstruction	2. Prevent aspiration by: • position on side • suction • insert oral/nasal airway Prevent respiratory failure: • prepare to intubate (nasal route preferred) • assist ventilations with ambu and O_2 if indicated	2. Document: • observations • interventions • duration of interrupted respiratory effort

3. Other data
• incontinence
• autonomic signs:
  flushing
  sweating
			3. Document:
			• observations
			  time
			  sequence
			  duration

dilatation of pupils
other

Postictal phase

1. Level of consciousness
   - confusion
   - agitation
   - somnolence

1. Potential for injury/violence
   related to:
   - confusion
   - agitation

1. Provide protection by:
   - reduce stimuli:
     lights
     noise
     voices
     manipulation
   - allow sleep
   - disturb only for essential
     care
   - continuous supervision

1. Document:
   - patient status
   - interventions
   - patient
     response
     time
     sequence

2. Vital signs for
   - respiratory status
     breath sounds
     color
     chest excursions:
       rate
       depth
   - temperature
   - blood pressure
   - pulse:
     rate
     rhythm

2. Impaired gas exchange
   related to:
   - aspiration
   - atelectasis
   Alteration in temperature
   related to:
   - presence of pyrogens
   - failure of central controls
   Cardiovascular instability
   related to:
   - autonomic dysfunction
   - associated cardiac
     abnormalities
   - circulatory collapse

2. Evaluate respiratory status:
   - obtain chest x-ray if
     indicated
   - obtain arterial blood gases
     if indicated
   Evaluate and control fever:
   - obtain culture, CBC
   - see Chapter 11 for
     management
   Evaluate and prepare to treat
   cardiovascular
   abnormalities
   - see Chapter 11 for
     management

2. Documentation:
   - begin flow chart
   - establish baseline
   - record all diagnostic data:
     time
     sequence
   - interventions
   - patient
     response
     time
     sequence

Table 16–1 continued

Assessment	Diagnoses (Medical/Nursing)	Rapid Response	Documentation, Planned Continuity

3. Neurological status for:
• motor function
  strength
  tone
• speech/language
• mental status
• nystagmus
• ataxia
• pupils
  size
  reactivity
	3. Residual neurological deficits related to:
	• Todd's palsy
	• aphasia
	• disorientation, confusion
	• autonomic dysfunction
	• slight nystagmus is common from anticonvulsant meds. Its absence may indicate noncompliance.
	• ataxia can be a side effect of anticonvulsant meds
		3. Monitor course of recovery by:
		• continuous supervision
		• routine neurological assessment every 5–15 minutes
			3. Document:
			• all signs, symptoms
			• residual deficits
			  duration
			  sequence of recovery
			• maintain neuro flow chart

4. Other datá
• examine for
  condition tongue/
    teeth/gums
  presence of bruises
  presence of fractures,
  .dislocations
  complaints of pain
	4. Injuries (actual) related to: related to:
	• tongue biting
	• gingival hyperplasia caused by phenytoin
	• falls/thrashing movements during seizure
		4. Manage injuries as indicated	4. Document
			• findings
			  negative or positive
			• interventions

5. History for:
   - previous seizure
   - last seizure
   - frequency of seizures
   - precipitating factors
   - medications
   - last dose
   - compliance
   - recent illnesses
   - alcohol/drug use
   - preceding events
   - other signs/symptoms

6. Record of compliance
   - history
   - signs of side effects
   - serum levels, anticonvulsant drugs

5. Known seizure disorder (treated)
   first seizure episode
   previous seizure (untreated)

6. Noncompliance related to:
   - ineffective coping
   - knowledge deficit
   - denial

5. Plan for follow-up:
   known seizure disorder (treated)
   - refer to usual source of medical care
   - contact responsible adult to escort from hospital
   - send all records
   First episode
   Untreated previous seizure
   - refer for immediate work-up and treatment
   - send all records

6. Reinforce compliance:
   - refer for counseling
     social worker
     psychiatric nurse
     physician
   - teach patient/family
     need for main-taining serum levels
     dosages, side effects
     appropriate medication schedule
   - discuss relationship of noncompliance to recurrent seizures
   - allow verbalization of reasons for noncompliance

5. Document:
   - history
   - usual treatment
   - complete all flow charts
   - record all observations
   - record all interventions and patient response
   - record all referrals
   - record name, relationship of responsible adult notified

6. Document:
   - history of noncompliance
   - observations
   - results of serum drug levels
   - interventions
   - patient/family response
   - referrals

Table 16–1 continued

Assessment	Diagnoses (Medical/Nursing)	Rapid Response	Documentation, Planned Continuity

7. Knowledge level of patient/family
• understanding of disease
• understanding of medications
• relationship of health patterns
• possible precipitating factors/events
• dangers
• carrying medical information
	7. Knowledge deficit related to:
	• disease/condition
	• medications
	• health patterns
	• precipitating factors/events
	• safety precautions
	• medical alert tags/cards
	   source
	   usefulness
		7. Instruct patient/family:
		• nature/cause of seizures
		• importance of regular medical care
		• medications
		   dose
		   side effects
		   schedule
		• related health patterns
		   rest/stress
		   diet
		   avoidance of drugs/ alcohol
		   exercise
		   menstruation
		   pregnancy
		   fever
		   metabolic abnormalities
		• common precipitating factors:
		   flashing lights
		   sudden change in illumination
			7. Document:
			• assessment of knowledge understanding
			• instruction given
			• response to instruction

sounds of certain
frequency
certain movements
or emotions
- safety precautions
driving
machinery
heights
unsupervised danger-
ous activities
- medical alert tags/cards

Table 16–2 Nursing Management of Status Epilepticus

Assessment	Diagnoses (Medical/Nursing)	Rapid Response	Documentation, Planned Continuity

1. Observe for
• onset
• sequence
• course
• frequency/duration
• interictal behavior
• type of seizure
   motor activity
   mental status
   other signs
	1. Potential for:
	• respiratory arrest
	• circulatory collapse
	• continued seizures
		1. Treat seizures by:
		• intravenous drugs
		  diazepam (fast acting)
		   5–10 mg. Repeat in
		   20–30 minutes if
		   needed (be prepared
		   to intubate)
		  phenytoin (slow acting)
		   up to 1000 mg over
		   20 minutes in saline
		   only, give no faster
		   than 50 mg/min
		   (monitor cardiac status
		   and blood pressure)
		  sodium phenobarbital
		   90–100 mg, slowly;
		   repeat up to 500 mg
		   (prepare to support
		   respirations)
		  pentothal sodium,
		   200–300 mg, slowly
		   (prepare to sup-
		   port respirations)
		• Other drugs
		  paraldehyde
		   2–4 ml (IV), up to
		   10 ml (rectal/
			1. Document:
			• all seizure activity
			   time
			   sequence
			   course
			   duration
			   frequency
			   type
			• interventions
			• patient response
			   time
			   sequence
			• respiratory status
			• cardiac status

2. Vital signs for
   - respiratory status
   - cardiovascular status
   - temperature

3. Other data
   - history
   - precipitating events
   - other illnesses
   - laboratory tests
     blood glucose
     drug/alcohol screen
     serum electrolytes

2. Potential for respiratory
   failure
   potential for cardiovascular
     collapse
   potential for failure of
     central control
     mechanisms-hyper-
     thermia
   (the above can result from
   the seizures or from the
   effects of emergency
   medications)

3. Undiagnosed seizures
   - therapeutic Dilantin
     (phenytoin) level is
     10–20 µg/mL

   nasogastric tube)
   (monitor respirations)
   ether
   pancuronium (only
     if on ventilator)

2. Support vital functions:
   - obtain arterial blood gases
   - prepare to intubate-nasal
     route preferred
   - prepare for ventilatory
     support
   - insert IV line(s)
   - begin glucose infusion after
     drawing serum glucose
   - add thiamine
   - insert indwelling catheter
   - control fever (see
     Chapter 11)
   - maintain electrolyte
     balance

3. Search for cause by:
   - obtaining complete data
   - obtaining and sending
     laboratory specimens
   - prepare for CT scan
   - other tests as indicated

2. Document:
   - begin flow chart
   - record I&O
   - all interventions
   - patient response

3. Document:
   - all tests
   - results of laboratory tests
     time
     sequence

Table 16–2 continued

Assessment	Diagnoses (Medical/Nursing)	Rapid Response	Documentation, Planned Continuity
BUN, creatinine CBC serum dilantin or other anticonvulsant level (if on medication) others as indicated • CT scan			
4. Assess for risk of injury • motor activity • changed mental status	4. Potential for injury related to: • uncontrolled motor activity • confusion/agitation	4. Prevent injury: • padded siderails • padded head/foot of bed • continuous presence • avoid restraints • control behavior by reducing stimuli restrain vests mitts	4. Document: • injuries • interventions • patient response
5. Other care needs • condition of skin • condition of mouth/teeth • condition of lungs	5. Altered mobility related to: continuous seizures lowered mental status impaired protective reflexes	5. Prevent secondary complications by: • meticulous nursing • mouth care • turning/positioning • skin care • chest hygiene	5. Document: • condition of mouth/teeth • condition of skin • condition of lungs • interventions • patient response

Reassessment (prior to transfer)

6. Review critical data
   - seizure activity
   - vital signs
       respiratory status
       cardiovascular status
       temperature
   - metabolic status
   - outstanding laboratory
     tests
   - intake and output
   - appearance and
     present signs and
     symptoms
   - ongoing therapy
       intravenous infusions
       medications
       other
   - patient response

6. Physiological stability related
   to
   - safety for transfer

6. Prepare to transfer patient:
   - rep enish all infusions
   - attach to portable monitor if
     indicated
   - suction to clear airway
   - remove excess equipment
   - clean patient, bed
   - review data with receiving
     nurse
   - transfer patient with
     documents

6. Record:
   - update all flow records
   - review all documents for:
       completeness
       medications
       infusions
       respiratory support
       laboratory data
       total intake and output
   - transfer all documents

BIBLIOGRAPHY

Adams R, Victor M: *Principles of Neurology*, ed 3. New York, McGraw-Hill, 1985.

Gumnit RJ, Leppek IE: The epilepsies, in Rosenberg RN (ed): *The Clinical Neurosciences*, vol I. New York, Churchill-Livingstone, 1983.

Hickey J: *The Clinical Practice of Neurological and Neurosurgical Nursing*. Philadelphia, Lippincott, 1981.

Hwang PA: Emergency management of seizures, in Earnest PA (ed): *Neurological Emergencies*. New York, Churchill-Livingstone, 1983.

Plum F, Posner JB: *The Diagnosis of Stupor and Coma*, ed 3. Philadelphia, FA Davis Co, 1980.

Taylor JW, Ballenger S: *Neurological Dysfunctions and Nursing Interventions*. New York, McGraw-Hill, 1980.

Chapter 17

Immediate Care of the Patient in Pain

DEFINITIONS

Pain	A subjective response to a noxious stimuli; a private, personal sensation of hurt
Pain threshold	The intensity of sensation required to be felt by the individual. It is relatively stable from person to person and from time to time. It can be measured, but is dependent on the report of the individual
Tolerance (pain)	The intensity of sensation that a particular individual will accept before seeking relief. Tolerance varies from person to person and in the same person at different times
Adaptation	The tendency for a continuously applied stimulus to cease to be appreciated. Adaptation does not appear to be operative with pain stimuli, but rather the painful sensation continues as long as the stimulus exists
Drug tolerance	The decreased responsiveness to a drug due to prolonged use
Dependence	Physiological state produced by repeated administration of a drug, which requires continued use of the drug to prevent the appearance of symptoms of withdrawal. Is treated by gradual reduction of the size or frequency of doses

Endorphins	Endogenous opiatelike compounds found in the central nervous system, which are believed to be capable of altering the sensation of pain. Their presence is believed to help explain phenomena such as delayed pain perception, physical addiction, and pain treatment modalities which use stimulation techniques (see Chapter 12 for further discussion)
Placebo	Any form of treatment that produces an effect in a patient because of its implicit or explicit intent, not because of its specific physical or chemical properties[1]
Placebo effect	The add-on effect of a supportive, healing relationship provided in conjunction with both placebos and with treatments believed by the care giver to be effective in treating the patient's disease[2]
Acute pain	Pain of sudden onset and limited duration due to an identifiable injury or illness (as burns, fractures, incisions)
Intractable pain	Pain that is constant, nonvarying, and persistent due to an incurable or untreatable progressing cause (such as from terminal cancer)
Chronic pain	Benign pain (that is, neither progressive nor due to terminal illness) that is without predictable time limit. There may or may not be an identifiable source or the original source may have been removed (as phantom limb pain, low back pain)
Localized pain	Occurs at the site of the stimulus
Radicular pain	Occurs along the pathway of a nerve root or within a dermatome
Radiating pain	Spreads from the site of origin to surrounding areas
Referred pain	Is felt by the patient in an area other than the site of origin
Dyesthesia	Unpleasant or painful sensation caused by a stimulus that is normally not painful (touch, mild pressure)
Paresthesia	Abnormal sensation without an obvious stimulus, such as burning, itching

ETIOLOGY

Free nerve endings found in the skin, deep tissues, arterial walls, periosteum, joint surfaces, and dura of the brain serve as pain receptors. They can be activated by the following:

1. direct cell damage
2. release of chemicals such as histamine from damaged cells
3. heat or cold in excess of what can be tolerated
4. ischemia
5. muscle spasm
6. stretching or pinching

Pain impulses travel from the receptors via axons to cell bodies located in the dorsal root ganglia of the spinal cord. Here the impulses pass through synaptic connections to fibers that terminate in the medulla, the reticular activating substance of the brainstem, and the thalamus. Exactly where the incoming impulse is perceived as painful is in dispute. However, it is generally believed that the interconnections with limbic structures as well as cortical influences affect both physiological and emotional responses to pain.

Discussion of the various theories used to explain the various pain syndromes can be found in Chapter 12. The recent research into the role of endogenous opiates (endorphins) in the perception and expression of pain has stimulated new interest in both the causative factors and the treatment of pain.

NURSING MANAGEMENT

Goals

- Rule out life-threatening illness
- Limit damage
- Find cause, if possible
- Interrupt the pain cycle
- Arrange for follow-up care

Process

- Pain assessment
- Diagnoses (medical/nursing)
- Rapid response
- Documentation and planned continuity

Table 17–1 Nursing Management of the Patient in Pain

Assessment	Diagnoses (Medical/Nursing)	Rapid Response	Documentation, Planned Continuity

1. Assessment of pain
 	
• history
   onset and chronology
   pain source
   other signs/
     symptoms
   preceding events
   precipitating factors
   variations in intensity
   variations in duration
     continuous
     episodic
   factors that relieve
     or exacerbate pain
   usual measures used
     to relieve pain:
     medications
     other therapies
     comfort measures
 	
• characteristics of pain
   location
     localized
     radicular
     radiating
     referred
	1. Alteration in comfort related to:
	
	• acute pain of *known* etiology
	• acute pain of *unknown* etiology
	• chronic/intractable pain of *known* origin
	• chronic pain of *unknown* origin
		1. Initiate comfort measures:
		
		• positioning
		• warmth
		• stimuli reduction
		• relaxation techniques
		• placebo effects
		   concern
		   reassurance
		   information
		• administer analgesics in dosages and at intervals to control pain
		• treat pain source
		• avoid masking symptoms with medications
		• explain to patient/family need to ascertain cause of pain
		• acknowledge patient's distress
		• allow verbalization of hopelessness/helplessness
		• reduce stressful, noxious stimuli
			1. Record:
			
			• pain assessment data
			• interventions
			• patient response

duration
  constant
  episodic
  length of episodes
intensity (subjective)
  intolerable
  severe
  moderate
  mild (dull)
quality (subjective)
  dull, aching
  sharp, shooting
  pressure,
    heaviness
  itching, burning
  cramping, twisting
  beating, pounding,
    throbbing

- keep patient informed of plan of care, purpose of interventions
- medications on regular schedule

2. Assessment of response (physiological)
- pulse
- respirations
- blood pressure
- diaphoresis
- pupil reactivity
- nausea, vomiting
- restlessness
- splinting
- limitation of movement

2. Immobility/self care deficit related to:
- pain
- splinting
- limitation of movement
- physiological instability

2. Facilitate mobility:
- assist into position of greatest comfort
- assist in frequent position change
- provide support for affected parts
- provide physical care
- maintain personal hygiene
- maintain nutrition/hydration

2. Record:
- physiological response
- interventions
- patient response

Table 17–1 continued

Assessment	Diagnoses (Medical/Nursing)	Rapid Response	Documentation, Planned Continuity
3. Assessment of response (psychological) • tense • anxious, fearful • depressed, hopeless • angry, hostile • apathetic • withdrawn	3. Ineffective coping, anxiety/fear related to: • pain intolerance • nature, duration of pain • threat to life, health • dread of increased pain	3. Assure ongoing support • provide continuous flow of information • reassure that pain can be controlled • reassure that help is/will be available • initiate self-help measures (put patient in control)	3. Record: • psychological response • interventions • patient response
4. Assessment of knowledge: • cause of pain • measures to control pain • medications, side effects • plan of care	4. Knowledge deficit related to: • pain syndrome • pain control • resources available for pain control	4. Teach patient/family: • nature of pain and pain resource • "cycle of pain" • relaxation techniques • distraction techniques • medications, dosage, side effects, intended effects • available resources	4. Refer for follow-up care • diagnostic work-up for unknown cause • pain center/experts for chronic/intractable pain

REFERENCES

1. McCaffery M: Would you administer placebos for pain? *Nursing 82,* February 1982, pp 80–85.
2. Brody H: The lie that heals: The ethics of giving placebos. *Ann Intern Med* 1982;97:112–118.

Chapter 18

Immediate Care of the Neuro-behavioral Patient

DEFINITIONS

Hypovigilance	A disturbance of consciousness resulting in reduced awareness of self and environment and difficulty in arousal
Hypervigilance	A disturbance of consciousness resulting in heightened awareness of self and environment and in abnormal processing of information (the content of consciousness)
Acute confusional state	Reduced wakefulness with hyperexcitability and irritability. Sudden onset of confusion, disorientation, restlessness, agitation
Delirium	Similar to acute confusional state but with autonomic signs (hypertension, tachycardia, diaphoresis, pupil dilation) and psychomotor signs (tremor, asterixis, myoclonus)
Dementia	Loss of intellectual capacity due to organic changes in the brain. Usually gradual onset and without change in the level of consciousness
Amnesia	Loss of ability to form memories with relative preservation of other mental functions
Korsakoff's syndrome	An amnestic confabulatory psychoses with loss of memory, confabulation, usually related to alcoholic malnutrition, but may be associated with other conditions that result in a lack of thiamine

Wernicke-Korsakoff's syndrome	Karsakoff's syndrome when associated with ataxia, nystagmus, and gaze palsy
Post-traumatic amnesia	Retrograde and anterograde amnesia (usually temporary) which may follow head injury, encephalitis, and other cerebral episodes
Transient global amnesia	A temporary retrograde amnesia of sudden onset and unknown cause seen most often in middle aged or older persons
Affective amnesia (fugue state)	Amnesia believed to result from situational stress. May be selective. There are usually no other cognitive deficits. The condition may be temporary or fairly long in duration
Pathological intoxication	Sometimes referred to as acute alcoholic paranoid state. Individual becomes violent after ingesting a small amount of alcohol without other symptoms of intoxication
Dyscontrol syndrome	Episodic violence in an individual (usually young males) who is normally peaceful and law abiding. May or may not follow ingestion of alcohol (see "Pathological intoxication"). Higher than average rate of abnormal EEGs in such individuals but not otherwise associated with seizure activity
Rage reaction	Probably a limbic system phenomenon characterized by violent and aggressive behavior elicited by any environmental stimuli. Individual is out of control and unreachable by reason or logic

ETIOLOGY

Behavioral changes may result from disturbances in the synthesis, release, storage, or inactivation of transmittor substances and changes in the dendritic receptor sites,[1] as well as from structural changes in the brain substance. Many patients who arrive in the emergency department due to behavioral abnormalities are alcohol or drug abusers, but many other diseases may begin with sudden or gradual changes in personality, memory, or cognition. The differential diagnosis for all such patients may be problematical, but since appropriate therapy and referral depend on accurate diagnosis, a careful work-up is essential. For further discussion of specific conditions see Chapter 13.

NURSING MANAGEMENT

Goals

- Prevent injury to patient, other patients and staff
- Assist with the medical diagnosis
- Document critical information
- Make appropriate referral

Process

- Initial screening assessment
- Rapid response (intervention)
- Documentation
- Planned continuity

Table 18–1 Nursing Management of Patients with Neuro-Behavioral Dysfunction

Assessment	Diagnoses (Medical/Nursing)	Rapid Response	Documentation, Planned Continuity

1. Level of consciousness
• hypovigilance
   impaired arousal
   excessive sleepiness
   slow to answer
     questions, obey
     commands
   confused, disoriented
     when aroused
• hypervigilance
   impaired cognition
   hyperexcitable
   restless, sleepless
   suspicious, fearful
   confused, disoriented
   inattentive, easily
     distracted
   visual, auditory
     hallucinations
   unable to follow
     commands
   resistive,
     uncooperative
• autonomic signs
   hypertension
   tachycardia
	1. Altered thought process
	related to:
	• obtundation
	• stupor
	• coma
	• acute confusional state
	• delirium
		1. Institute appropriate
		interventions:
		• see Chapter 14
		• reduce environmental
		  stimuli (lights, noise,
		  voices)
		• calm, reassuring presence
		• short words, short
		  sentences
		• siderails, restraint vest,
		  mitts if necessary for safety
		• avoid sedation and
		  neuraleptics
		• frequent vital signs
		• maintain hydration
		• maintain, correct
		  electrolytes
		• determine and treat cause
		  paradoxical, idiosyncratic
		    effect of medication
		    use of illicit drugs
		    fever
		    hypoglycemia
		    dehydration
			1. Record:
			• onset
			   sudden
			   gradual
			• behavior
			• preceding events
			• drug history
			• initiate flow chart:
			   vital signs
			   intake and output
			• interventions
			• patient response

diaphoresis
pupil dilatation
fever

- psychomotor signs
  tremors
  asterixis
  myoclonus

electrolyte imbalance
anoxia
subdural hematoma
alcoholic withdrawal
  (delirium tremens)
other

2. Cognition (normal level of consciousness)

- immediate recall
- recent memory
- personality change
- decreased ability to:
  make judgments
  grasp ideas
  abstract
  conceptualize
  calculate
- delusions, paranoid ideation
- increased or reduced motor activity
- altered sleep patterns
  nighttime confusion
  reversed sleep cycles
- speech abnormalities

2. Altered thought process related to:

- dementia
- psychotic depression (differential diagnosis)

2. Institute appropriate interventions:

- provide familiar, meaningful stimuli (remembered from past)
- provide information, explanations at time needed
- repeat information at frequent intervals
- calm, reassuring presence
- avoid sedatives, neuraleptics; if used, give small dose in evening
- avoid restraints
- maintain hydration, nutrition, personal hygiene

2. Record:

- onset
- course
- other signs, symptoms
- previous medical information

Refer:

- work-up
- medical follow-up
- possible long-term care

Table 18–1 (continued)

Assessment	Diagnoses (Medical/Nursing)	Rapid Response	Documentation, Planned Continuity

3. Memory deficit (other cognition normal)
• anterograde amnesia
• retrograde amnesia
• unable to retain new information
• confabulation
• affect
• other cognitive abilities
• language skills
• social skills
	3. Altered thought process related to:
	• amnestic states (organic)
	  Korsakoff's syndrome
	  post-traumatic amnesia
	  transient global amnesia
	• amnestic states (psychiatric)
		3. Institute appropriate interventions:
		• establish patient's identity
		• obtain history (from relatives, others)
		• establish last events remembered
		• provide familiar, meaningful stimuli
		• provide visual clues as to time, place, person
		• give information, instructions at time needed
		• calm, reassuring presence
			3. Record:
			• source of all information
			• history, when available
			• last remembered event
			• behavior
			• interventions
			• patient's response

4. Aggressivity
• history of aggressive behavior
• angry, hostile affect
• frightened, suspicious
• verbally aggressive, abusive
• fighting, striking, biting, spitting
	4. Violence (actual, potential) related to:
	• intoxication
	• pathological intoxication
	• alcohol withdrawal
	• use of psychedelic drugs
	• limbic lobe phenomena
	  rage reactions
	  dyscontrol syndrome
		4. Initiate appropriate safety precautions:
		• isolate (away from other patients, staff)
		• reduce total environmental stimuli
		• reduce, avoid physical contact
		• retreat in face of escalating agitation
			4. Record:
			• behavior
			• appearance
			• history
			• interventions
			• patient response
			Notify receiving nurse
			Advise on appropriate precautions

- other aggressive
  behavior

- complex partial seizures

- avoid bargaining,
  reasoning, arguing,
  scolding
- approach with planned and
  adequate force
- calm, reassuring,
  nonpunitive presence
- use restraints with care
- determine and treat cause
- see Chapters 10 and 16

REFERENCE

1. Pincus JH, Tucker GJ: *Behavioral Neurology,* ed 2. New York: Oxford University Press, 1978.

BIBLIOGRAPHY

Adams RD, Victor M: *Principles of Neurology,* ed 3. New York, McGraw-Hill, 1985.

Brigman C, Dickey C, Zegeer J: The agitated aggressive patient. *Am J Nurs,* Oct 1983, pp 1409–1411.

Misik I: About using restraints. *Nursing '81,* August 1981, pp 50–55.

Plum F, Posner JB: *The Diagnosis of Stupor and Coma,* ed 3. Philadelphia: FA Davis Co, 1980.

Taylor JW, Ballenger S: *Neurological Dysfunctions and Nursing Interventions.* New York, McGraw-Hill, 1980, chaps 7 and 12.

Index

C

T

U

Uncal herniation, intracranial pressure dynamics and, 135-38

Uniform Anatomical Gift Act, 165, 170-171

Uniform Determination of Death Act, 166. *See also* Brain death

Urinary retention prevention, intracranial hypertension and, 143

Urination problems, spinal cord injury and, 237-38, 239-40

V

Vagus nerve, 92

Vascular blood supply to CNS, 52-58

Vascular injury, 210

Vasodilation therapy (stroke), 253

Vasogenic cerebral edema, 134, 142

Vasospasm (stroke), 256, 257, 259

Vasovagal reflex, cardiac hemodynamic changes and, 292

Vegetative state, 216

Veous blood flow from brain, 52-55

Venous drainage obstruction, intracranial blood volume increase and, 133-34

Venous return, intracranial hypertension control and, 141

Venous thrombosis, 237

Vertebral column, CNS and, 42-44, 45-47

Vertical compression injuries, 192

Vertebral injury, 46-47, 217-20

Vertigo, 102

Victor, M., 186, 315

Viral encephalitis, 185-86

Vital signs, 18-19
testing for, 121-24

Volume-pressure responses, intracranial pressure monitoring, 146-47

Vomiting
alcoholic coma and, 318
botulism and, 284
concussion and, 205
cranial nerve injury and ,196
hypertensive intracranial hemorrhage and, 254
ICP increase and, 143
seizure and, 277
spinal cord injury and, 230, 237
subtentorial lesions and, 248

W

Walking difficulty, 103

Wernicke-Korsakoff's syndrome, 316, 374

Withdrawal syndromes, 319-20

X

X-rays
cervical spine, 19-20
skull, 20-21
fracture, 193, 196
stroke and, 250
spinal cord injury, 233